99/872

616.853 SCH

D0228934

50p

Withdrawn 06/04/22

THE COMPREHENSIVE

EVALUATION

AND

TREATMENT OF EPILEPSY

GWENT HEALTHCARE NHS TRUST
LIBRARY
ROYAL GWENT HOSPITAL
NEWPORT

THE COMPREHENSIVE EVALUATION AND TREATMENT OF EPILEPSY

A PRACTICAL GUIDE

Edited by

Steven C. Schachter, M.D. and Donald L. Schomer, M.D.

Comprehensive Epilepsy Center
Department of Neurology
Beth Israel Deaconess Medical Center
Harvard Medical School
Boston, Massachusetts

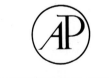

ACADEMIC PRESS

San Diego   London   Boston   New York   Sydney   Tokyo   Toronto

Front cover graphic by Isabelle Delmotte, taken from a larger work entitled *Epileptograph: The Internal Journey*. Ms. Delmotte, an Australian artist with epilepsy, writes that "this work focuses on the visceral, primal, frightful non-lingual reality of the postictal state."

This book is printed on acid-free paper. ∞

Copyright © 1997 by ACADEMIC PRESS

All Rights Reserved.
No part of this publication may be reproduced or transmitted in any form or by any means, electronic or mechanical, including photocopy, recording, or any information storage and retrieval system, without permission in writing from the publisher.

Academic Press
a division of Harcourt Brace & Company
525 B Street, Suite 1900, San Diego, California 92101-4495, USA
http://www.apnet.com

Academic Press Limited
24-28 Oval Road, London NW1 7DX, UK
http://www.hbuk.co.uk/ap/

Library of Congress Cataloging-in-Publication Data

The comprehensive evaluation and treatment of epilepsy : a practical
    guide / edited by Steven C. Schachter, Donald L. Schomer.
            p.   cm.
    Includes bibliographical references and index.
    ISBN 0-12-621355-0 (alk. paper)
    1. Epilepsy.   I. Schachter, Steven C.   II. Schomer, Donald L.
    [DNLM: 1. Epilepsy--therapy.   2. Epilepsy--diagnosis.
    3. Epilepsy--classification.   WL 385 C7376 1997]
    RC372.C63   1997
    616.8'53--dc21
    DNLM/DLC
    for Library of Congress   97-10913
                                                               CIP

PRINTED IN THE UNITED STATES OF AMERICA
97 98 99 00 01 02 BC 9 8 7 6 5 4 3 2 1

CONTENTS

CHAPTER 1

Classification of Seizures and the Epilepsies

Gregory L. Holmes

CHAPTER 2

Radiographic Assessment of Patients with Epilepsy

Gottfried Schlaug and Mahesh Patel

CHAPTER 3
Treatment of Seizures

Steven C. Schachter

CHAPTER 4
Definition and Overview of Intractable Epilepsy

Orrin Devinsky

CHAPTER 5
Psychosocial Aspects of Epilepsy
Patricia O. Shafer and Eileen Salmanson

CHAPTER 6
Neuropsychological Assessment and Application to Temporal Lobe Epilepsy
Peter J. Hayashi and Margaret O'Connor

CHAPTER 7
Psychiatric Considerations in Patients with Epilepsy
Jacob C. Holzer and David M. Bear

CHAPTER 8
Status Epilepticus
Frank W. Drislane

CHAPTER 9
Diagnosis and Management of Nonepileptic Seizures
A. James Rowan

CHAPTER 10

Ambulatory Electroencephalographic Monitoring: Technology and Uses

John R. Ives

CHAPTER 11

The Surgical Treatment of Epilepsy

Howard Blume

CHAPTER 12
Endocrine Aspects of Partial Seizures
Pavel Klein and Andrew G. Herzog

CHAPTER 13
Epilepsy and the Elderly
Edward B. Bromfield

CHAPTER 14

The Team Approach to the Treatment of Epilepsy

Donald L. Schomer

CONTRIBUTORS

Numbers in parentheses indicate the pages on which the authors' contributions begin.

David M. Bear, M.D. (131), Department of Psychiatry, University of Massachusetts Medical Center, Worcester, Massachusetts 01605

Howard Blume, M.D., Ph.D. (197), Department of Surgery, Division of Neurosurgery, Beth Israel Deaconess Medical Center, Harvard Medical School, Boston, Massachusetts 02215

Edward B. Bromfield, M.D. (233), EEG Laboratory, Brigham and Women's Hospital, Boston, Massachusetts 02115

Orrin Devinsky, M.D. (75), Department of Neurology, New York University School of Medicine, Hospital for Joint Diseases, New York University Comprehensive Epilepsy Center, New York, New York 10003

Frank W. Drislane, M.D. (149), Beth Israel Deaconess Medical Center, Boston, Massachusetts 02215

Peter J. Hayashi, Ph.D. (111), Behavioral Neurology Unit, Beth Israel Deaconess Medical Center, Harvard Medical School, Boston, Massachusetts 02215

Andrew G. Herzog, M.D., M.Sc. (207), Neuroendocrine Unit, Department of Neurology, Beth Israel Deaconess Medical Center, Boston, Massachusetts 02215

Gregory L. Holmes, M.D. (1), Department of Neurology, Harvard Medical School, Clinical Neurophysiology Laboratory, Children's Hospital, Boston, Massachusetts 02115

Jacob C. Holzer, M.D. (131), Department of Psychiatry, Tufts School of Medicine, Boston, Massachusetts 02111

John R. Ives, B.Sc. (185), Beth Israel Deaconess Medical Center, Boston, Massachusetts 02215

Pavel Klein, M.B., B.Chir. (207), Neuroendocrine Unit, Department of Neurology, Beth Israel Deaconess Medical Center, Boston, Massachusetts 02215

Margaret O'Connor, Ph.D. (111), Behavioral Neurology Unit, Beth Israel Deaconess Medical Center, Harvard Medical School, Boston, Massachusetts 02215

Mahesh Patel, M.D. (37), Department of Radiology, Beth Israel Deaconess Medical Center, Boston, Massachusetts 02215

A. James Rowan, M.D. (173), Department of Neurology, Mount Sinai School of Medicine, Neurology Service, Bronx Veteran's Administration Medical Center, New York, New York 10468

Eileen Salmanson, M.S.W., L.I.C.S.W. (91), Sleep Epilepsy Program and Brigham Behavioral Neurology Group, Brigham and Women's Hospital, Boston, Massachusetts 02115

Steven C. Schachter, M.D. (61), Comprehensive Epilepsy Center, Department of Neurology, Beth Israel Deaconess Medical Center, Harvard Medical School, Boston, Massachusetts 02215

Patricia O. Shafer, R.N., M.N. (91), Comprehensive Epilepsy Center, Beth Israel Deaconess Medical Center, Boston, Massachusetts 02215

Gottfried Schlaug, M.D., Ph.D. (37), Department of Neurology, Beth Israel Deaconess Medical Center, Boston, Massachusetts 02215

Donald L. Schomer, M.D. (255), Comprehensive Epilepsy Center, Department of Neurology, Beth Israel Deaconess Medical Center, Harvard Medical School, Boston, Massachusetts 02215

PREFACE

The primary objective of caring for patients with epilepsy is to restore their functional capacity to its maximal potential. In diagnosing epilepsy in patients, planning treatment, and providing follow-up care, it is important that the physician be familiar with current diagnostic and therapeutic protocols. Often this information is not included in textbooks of general neurology beyond an overview. Further, the care of patients with epilepsy often requires a team approach, utilizing medical and social service professionals in addition to the patient's family, friends, and co-workers. In these cases, the physician must take into account psychosocial, cognitive, educational, and vocational issues in addition to pharmacologic considerations. Guidelines for this process are generally unavailable in neurology textbooks.

The purpose of this book, therefore, is to provide current information about epilepsy in a comprehensive, easy-to-use, and practical form. It is particularly intended for general neurologists and neurologically oriented primary care physicians.

Each chapter is organized under headings presented as commonly asked clinical questions pertaining to the subject of the chapter. Each of these questions is listed in the contents of the book, a feature that should help the busy practitioner find the answer to a particular question in the midst of a hectic clinic session.

The first three chapters cover the initial management of patients with seizures. Chapter 1 discusses the classification of seizures and epilepsy syndromes and the spectrum of EEG abnormalities associated with seizure disorders. Chapter 2 addresses the optimal radiographic evaluation of epilepsy patients. Chapter 3 presents the medical therapy of seizures.

Subsequent chapters detail the factors that contribute to intractable seizures (Chapter 4), including psychosocial aspects of epilepsy (Chapter 5), neuropsychologic problems associated with temporal lobe epilepsy (Chapter 6), and related psychiatric disorders (Chapter 7). The diagnosis and treatment of status epilepticus (Chapter 8) and nonepileptic seizures (Chapter 9) are then presented, followed by discussions of ambulatory EEG monitoring (Chapter 10), epilepsy surgery (Chapter 11), endocrine aspects of partial seizures (Chapter 12), and epilepsy in the elderly (Chapter 13). Chapter 14 provides guidelines for referring patients to comprehensive epilepsy centers.

In summary, this book represents our current body of knowledge about epilepsy, formulated for general neurologic or medical practice. The field of epilepsy is rapidly changing as new therapies are introduced, genetic breakthroughs are announced, and new imaging modalities are invented. The editors hope that the clinical approach to epilepsy reflected in this book will provide a foundation on which the reader can integrate these new advances with compassionate care of patients with seizures.

The editors express their appreciation to Cathy Somer and Loraine Karol for editorial assistance.

Steven C. Schachter, M.D.
Donald L. Schomer, M.D.

CHAPTER 1

Classification of Seizures and the Epilepsies

Gregory L. Holmes, M.D.

HOW ARE SEIZURES CLASSIFIED?

One of the first priorities facing the physician when evaluating a patient with epileptic seizures is to determine seizure type and, when possible, the epileptic syndrome. This determination is critical because seizure type and epileptic syndrome to a great extent determine the type of evaluation the patient will receive, as well as the type of therapy.

Seizures are classified into two basic groups: partial and generalized (Table 1.1).[1] Partial seizures involve only a portion of the brain at the onset. Seizures can be further divided into those in which consciousness is not impaired (simple partial) and those in which it is (complex partial). Both types of partial seizures can spread, resulting in 2° generalized tonic-clonic seizures. Primary generalized seizures are those in which the first clinical changes indicate the initial involvement of both hemispheres. There is usually impairment of consciousness during generalized seizures, although some seizures, such as the myoclonic type, may be so brief that impairment of consciousness cannot be assessed. Space limitations do not permit detailed descriptions of all the seizure types.

HOW CAN THE PHYSICIAN DISTINGUISH BETWEEN SIMPLE PARTIAL AND COMPLEX PARTIAL SEIZURES?

Simple partial seizures (SPS) can occur at any age. The signs or symptoms of this type of seizure depend on the location of the focus of the seizure.[2] Seizures involving the motor cortex most commonly consist of rhythmic to semirhythmic clonic activity of the face, arm, or leg. Diagnosing this type of seizure is usually not difficult. Seizures with somatosensory, autonomic, and psychic symptoms (hallucinations, illusions, déja vu) may be more difficult to diagnose.[3] Psychic symptoms usually occur as a component of a complex partial seizure.

Complex partial seizures (CPS), formerly termed temporal lobe or psychomotor seizures, are one of the most common seizure types encountered in both

The Comprehensive Evaluation and Treatment of Epilepsy
Copyright © 1997 by Academic Press. All rights of reproduction in any form reserved.

Table 1.1

International Classification of Epileptic Seizures[a]

I. Partial Seizures
  A. Simple partial seizures
    1. With motor signs
      a. Focal motor without march
      b. Focal motor with march (Jacksonian)
      c. Versive
      d. Postural
      e. Phonatory
    2. With somatosensory or special-sensory symptoms
      a. Somatosensory
      b. Visual
      c. Auditory
      d. Olfactory
      e. Gustatory
      f. Vertiginous
    3. With autonomic symptoms or signs
    4. With psychic symptoms
      a. Dysphasia
      b. Dysmnesic
      c. Cognitive
      d. Affective
      e. Illusions
      f. Structured hallucinations
  B. Complex partial seizures
    1. Simple partial seizures
      a. With simple partial features
      b. With automatisms
    2. With impairment of consciousness at onset
      a. With impairment of consciousness only
      b. With automatisms
  C. Partial seizures evolving to secondarily generalized seizures
    1. Simple partial seizures evolving to generalized seizures
    2. Complex partial seizures evolving to generalized seizures
    3. Simple partial seizures evolving to complex partial seizures evolving to generalized seizures
II. Generalized Seizures
  A. Absence seizures
    1. Typical absence seizures
      a. Impairment of consciousness only
      b. With mild clonic components
      c. With atonic components
      d. With tonic components
      e. With automatisms
      f. With autonomic components
    2. Atypical absence seizures
  B. Myoclonic seizures
  C. Clonic seizures
  D. Tonic seizures
  E. Tonic-clonic seizures
  F. Atonic seizures

[a] Modified from Ref. 1.

children and adults.[3] This type of seizure may be preceded by a simple partial seizure that may serve as a warning to the patient (i.e., aura) of a more severe seizure to come. It is important to realize that the aura may enable the clinician to determine the cortical area in which the seizure is beginning.

By definition, all patients with CPS have impaired consciousness; thus the patient either does not respond to commands or responds in an abnormally slow manner. Although CPS may be characterized by simple staring and impaired responsiveness, behavior is usually more complex during the seizure. Automatisms (involuntary motor activity) are common during the period of impaired consciousness in CPS. Automatic behavior is variable and may consist of activities such as facial grimacing, gesturing, chewing, lip smacking, finger snapping, and repeating phrases; the patient does not recall this activity after the seizure.[4,5] Although variable, CPS usually last from 30 s to several minutes. In contrast, absence seizures (described later) usually last less than 15 s.[6] Most patients have some degree of postictal impairment, such as tiredness or confusion.

WHAT ARE THE TYPES OF GENERALIZED SEIZURES?

GENERALIZED TONIC-CLONIC SEIZURES

There is rarely any difficulty in correctly diagnosing generalized tonic–clonic (GTC) seizures (formerly termed *grand mal seizures*). The only caution is that toddlers with breath-holding attacks and adults and children with syncope may have brief generalized tonic–clonic seizures at the end of the attack.[7] Those brief seizures should not be treated with antiepileptic drugs.

Some patients may have a simple partial seizure (aura) preceding the loss of consciousness. As previously described, this indicates that the seizure was simple partial in onset. As the seizure spreads in the cortex, the seizure develops into a GTC seizure. The seizure would then be classified as a simple partial seizure with secondary generalization.[8] The loss of consciousness usually occurs simultaneously with the onset of a generalized stiffening of the flexor or the extensor muscles (termed *tonic phase*). After the tonic phase, generalized jerking of the muscles (clonic activity) occurs. A GTC seizure is almost always associated with deep postictal sleep.

ABSENCE SEIZURES

The revised classification of epileptic seizures by the International League against Epilepsy categorizes absence seizures as generalized seizures, indicating bihemispheric initial involvement clinically and electroencephalographically. Many children with absence seizures can be further categorized as having a characteristic epileptic syndrome.

The terms *typical* and *atypical absence seizures* were used in the International Classification of Epileptic Seizures to describe and categorize the various absence types. The simple typical absence consists of the sudden onset of impaired consciousness, usually associated with a blank facial appearance without other motor or behavioral phenomena. This subtype is actually relatively rare and comprised only 9% of 374 absence seizures video-recorded from 48 patients by Penry *et al.*[9] The complex typical absence, alternatively, is accompanied by other motor, behavioral, or autonomic phenomena.

Clonic components may be subtle and most frequently consist of eye blinking. Clonic activity may range from nystagmus to rapid jerking of the arms. Changes in tone often include a tonic postural contraction leading to flexion or hypertonic extension. Although a decrease in tone rarely causes a fall, the decrease may lead to nodding of the head or the dropping of objects.

Automatisms are the most common clinical accompaniment, occurring in 44% of 476 typical absence seizures studied by simultaneous video-electroencephalography radiotelemetry in 27 patients.[6] Automatisms are semipurposeful behaviors of which the patient is unaware and subsequently cannot recall. They may be either perseverative, reflecting the continuation of preictal activities, or de novo. Simple behaviors, such as rubbing the face or hands, licking the lips, chewing, grimacing, scratching, or fumbling with clothes, tend to be de novo automatisms. Complex activities, such as dealing cards, playing patty-cake, or handling a toy, are generally perseverative. Speech, if it occurs, is usually perseverative and is often slowed and dysarthric, but speech may be totally normal and may include both expressive and receptive aspects.

Autonomic phenomena associated with absence seizures include pupil dilatation, pallor, flushing, sweating, salivation, piloerection, and even urinary incontinence. Neither the autonomic changes nor the automatisms distinguish absence from other seizure types.

Atypical absence seizures have traditionally been characterized as having less abrupt onset or cessation, more pronounced changes in tone, and longer duration than typical absence seizures.[6,10,11] They usually begin before 5 years of age and are associated with other generalized seizure types and mental retardation.

Holmes *et al.*[6] compared 426 typical and 500 atypical absence seizures in 54 children. The atypical absence seizure lasted significantly longer, on average, than the typical absence seizure. A change in facial expression or the appearance of a blank stare was the most common initial clinical manifestation in either type. A pause or slowing of motor activity was also frequently noted as the initial finding in either seizure type. Either diminished postural tone or tonic or myoclonic activity was significantly more likely to be the initial clinical feature in atypical than in typical absences.

A blank stare or change in facial expression was the sole clinical finding in only 16% of typical and 28% of atypical absences. Automatisms, eye blinking, and lip smacking occurred more commonly in typical absences. A change in postural tone—either an increase or a decrease—was more commonly seen in atypical absences. Automatisms were more common in typical than in atypical absences and were usually perseverative, often consisting of playing with a toy or game. De novo automatisms were associated with longer spells and most commonly consisted of rubbing the face or hands or smiling.

Both typical and atypical absences started abruptly without an aura, lasted from a few to 30 s, and ended abruptly. Both were frequently associated with eye blinking, lip smacking, a decrease in tone, and automatisms. Although statistically significant differences can be identified, there is considerable overlap between the two seizure types and they most likely represent a clinical continuum. This overlap pertains to the electroencephalogram (EEG) and proposed pathophysiology as well.

Electroencephalography

The EEG signature of a typical absence seizure is the sudden onset of 3-Hz generalized symmetrical spike- or multiple spike-and-slow wave complexes (Fig. 1.1, A–C). The voltage of the discharges is often maximal in the frontocentral regions. The frequency tends to be faster (about 4 Hz) at the onset and slower (down to 2 Hz) toward the end of discharges if they persist longer than 10 s. The spike-and-wave discharge may be precipitated by hyperventilation or photic stimulation. The ictal discharges during an atypical absence seizure are more variable. They occur at frequencies between 1.5 and 2.5 Hz or may be faster than 2.5 Hz, but they are irregular or asymmetric in voltage.

The interictal EEG background is generally normal in typical and abnormal in atypical absences. Utilizing the preceding ictal EEG criteria to classify absence seizures, Holmes et al.[6] found that only 44% of 27 patients with typical absences had normal EEG backgrounds. Diffuse slowing was seen in 22% and paroxysmal spikes or sharp waves were seen in 37%. Conversely, only 11% of 27 patients with atypical absences had a normal interictal EEG. Diffuse slowing and focal or multifocal spikes or sharp waves were seen in 85% of patients.

The discharges are more numerous during all sleep states except rapid eye movement (REM) sleep. The bursts have a modified appearance in sleep: they are briefer and are irregular and they slow to 1.5–2.5 Hz. Hyperventilation, photic stimulation, and hypoglycemia will activate typical absence seizures, but hyperventilation is the most effective procedure.

Clinical effects are generally perceived to accompany discharges lasting longer than 3 seconds. Detailed neuropsychologic investigations have demonstrated functional impairment from a spike-and-wave burst of any duration. Auditory reaction times were delayed 56% of the time when a stimulus was presented at the onset

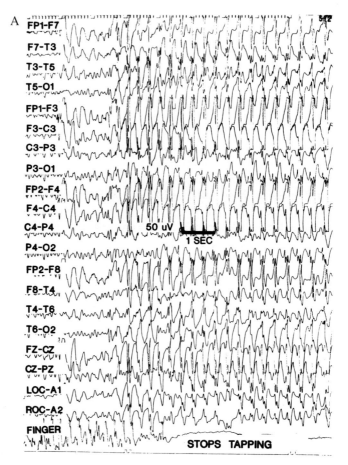

Figure 1.1 (A) Typical absence seizure. Note generalized onset of seizure. The child stops tapping her finger shortly after the onset of the seizure.

of the EEG paroxysm[12] and were abnormal 80% of the time when the stimulus was delayed 0.5 s. Responsiveness may improve as the paroxysm continues.

In atypical absences, the ictal EEG is more heterogeneous, showing 1.5- to 2.5-Hz slow spike-and-wave or multiple spike-and-wave discharges that may be irregular or asymmetric (Fig. 1.2). The interictal EEG is usually abnormal, reflecting slowing and multifocal epileptiform features.

CLONIC SEIZURES

Clonic seizures are similar to GTC seizures but consist only of rhythmic or semirhythmic contractions of a group of muscles. These jerks can involve any

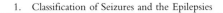

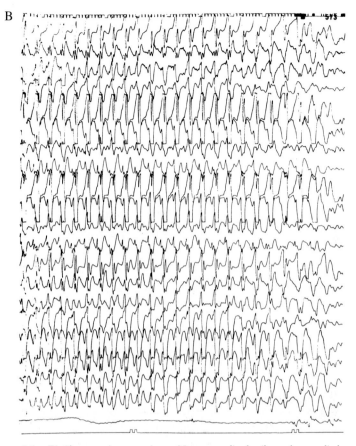

Figure 1.1 (B) Absence seizure continues. Note generalized spike-and-wave discharges.

muscle group, although the arms, neck, and facial muscles are most commonly involved. Clonic seizures are more common in children than adults.

MYOCLONIC SEIZURES

Myoclonic seizures are characterized by sudden, brief (<350 milliseconds), shocklike contractions that may be generalized or confined to the face and trunk or to one or more extremities, or even to individual muscles or groups of muscles.[3] Myoclonic seizures result in short bursts of synchronized electromyographic activity, which often involves simultaneous activation of agonist and antagonist muscles. The contractions of muscles are quicker than the contractions with clonic seizures. Any group of muscles can be involved in the jerk. Myoclonic seizures may be

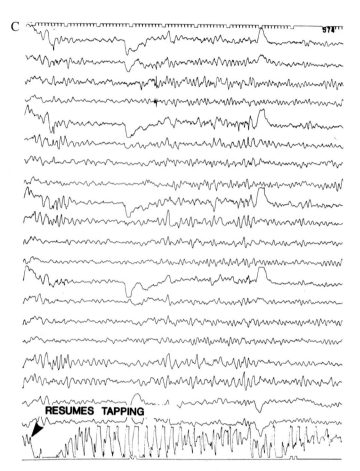

Figure 1.1 (C) End of absence seizure. Note that the child begins tapping finger again.

dramatic, causing the patient to fall to the ground, or they may be subtle, resembling tremors. Because of the brevity of the seizures, it is not possible to determine if consciousness is impaired. Myoclonus may occur as a component of an absence seizure or at the beginning of a GTC seizure. Myoclonic seizures are usually associated with generalized spike-and-wave activity.

TONIC SEIZURES

Tonic seizures are brief seizures (usually <60 s) consisting of the sudden onset of increased tone in the extensor muscles.[13-15] If standing, the patient typically

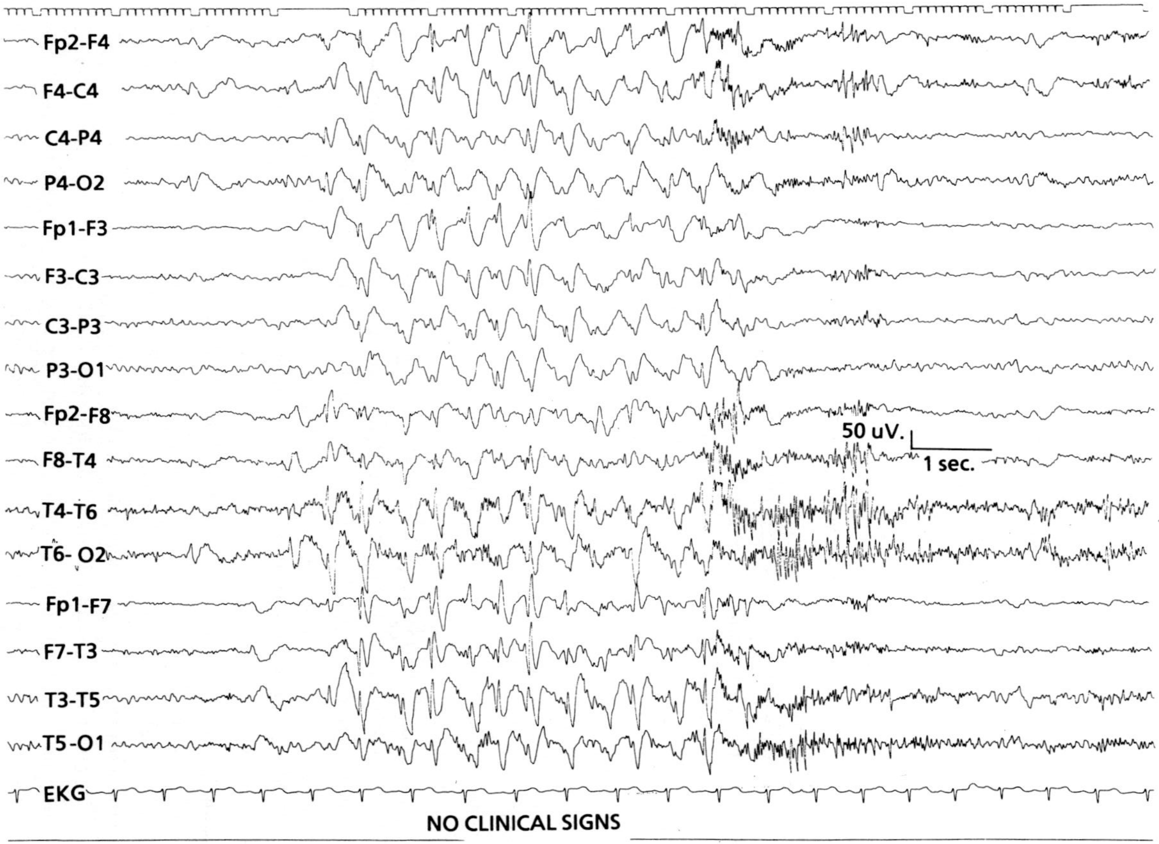

Fp2-F4
F4-C4
C4-P4
P4-O2
Fp1-F3
F3-C3
C3-P3
P3-O1
Fp2-F8
F8-T4
T4-T6
T6-O2
Fp1-F7
F7-T3
T3-T5
T5-O1
EKG

50 uV.
1 sec.

NO CLINICAL SIGNS

Figure 1.2 Atypical absence seizure with slow spike-and-wave.

falls to the ground. These seizures are invariably longer than myoclonic seizures. Electromyographic activity is dramatically increased in tonic seizures.

Impaired consciousness occurs during tonic seizures, although in short seizures it may be difficult to assess. Tonic seizures are frequently seen in patients with the Lennox–Gastaut syndrome, which is a disorder consisting of a mixed seizure disorder, mental retardation, and the EEG findings of a slow spike-and-wave pattern.[16-18] The seizures are usually more frequent at night.

Tonic seizures have been divided into four types: axial, axorhizomelic, global, and asymmetric. Axial tonic seizures begin with a tonic contraction of the neck muscles, leading to the fixation of the head in an erect position, widely opened eyes, and jaw clenching or mouth opening.[14,15] Contraction of the respiratory and abdominal muscles often follows and may lead to a high-pitched cry and brief periods of apnea.

Tonic axorhizomelic seizures begin with a sequence similar to the axial type, but then the tonic contractions extend to the proximal musculature of the upper limbs, elevating the shoulders and abducting the arms. In global tonic seizures, the tonic contractions extend to the periphery of the limbs. The arms are pulled upward to a semiflexed position in front of the head, and the fists are clenched, producing a body position similar to that of a child defending himself against a facial blow. Involvement of the lower extremities can also occur, leading to falls if the child is in a standing position. Asymmetric tonic seizures vary from a slight rotation of the head to a tonic contraction of all the musculature of one side of the body. Occasionally tonic seizures terminate with a clonic phase.

In a study of epileptic falls in children, Ikeno et al.[19] described two types of tonic seizures. The first type, termed the *tonic type,* is characterized by excessive flexion or extension of fingers, forced flexion of hand joints, jaw protrusion, shoulder elevation, upper arm abduction, and tonic flexion of the trunk. This hypertonic state continues unchanged even after the patient falls down. The second type, termed *flexor spasms,* is differentiated from the tonic type by the different distribution of hypertonicity. Flexor spasms are characterized by forward flexion of the head, elevation of the shoulders, flinging of the arms outward and forward, and flexion of the thighs at the hip. Unlike the tonic seizure type, fingers, hand joints, and elbows remain neither tonic nor atonic. The flexor spasms were noted by the authors to resemble infantile spasms.

Egli et al.[13] described tonic seizures that lead to falls as "axial spasms." Reflecting a uniform pattern of movement, these seizures consist of moderate flexion of the hips, upper trunk, and head, lasting from 0.5–0.8 s. The arms are almost always abducted, elevated, and in a semiflexed position. The fall is provoked by the rapidity and violence of the flexion in the hips.

Degree of consciousness impairment is often difficult to assess. In seizures lasting longer than a few seconds, impairment of consciousness is usually apparent.

Postictal impairment with confusion, tiredness, and headache is common. The degree of postictal impairment is usually related to the duration of the seizure.

The EEG ictal manifestations of tonic seizures usually consist of bilateral synchronous spikes of 10–25 Hz of medium to high voltage with a frontal accentuation (Fig. 1.3). Simple flattening or desynchronization may also occur. Occasional multiple spike-and-wave or diffuse slow activity may occur during a tonic seizure.

ATONIC SEIZURES

Atonic (astatic) seizures, or drop attacks, are characterized by a sudden loss of muscle tone. They begin suddenly and without warning and cause the patient, if standing, to fall quickly to the floor. Because there may be total lack of tone, the child has no means to protect himself or herself and injuries often occur. The attack may be fragmentary and lead to dropping of the head with slackening of the jaw or dropping of a limb. In atonic seizures there is a loss of electromyographic activity. Consciousness is impaired during the fall, although the patient may regain alertness immediately upon striking the floor. Atonic attacks are frequently associated with myoclonic jerks either before, during, or after the atonic seizure.[13,20] This combination has been described as myoclonic–astatic seizures (discussed later in this chapter). Atonic seizures are rare and are usually confined to childhood.[13,15,19] The majority of children with drop attacks have myoclonic or tonic seizures.[19] Atonic seizures are usually associated with rhythmic spike-and-wave complexes varying from slow (1–2 Hz) to more rapid, irregular spike- or multiple spike-and-wave activity.

WHAT IS AN EPILEPTIC SYNDROME?

After identifying the epileptic seizure type, it is important for the clinician to determine whether the patient has an epileptic syndrome. An epileptic syndrome is defined by a cluster of signs and symptoms customarily occurring together.[3,21] Identification of an epileptic syndrome may allow the physician to determine genetic risk; that is, certain epileptic syndromes are associated with specific genotypes. In addition, syndrome identification helps determine appropriate therapy and prognosis.

Two dichotomies are used to shape the major classes of epilepsy. One separates epilepsies with generalized seizures (generalized epilepsies) from epilepsies with partial or focal seizures (localization-related partial or focal epilepsies); the other separates epilepsies of known etiology (symptomatic or secondary epilepsies) from those that are idiopathic (primary) or cryptogenic (Table 1.2).

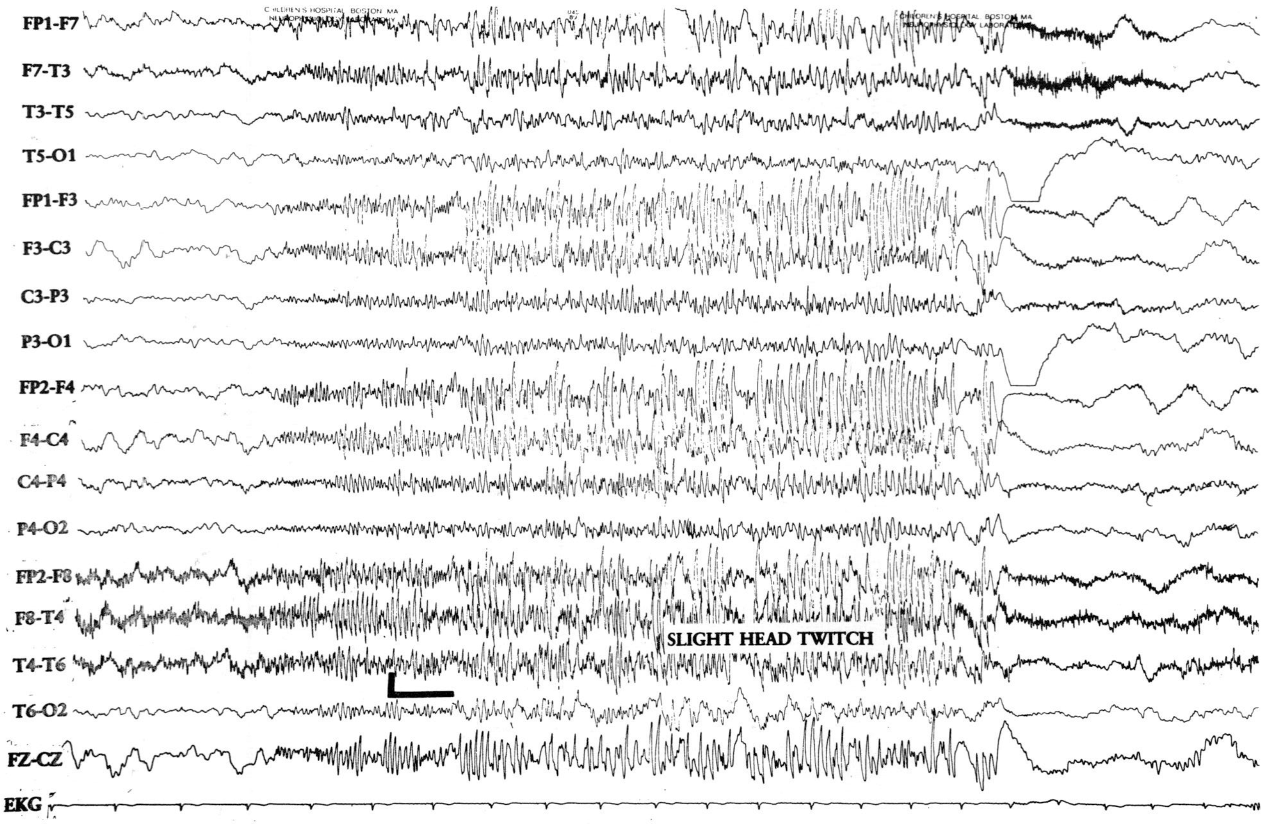

Figure 1.3 Rapios spikes in a child with tonic seizures.

Table 1.2

International Classification of Epilepsies and Epileptic Syndromes[a]

I. Localization-Related (Focal, Local, Partial) Epilepsies and Syndromes
  A. Idiopathic with age-related onset
    1. Benign childhood epilepsy with centrotemporal spikes
    2. Childhood epilepsy with occipital paroxysms
  B. Symptomatic
II. Generalized Epilepsies and Syndromes
  A. Idiopathic with age-related onset listed in order of age
    1. Benign neonatal familial convulsions
    2. Benign idiopathic convulsions
    3. Benign myoclonic epilepsy in infancy
    4. Childhood absence epilepsy (pyknolepsy)
    5. Juvenile absence epilepsy
    6. Juvenile myoclonic epilepsy (impulsive petit mal)
    7. Epilepsy with grand mal seizures on awakening
  C. Idiopathic and/or symptomatic, in order of appearance
    1. West syndrome (infantile spasms)
    2. Lennox–Gastaut syndrome
    3. Epilepsy with myoclonic–astatic seizures
    4. Epilepsy with myoclonic absences
  D. Symptomatic
    1. Nonspecific etiology
      a. Early myoclonic encephalopathy
    2. Specific etiology
      a. Epileptic seizures may complicate many disease states
III. Epilepsies and syndromes undetermined as to whether they are focal or generalized
  A. With both generalized and focal seizures
    1. Neonatal seizures
    2. Severe myoclonic epilepsy in infancy
    3. Epilepsy with continuous spike waves during slow-wave sleep
    4. Acquired epileptic aphasia (Landau–Kleffner syndrome)
  B. Without unequivocal generalized focal features
IV. Special syndromes
  A. Situation-related seizures
    1. Febrile convulsions
    2. Seizures related to other identifiable situations such as stress, hormonal changes, drugs, alcohol, or sleep deprivation
  B. Isolated, apparently unprovoked epileptic events
  C. Epilepsies characterized by specific modes of seizure precipitation

[a] Modified from Ref. 21.

WHAT ARE THE CATEGORIES OF IDIOPATHIC-RELATED PARTIAL EPILEPSIES?

BENIGN ROLANDIC EPILEPSY

Originally described by Marinus Rulandus in 1597,[22] benign rolandic epilepsy is a genetic disorder confined to children that is characterized by nocturnal generalized seizures of probable focal onset, diurnal partial seizures arising from the lower rolandic area, and an EEG pattern consisting of a midtemporal–central spike focus.[23-36] Diagnosis of the syndrome, which depends on the patient's history and EEG features, allows the clinician to offer the patient and parents a rational plan for treatment, genetic counseling, and prognosis.

The disorder always begins during childhood. The age range is from 3 to 13 years, the peak incidence occurring between the seventh and eighth years of life.[34] The disorder occurs more frequently in boys than in girls.[24,25,37,38] Most affected children have normal intelligence and normal neurologic examination findings.[38]

The syndrome is termed *rolandic epilepsy* because of the characteristic feature of partial seizures involving the region around the lower portion of the central gyrus of Rolando. Although a nocturnal seizure is the most dramatic and common mode of initial presentation, diurnal seizures may also lead to a neurologic evaluation.

Lombroso[39] described the characteristic features of benign rolandic epilepsy: (1) somatosensory stimulation of the oral-buccal cavity; (2) speech arrest; (3) preservation of consciousness; (4) excessive pooling of saliva; (5) tonic or tonic-clonic activity of the face. Less often the somatosensory sensation will spread to the face or arm. On rare occasions a typical Jacksonian march of tonic or tonic-clonic activity will occur.

Although the somatosensory aura is common, a history of this symptom is frequently not elicited, especially in young patients.[39] Motor phenomena during daytime attacks are usually restricted to one side of the body and include tonic, clonic, or tonic-clonic events. These attacks most frequently involve the face, although the arm and leg may be involved. Although seizures rarely generalize when the patient is awake, the sensory or motor phenomena may change sides during the course of the attack.[37] Arrest of speech may initiate the attack or occur during its course. Consciousness is rarely impaired during daytime attacks. After the seizure the child may feel numbness, pins and needles, or "electricity" in his tongue, gums, and cheek on one side. Postictal confusion and amnesia are unusual in benign rolandic epilepsy.

In nocturnal seizures the initial event is typically clonic movements of the mouth along with salivation and gurgling sounds from the throat. Secondary generalization of the nocturnal seizure is common. The initial focal component of the seizure may be brief and it is surmised that this portion of the seizure may not be seen by the parents. Some nocturnal seizures remain partial and do not generalize. It is likely that the frequency of seizures during sleep is underreported.

Seizure frequency in benign rolandic epilepsy is typically low.[24,37,38] Lerman[37] states that 10–13% of children will have only one seizure, regardless of drug therapy. In a study of 100 patients with benign rolandic epilepsy, Lerman and Kivity[38] found that 13 of the patients had only one seizure and 66 had infrequent seizures. However, 21% of the patients had frequent seizures.

Status epilepticus is extremely rare in this disorder. Fejerman and Di Blasi[40] described two children who had clinical and EEG features consistent with benign rolandic epilepsy and in whom status epilepticus developed. The status epilepticus in both children consisted of facial clonus, anarthria, and sialorrhea. However, both children had features that were somewhat unusual for benign rolandic epilepsy: the first had atypical absences and the second had recurrent seizures despite trials of phenobarbital and of combination therapy with phenytoin and carbamazepine. Calamaria et al.[41] reported on a child who had seizures that lasted 4–5 h and that were characterized by speech arrest, sialorrhea, and facial weakness, along with occasional facial and tongue clonic activity. The interictal EEG demonstrated typical centrotemporal spikes. Roulet et al[42] described a child with prolonged but intermittent drooling, lingual dyspraxia, and other clinical and EEG features of benign rolandic epilepsy. The fluctuating course of the symptomatology and correlation with the intensity of paroxysmal discharges on the EEG were consistent with epileptic dysfunction in the lower rolandic area.

Both daytime and nighttime seizures may occur, although in most children the seizures usually occur during sleep. More than half of the children with benign rolandic epilepsy have nocturnal seizures only.[34] Approximately 15% have seizures during sleep and while awake and 10–20% have them in the waking state alone.[37] The increase in seizure incidence during sleep parallels the increase in spikes seen during drowsiness and sleep.

Electroencephalography

Benign rolandic epilepsy is characterized by a distinctive EEG pattern. The characteristic interictal EEG abnormality is a high-amplitude, usually diphasic spike with a prominent following slow wave (Fig. 1.4). The spikes (<70 milliseconds) or sharp waves (<200 milliseconds) appear singly or in groups at the midtemporal (T3, T4) and central (rolandic) regions (C3, C4). When bipolar recording montages are used, the spikes may appear most prominent in the central or midtemporal region and usually occur synchronously in both regions. Although typically present in both regions, at times the spikes may shift from one to the other or may be seen only in the midtemporal or central region. As will be discussed, the rolandic discharges typically occur only during childhood, peaking at about age 10.

The spikes may be confined to one hemisphere or may occur bilaterally. In approximately 60% of patients, the spike focus is unilateral, whereas in 40% there are bilateral spike foci either on the initial EEG or on subsequent recordings.[37] When the spikes are unilateral, they are equally represented in the left and right hemispheres. When bilateral, the spikes can be synchronous or asynchronous and symmetric or asymmetric. Rolandic spikes usually occur on a normal background. However, when the spikes occur frequently, focal slowing may appear to occur

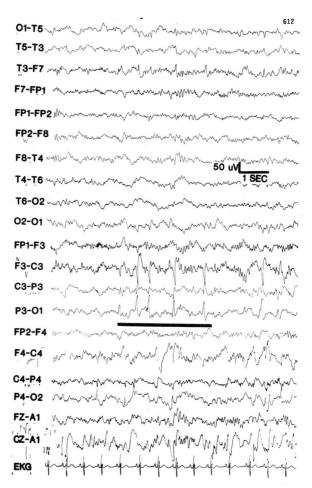

Figure 1.4   Central spikes in a patient with benign rolandic epilepsy.

in the region of the spikes. This "pseudoslowing" is secondary to the slow waves accompanying the spikes. The spikes are often activated by sleep.[43-49] In approximately 30% of children with benign rolandic epilepsy, spikes appear only in sleep.[43] Sleep states are usually normal in benign rolandic epilepsy. Some records show generalized spike-wave discharges without any concomitant clinical signs of absence seizures.[46] These diffuse spike-and-wave discharges, which can occasionally occur during the awake state, are strongly activated by sleep.[46] Most children with benign rolandic epilepsy who have spike-wave discharges during sleep do not have typical absence seizures.

BENIGN OCCIPITAL EPILEPSY

Benign occipital epilepsy was described by Gastaut as a benign form of partial epilepsy in childhood in which seizures characteristically began with visual ictal symptoms and in which interictal occipital rhythmic spikes appeared only after eye closure.[50-53] Numerous other authors have subsequently presented additional cases and, as is the case for benign rolandic epilepsy, the clinical and EEG features of the syndrome are stereotypical enough to warrant its classification as a syndrome.[54]

In a large series, Gastaut[52] reviewed the clinical and EEG features of 53 patients with the syndrome. However, only 55% of the patients had the "complete" syndrome. Twenty-five percent of the patients either lacked the ictal visual symptoms or the interictal occipital EEG abnormality.

The age of onset of benign occipital epilepsy is from 15 months to 17 years, the peak age of onset being between 5 and 7 years.[52,55] Both the clinical manifestations and frequency of the seizures are variable, depending on when the seizure occurs.[56] In nocturnal seizures motor symptoms predominate, whereas in diurnal seizures visual symptoms are most common. Nocturnal seizures are more common in younger children and appear to bear a good prognosis. Seizures starting after the age of 8 years are more likely to be frequent and diurnal and to continue for longer periods of time.[55]

The visual symptoms consist of amaurosis and elementary visual hallucinations (i.e., phosphenes, complex visual hallucinations, or visual illusions including micropsia, metamorphopsia, or palinopsia). Although Gastaut described the ictal visual symptoms as common, Beaumanoir[57] found that only 44% of her patients had these symptoms, a finding similar to those of Newton and Aicardi.[58] Panayiotopoulos[55] found that visual phenomena were rare in children and that the age of onset was younger than 8 years. However, it is possible that young children underreport visual phenomena.

A variety of motor activities are seen in this disorder. Hemiclonic seizures occurred in 43% of the patients, complex partial seizures in 14%, generalized tonic-clonic seizures in 13%, and other types of ictal manifestations, including dysphasia, dysesthesia, and adversive seizures, in 25% in Gastaut's series.[52] Other authors have emphasized that adversive seizures, usually contraversive, are the most common of the ictal motor phenomena that occur in this disorder.[55,59-61] Talwar et al.[53] reported that 75% of their patients had partial seizures and 25% had absence seizures.

Seizure duration and frequency in benign occipital epilepsy are variable. Panayiotopoulos[55] reported seizure durations lasting minutes to hours. Seizure frequency also varies from many attacks daily to occasional seizures.[52,55]

Headache and vomiting may occur after benign occipital epilepsy. Following their seizures, 33% of Gastaut's patients[52] had diffuse headache and 17% had postictal migraine-like nausea and vomiting. Talwar et al.[53] reported that 40% of their patients had migraine. Lerman and Kivity[56] and Terasaki et al.[62] noted that headaches can occur at variable times around the seizure, sometimes preceding the visual phenomena.

Electroencephalography

The interictal EEG is characterized by normal background activity and well-defined occipital discharges.[52] The occipital spikes are typically high in voltage (200–300 μV) and diphasic, having a main negative peak followed by a relatively small positive peak and a negative slow wave.[55] An important feature is the prompt disappearance of the discharges with eye opening, along with their reappearance 1–20 s after eye closure. The spike component is typically higher in amplitude than the negative slow wave, often exceeding 100 μV and a duration of less than 70 milliseconds.[55] The amplitude is highest over the occipital and posterotemporal regions and can be unilateral or bilateral. When occurring bilaterally, the spikes are frequently asymmetric.[55] The location of the spikes may change over time and serial EEGs may show that the spikes "migrate" from the occipital region to the centrotemporal region.[63] The spikes may persist long after the child stops experiencing seizures.[55] Like rolandic spikes, occipital spikes are usually confined to childhood, peaking at about 3–5 years of age. The spikes usually appear rhythmically at a frequency of 1–3 Hz in bursts or trains.

WHAT ARE THE CATEGORIES OF GENERALIZED EPILEPSIES AND SYNDROMES?

BENIGN FAMILIAL NEONATAL SEIZURES

There is general agreement among authors that the diagnosis of benign familial neonatal seizures in a child with seizures is based on five criteria: (1) normal neurologic examination; (2) negative evaluation for another etiology of the seizures; (3) normal developmental and intellectual outcome; (4) positive family history of newborn or infantile seizures with benign outcome; (5) onset of seizures during the neonatal or early infantile period.[64–66] Although early reports indicated that the seizures had their onset during the first week of life—usually on the third day—in some patients the onset has occurred after the first week. Whether these infants should be considered to have a distinct syndrome is not yet settled.

The seizures usually occur frequently for a few days and then stop. The infant is usually alert and vigorous during the interictal period. Focal or multifocal clonic seizures are the most frequent type of seizure, although generalized seizures have also been reported. The seizures are generally brief, lasting for approximately 1–2 min, but may occur as many as 20 to 30 times a day.

Electroencephalography

The interictal EEG is of little assistance in diagnosing benign familial neonatal seizures, because it may or may not be abnormal interictally. No diagnostic features have been reported. When abnormal, the findings are frequently transient. Unfortunately, in many of the case reports that have been published, electroencephalography was not performed or the results were not described in sufficient detail. Abnormalities reported include spikes, sharp waves, "epileptiform" patterns, "generalized periodicity," and slowing. The ictal EEG has been reported to demonstrate bilateral, symmetrical flattening followed by bilateral discharges of spikes and sharp waves.[67]

BENIGN NEONATAL CONVULSIONS

Benign neonatal convulsions, also called *benign neonatal idiopathic seizures,* are notable for occurring in term, otherwise healthy infants.[64,65,68] Criteria used by Plouin[65-66] and Dehan *et al.*[69] to make the diagnosis include: (1) birth after 39 weeks of gestation; (2) an APGAR score of 9 or above, 5 minutes after birth; (3) the presence of a seizure-free interval between birth and the onset of seizures; (4) clonic or apneic seizures; (5) negative evaluations for etiology; (6) a favorable outcome in regard to neurologic development; (7) lack of seizures outside the neonatal period. Some authors have reported such seizures as being "fifth-day fits."[65] It is likely that benign idiopathic neonatal seizures and fifth-day fits are identical syndromes.

Typically the seizures begin on the fifth day of life. In a review of six different series of patients with benign idiopathic neonatal seizures, Plouin[65] noted that in all 182 patients described, the onset of seizures occurred between the first and seventh day of life. The initial seizure occurred on the fourth, fifth, or sixth day of life in 80% of cases. In 153 of the 182 cases reported, the exact day that seizure activity began was given; it was found that one-half of these patients had their first seizure on day 5 of life.

The seizures are usually partial clonic and may be confined to one body part or may migrate from one region to another. Apnea may occur with the clonic activity or may be the sole manifestation of the seizure. Tonic seizures are rare. The seizures often occur in a crescendo of activity. Initially the patient is normal between seizures. The seizures then increase in frequency until the child goes into status epilepticus. The flurry of seizures usually lasts less than 24 h but may continue for a few days.[65,66]

Electroencephalography

As for benign familial neonatal seizures, EEG findings in benign idiopathic neonatal seizures have been variable. In a survey of 101 EEGs from infants with the disorder, the interictal EEG was normal in 10 of the infants, was excessively discontinuous in 6, showed "focal" or "multifocal" abnormalities in 25, and demonstrated the theta pointu alternant pattern in 60.[65] The theta pointu alternant pattern consists of dominant theta activity that is discontinuous, unreactive, and often asynchronous and that has intermixed sharp waves. It is present throughout sleep and throughout the awake state and may persist up to the twelfth day of life, even after the seizures have ceased.

The theta pointu alternant pattern is not specific for benign seizures and can be seen after a variety of neonatal encephalopathies. However, Plouin[65] claims that the EEG pattern is associated with a favorable prognosis regardless of etiology.

BENIGN MYOCLONIC EPILEPSY IN INFANCY

Benign myoclonic epilepsy in infants is a rare syndrome in which brief bouts of generalized myoclonus occur during the first or second year of life.[70,71] The EEGs typically show generalized spike-waves occurring in brief bursts during the early stages of sleep. The infants do not have other seizure types, although generalized tonic-clonic seizures may occur during adolescence. Usually, the seizures are easily controlled with epileptic drugs and are limited to the first few years of life.

CHILDHOOD ABSENCE EPILEPSY (PYKNOLEPSY)

Pyknolepsy refers to typical absence seizures (i.e., both simple and complex) in children between the ages of 3 years and puberty who are otherwise healthy. There is a strong genetic predisposition and girls are more frequently affected. The absences are frequent, occurring at least several times daily, and tend to cluster. The EEG reveals a bilateral, synchronous symmetric 3-Hz spike-and-wave discharge with normal interictal background activity. The absences may remit during adolescence, but generalized tonic-clonic seizures may develop.

JUVENILE ABSENCE EPILEPSY

Juvenile absence epilepsy begins around puberty and differs from pyknolepsy in that the seizures are more sporadic and retropulsive movements are less common. This syndrome blurs with juvenile myoclonic epilepsy, because generalized tonic-clonic seizures and myoclonic seizures are often seen upon awakening. Sex distribution is equal and the EEG reveals the spike-waves to be often slightly faster than 3 Hz.

In the author's experience, childhood and juvenile absence seizures do not have distinct distinguishing features.

JUVENILE MYOCLONIC EPILEPSY

Juvenile myoclonic epilepsy (JME) is a familial disorder that typically begins in the second decade of life and is characterized by mild myoclonic seizures, generalized tonic-clonic or clonic-tonic-clonic seizures (clonic-tonic-clonic seizures are a variation of GTC seizures in which there is an initial clonic phase), and occasionally absence seizures. The syndrome is named after Janz, who described a familial disorder of myoclonic epilepsy associated with an excellent prognosis in patients who were otherwise mentally and neurologically healthy. Janz initially termed the syndrome *impulsive petit mal* to indicate that the myoclonic jerks are a type of minor seizure.[72]

The myoclonic seizures are usually mild to moderate in intensity and involve the neck, shoulders, and arms. The movements involve an entire extremity or body part rather than an isolated muscle contraction. They can occur either singularly or repetitively and may cause the patient to drop objects. They are generally bilateral, although sometimes they are asymmetric with changing left–right accentuation. The jerks may rarely involve the legs and cause the patient to fall to the ground. More commonly they are mild, and the patient may attribute them to nervousness or clumsiness.[62] Occasionally, however, the jerks become more severe and violent jerks occur in rapid succession, in a chorea-like episode. Myoclonic status, a state in which the patient has myoclonic jerks every few seconds or in salvos of three to five jerks, can occur. Despite preserved consciousness, the patient is often incapacitated by the continuous myoclonic jerks. The myoclonic seizures are usually confined to the period several hours after awakening from a night's sleep or a nap, however in some patients the seizures may continue all day, although less frequently. In these patients the seizures may increase in frequency again at the end of the day when the patient is fatigued. They are typically aggravated by sleep deprivation.

The vast majority of patients with JME have tonic-clonic or clonic-tonic-clonic seizures.[73,74] Only 2 of 43 of Delgado–Escueta and Enrile–Bascal's[74] patients were free from these seizure types. Ten of a series of 12 patients reported by Asconape and Penry[73] had generalized tonic-clonic seizures. Although there are cases in which the myoclonic and generalized tonic-clonic seizures begin simultaneously and others in which the generalized tonic-clonic seizures occur before the onset of the myoclonic seizures, in the large majority of cases the myoclonic jerks precede the onset of the generalized tonic-clonic seizures. Like the myoclonic seizures, the tonic-clonic seizures often occur shortly after awakening or during early-morning sleep. At times patients will experience a series of myoclonic seizures culminating in a generalized seizure. In addition, some patients will have several days of an increasing number of myoclonic seizures, followed by generalized tonic-clonic seizures.

Absence seizures also occur in a substantial number of patients. Delgado–Escueta and Enrile–Bascal[74] reported that 40% of patients also had absences, usually in association with tonic-clonic or clonic-tonic-clonic seizures. As with other seizure types, these often occur shortly after awakening.

Juvenile myoclonic epilepsy begins in childhood; onset occurs in the second decade in most patients. In a study of 43 patients, the average age of seizure onset was 13.6 years with the range being 8–24 years.[74] The general findings from physical and neurologic examinations of these patients are usually normal. In addition, normal intelligence is the rule. A positive family history of epilepsy is common. The mode of inheritance appears to be polygenic with females having a lower threshold than males.[74]

Electroencephalography

The interictal EEG in this disorder is reported to be distinctive and easily distinguished from those of other forms of generalized epilepsy.[74] The characteristic feature of the EEG is the fast (3.5–6-Hz) spike-and-wave and multiple spike-and-wave complexes (Fig. 1.5). This pattern is in contrast with the 3-Hz spike-and-wave complexes seen in classic absence and the slow (1.5–2.5-Hz) spike-and-wave complexes of the Lennox–Gastaut syndrome (LGS). During myoclonic seizures, the ictal EEG consists of 10–16-Hz rapid spikes, followed by irregular slow waves. Photosensitivity may activate the epileptiform discharges. If the diagnosis is suspected and the awake EEG is normal, it is imperative that a sleep-deprived EEG be obtained, because this may be the only time the abnormality is present.

EPILEPSY WITH GRAND MAL SEIZURES ON AWAKENING

Epilepsy with grand mal seizures on awakening is a syndrome in which generalized tonic-clonic seizures occur, either exclusively or predominantly, a short time after awakening.[75] The onset is usually in the second decade of life. If patients have other seizure types, they are usually absence or myoclonic. The EEG typically shows generalized spike-wave activity. Photosensitivity is a common feature.

INFANTILE SPASMS

Infantile spasms constitute a unique and frequently malignant epileptic syndrome confined to infants. The usual characteristic features of this syndrome are

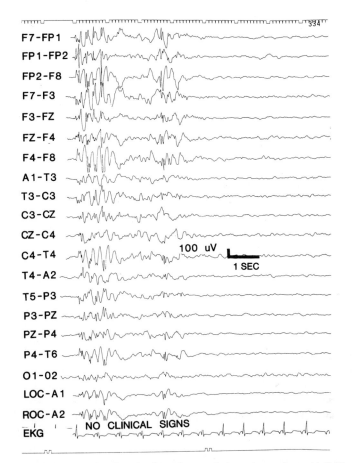

Figure 1.5   Example of rapid spike-and-wave discharge in a patient with JME.

tonic or myoclonic seizures, hypsarrhythmic EEGs, and mental retardation. The triad of infantile spasms, hypsarrhythmic EEG, and mental retardation is referred to as West's syndrome. Not all cases of infantile spasms conform strictly to this definition. The disorder is also referred to in the literature as massive spasms, salaam seizures, flexion spasms, jackknife seizures, massive myoclonic jerks, or infantile myoclonic seizures, and in the German literature it is called Blitz–Nick–Saalam Krampfe.

Infantile spasms are an age-specific disorder beginning during the first two years of life. The peak age of onset is between 4 and 6 months. Approximately 90% of infantile spasms begin before 12 months of age.[76] It is rare for infantile spasms to begin during the first 2 weeks of life or after 18 months of age.

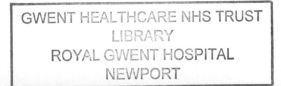

GWENT HEALTHCARE NHS TRUST
LIBRARY
ROYAL GWENT HOSPITAL
NEWPORT

Infantile spasms may vary considerably in their clinical manifestations. Some seizures are characterized by brief head nods, whereas other seizures consist of violent flexion of the trunk, arms, and legs. Infantile spasms can be classified into three major groups: flexor, extensor, and mixed flexor–extensor types.[77] Flexor spasms consist of flexion of the neck, trunk, arms, and legs. Spasms of the muscles of the upper limbs result in either adduction of the arms or a self-hugging motion or in adduction of the arms to either side of the head with the arms flexed at the elbows. Extensor spasms consist of a predominance of extensor muscle contractions that produce abrupt extension of the neck and trunk, along with extensor abduction or adduction of the arms, legs, or both. Mixed flexor–extensor spasms include flexion of the neck, trunk, and arms and extension of the legs or flexion of the legs and extension of the arms with varying degrees of flexion of the neck and trunk. Asymmetric spasms occasionally occur and consist of the maintenance of a "fencing" posture. Variations in infantile spasms occur frequently with the majority of patients having more than one seizure type. Infantile spasms may also be associated with autonomic dysfunction characterized by pallor, flushing, sweating, pupillary dilation, lacrimation, and changes in respiratory and heart rate.[78,79]

Infantile spasms frequently occur in clusters and the intensity and frequency of the spasms in each cluster may increase to a peak before progressively decreasing. The seizures are brief and single seizures may be missed by the casual observer. The number of seizures per cluster varies considerably with some clusters having as many as 150 seizures. The number of clusters per day also varies; some patients have as many as 60 clusters per day. Clusters can occur during sleep or shortly after awakening. Crying or irritability during or after a flurry of spasms is commonly observed. The number of infantile spasms that occur at night are similar to the number that occur during the day.[78]

Infantile spasms are frequently associated with developmental delay. In a review of the literature, Lacy and Penry[78] reported that only 10% of patients were developmentally normal at the time their infantile spasms were diagnosed. Patients whose symptomatic infantile spasms have identifiable causes have a higher incidence of retardation than patients whose spasms have idiopathic causes.[79] Abnormal neurologic findings upon physical examination are also commonly reported. Lacy and Penry[78] reported that 70% of patients with infantile spasms have abnormal findings upon neurologic examination. Children with identifiable etiologies for the spasms are more likely to have neurologic impairment than those in the idiopathic group.[79,80]

Electroencephalography

Infantile spasms are usually associated with markedly abnormal EEGs. The most commonly found EEG pattern is hypsarrhythmia (Fig. 1.6).[78,80–83] Variations of hypsarrhythmia include hypsarrhythmia with interhemispheric synchrony, hypsarrhythmia with a consistent focus of abnormal discharge, hypsarrhythmia with episodes of attenuation, and hypsarrhythmia consisting primarily of high-voltage slow activity with few sharp waves or spikes.[84] During sleep, especially REM sleep, the hypsarrhythmic pattern may be markedly reduced or may totally disappear.[84] A hypsarrhythmic or modified hypsarrhythmic pattern is the most common type of interictal abnormality seen in infantile spasms, although this pattern may not be present in some patients with infantile spasms.[81] Some patients with infantile spasms do not have hypsarrhythmia early in the course of the disorder but go on to develop the pattern. Although hypsarrhythmia is associated primarily with infantile spasms, it occurs in other disorders as well.[85]

The ictal EEG changes during infantile spasms are variable.[77,86] Although Kellaway et al.[77] found 11 different types of ictal EEG patterns that accompanied the clinical seizures, a marked generalized attenuation of electrical activity was a feature of 72% of the seizures.[17,82] Ictal EEG abnormalities and clinical seizure type were not closely correlated.

LENNOX–GASTAUT SYNDROME

Lennox–Gastaut syndrome (LGS) is characterized by a mixed seizure disorder with tonic seizures and a slow spike-and-wave EEG pattern being major components. The syndrome always begins in childhood. Mental retardation is considered a component by some authors.[3]

The child with LGS typically exhibits a mixture of seizure types; the most frequently occurring are tonic, tonic-clonic, myoclonic, atypical absences, and "head drops," which represent forms of atonic, tonic, or myoclonic seizures.[13,15–18,20,87]

Tonic seizures, a key component of this syndrome,[17,87] are typically activated by sleep and may occur repetitively throughout the night. They occur more frequently during non-REM sleep than they do during the awake state and they usually do not occur during REM sleep. In LGS, tonic seizures are usually brief, lasting from a few seconds to 1 min, with an average duration of about 10 s. The seizures may cause falls and injury. Eyelid retraction, staring, mydriasis, and apnea are commonly associated with this syndrome and they may be the most prominent features.[17] During tonic seizures the patient is unconscious, although arousal from light sleep may occur. Because they are often brief, the seizures frequently go undetected.

Although atonic seizures are common in LGS, they occur less frequently than tonic and myoclonic seizures. Most such seizures last only 1–4 s. In the shortest attacks, patients may show only head nodding or sagging at the knees. The seizures are so brief that it is difficult to determine if consciousness is lost. If a fall occurs, the patient usually gets up immediately and resumes what he or she was doing. Many children with drop attacks will have myoclonic or tonic seizures. In a study of 48 drop attacks in 15 children with LGS,[19] only 4% of the seizures were of the atonic type.

Myoclonic seizures, occurring either in isolation or as a component of absence seizures, are common in this disorder. Occasionally in a patient, the myoclonus may be so prominent that some investigators have described a myoclonic variant

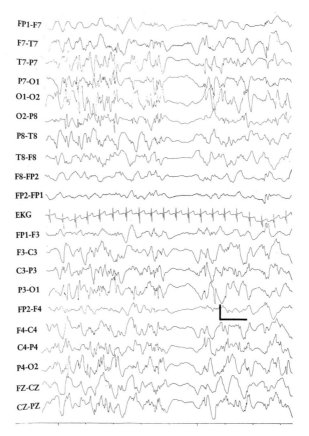

Figure 1.6 Hypsarrhythmia in infant with infantile spasms. There are multifocal spikes and sharp waves. In addition, brief periods of suppression are noted. (Calibration 50 μv and 1 sec)

of LGS.[17] Atypical absence and generalized tonic-clonic seizures are seen in more than half of the patients with LGS.[18,20] Generalized tonic-clonic seizures usually cause the most concern to parents and are often the seizure type that precipitates hospitalization. Atypical absences are generally longer than typical absences and have a higher association with changes in postural tone and myoclonic jerks.[3]

Patients with LGS typically have frequent seizures. Markand[18] found that 60% of his patients had seizures daily, whereas Papini *et al.*,[88] in a longitudinal study of 16 patients with LGS, found that the mean daily frequency of seizures ranged from 9–70. Some children with this syndrome have hundreds of seizures daily.

Mental retardation is present before seizure onset in 20–60% of patients.[17] Some patients whose seizures have idiopathic or cryptogenic etiologies have normal

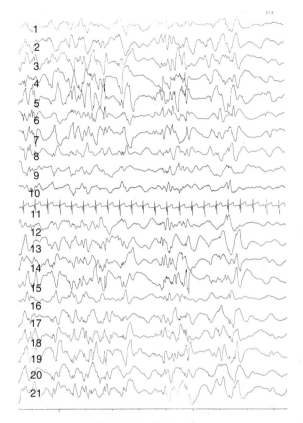

Figure 1.6 (*Continued*)

IQ scores or developmental histories before the onset of their seizures. The proportion of retarded patients increases with age because of the deterioration that often occurs in LGS.[17] Rarely, a few patients escape mental retardation.[17] Marked fluctuations in cognitive abilities occur in LGS patients and are, to some degree, correlated with the intensity of EEG abnormalities. In addition to cognitive difficulties, behavioral problems are common in LGS, ranging from hyperactivity with aggressive behavior to frank psychotic and autistic behavior. In addition to mental retardation and behavioral problems, neurologic abnormalities have been reported in 30–88% of patients with LGS.[18,20,89]

Electroencephalography

The sine qua non of EEG findings in LGS is a slow spike-and-wave discharge superimposed on an abnormal, slow background. The slow spike-and-wave or sharp-and-slow-wave complexes consist of generalized discharges occurring at a frequency of 1.5–2.5 Hz (see Fig. 1.2). The morphology, amplitude, and repetition rate may vary both between bursts and during paroxysmal bursts of spike-and-wave activity. Transient and shifting asymmetries of the discharge frequently occur. The area of maximum voltage, although variable, is usually frontal or temporal. Sleep increases the frequency of the discharges, but hyperventilation and photic stimulation rarely activate them. During non-REM sleep, slow spike-and-wave discharges may be replaced by multiple spike-and-wave discharges, whereas in REM sleep, the paroxysmal activity decreases markedly. The typical EEG manifestation of tonic seizures is the occurrence of fast-rhythm discharges of 10 to 20 Hz (see Fig. 1.3). Patients may also have bursts of multiple spike-and-wave discharges during tonic seizures. In atonic seizures the EEG pattern is most frequently a fast-rhythm discharge, but bursts of slow spike-wave complexes or high-amplitude 10-Hz discharges are sometimes recorded. The EEG correlate of myoclonic seizures consists of bursts of arrhythmic multiple spike-wave or irregular spike-wave activity. Atypical absence seizures are associated with slow (<2.5 Hz), and often asymmetric and irregular, spike-and-wave activity.[6]

EPILEPSY WITH MYOCLONIC–ASTATIC SEIZURES

Doose[90] described a group of children with myoclonic and astatic seizures, often in combination with absence, generalized tonic-clonic, and tonic seizures. In this syndrome, astatic seizures (defined as seizures during which the patient is unable to stand) occurred suddenly, without warning, and the child collapsed onto the floor as if his or her legs had been pulled from under the child. No apparent loss of consciousness accompanies these seizures. At times the astatic seizures are so short that only a brief nodding of the head and slight flexion of the knees are apparent. From the clinical description of these seizures, it appears that they are atonic. The myoclonic seizures in this disorder are characterized by symmetric jerking of the arms and shoulders with simultaneous nodding of the head. Some myoclonic jerks are violent, causing the arms to fling upward, and some are so mild that they are easier to feel than to see. A combination of myoclonic and astatic seizures were frequently observed. In these children, the loss of postural tone is immediately preceded by myoclonic jerks—hence the term *myoclonic–astatic seizures*.

The onset of the disorder, which is more common in boys than in girls, occurs between the ages of 1 and 5. The EEG pattern consists of bilaterally synchronous, regular or irregular 2–3-Hz spike-and-wave discharges, whereas the background activity exhibits an excess of monomorphic theta activity.

With few exceptions, mental and motor development is normal before the onset of the illness. However, the prognosis is generally unfavorable and dementia develops in most patients. Absence status is reported to play a role in the pathogenesis of the dementia.

Epilepsy with Myoclonic Absences

Myoclonic seizures often occur as a component of absence seizures. In a study of 426 typical and 500 atypical absence seizures in 54 children, in which simultaneous electroencephalography frequency modulation radiotelemetry and videotape monitoring were deployed, Holmes et al.[6] found myoclonic jerks in 13% of typical absences and 12% of atypical absences. Myoclonus was never seen as the initial manifestation in typical absences but was occasionally seen as the first manifestation of atypical absences. In this study,[6] absence seizures were classified by EEG criteria. Seizures with generalized, regular, symmetric spike-and-wave discharges were classified as typical absences, whereas absences with slow (<2.5 Hz), irregular, or asymmetric spike-and-wave discharges were classified as atypical absences.

Early Myoclonic Encephalopathy

Early myoclonic encephalopathy, or neonatal myoclonic encephalopathy, is a seizure disorder that begins in the neonatal period and consists of partial or fragmentary erratic myoclonic seizures, massive myoclonia, partial motor seizures, and tonic seizures.[91] The EEGs demonstrate bursts of spikes, sharp waves, and slow waves separated by suppression of the background activity. Affected infants are usually severely impaired neurologically and more than half of them die before 1 year of age. Early myoclonic encephalopathy is associated with a variety of different etiologies, including nonketotic hyperglycinemia.

Epilepsy with Continuous Spikes and Waves during Slow Sleep

A condition characterized by continuous spikes and waves occurring during sleep was described in 1971 under the name of *subclinical electrical status epilepticus induced by sleep in children* and later under the name of *electrical status epilepticus during sleep*.[92] The original description stressed the importance of defining the syndrome by the amount of spike-wave activity during sleep. To meet the requirements of the syndrome, spike-wave activity should occupy no less than 85% of the time of slow sleep.

The types of clinical seizures that occur in this syndrome are variable. Epilepsy appeared in the series of 18 patients by Tassinari et al.[92,93] at a mean age of 4 years, 6 months. In this series, seizures at the onset consisted of unilateral seizures in five patients; generalized motor seizures in eight patients; motor manifestations involving the facial muscles, along with mandibular contraction and loss of consciousness, in four patients; and myoclonic absences in one patient. In 9 of 18 patients, the first seizure occurred during sleep. Morikawa et al.[94] reported that in five children with continuous spike-wave discharges during sleep, atypical absence seizures and partial seizures were observed.

The syndrome can be differentiated from LGS by the total amount of sleep occupied by spike-wave discharges. In children with continuous spike-wave discharges during sleep (CSWDS), generalized spike-wave activity occurs during more than 85% of sleep time. But in LGS, this epileptiform activity occurs during less than 50% of sleep time. In addition, tonic seizures, which are so common with LGS, are rare in children who have continuous spike-wave discharges during sleep.[92,94]

There appears to be an overlap between CSWDS and the Landau–Kleffner syndrome. Tassinari et al.[93] found that 11 children who had been normal before the development of CSWDS experienced a decrease in IQ (ranging from 45–78 points) after the onset of the disorder. A marked reduction in language function occurred in six children. In 10 cases disturbances in behavior were found, including decreased attention, hyperactivity, and aggressiveness. In seven patients who had abnormal psychomotor development before the occurrence of CSWDS, a worsening of mental deficiency was observed. Morikawa et al.[94] also found that the onset of CSWDS was associated with a deterioration in the behavior and speech in children.

Hirsch et al.[95] reported on five children in whom the Landau–Kleffner syndrome developed when they were between the ages of 3 and 7. The EEG in the awake state demonstrated focal and generalized spike-wave activity on a normal background. During sleep the discharges always increased. At some point during the development of the syndrome, the patients had bilateral spike-wave activity lasting for >75% of their sleep time. The authors suggested that the Landau–Kleffner syndrome and epilepsy with continuous spike-wave activity cannot be clearly differentiated and that they represent different points on a single spectrum. Patry et al.[96] reported on six children with subclinical "electrical status epilepticus" during sleep. In five of the six children, the electrical status subsided during REM sleep. All the children were mentally retarded and two of them failed to acquire speech.

As with the Landau–Kleffner syndrome, there appears to be variable improvement in affected children as CSWDS resolves.[92,94] Tassinari et al.[92] found that seven children who were normal before the onset of CSWDS improved in performance or behavior after CSWDS resolved. Two children totally recovered. In the other patients there was a slight degree of recovery. This variability in recovery was also noted by Morikawa et al.[94]

SEVERE MYOCLONIC EPILEPSY IN INFANCY

Severe myoclonic epilepsy in infants begins during the first year of life.[97] The first seizure, which is frequently febrile, is either generalized or unilateral. The febrile seizures tend to be long and recurrent. When the children are between 1 and 4 years of age, either generalized or partial myoclonic seizures develop. Partial seizures often occur as well. EEG recordings show generalized spike-waves or multiple spike-and-waves, early photosensitivity, and focal abnormalities. Retardation in psychomotor development, including ataxia, corticospinal tract dysfunction, and non-ictal myoclonus, is evident from the second year of life. This type of epilepsy is resistant to all forms of treatment and all affected children are mentally retarded.

LANDAU–KLEFFNER SYNDROME

The Landau-Kleffner syndrome is a childhood disorder consisting of acquired aphasia and epileptiform discharges involving the temporal or parietal regions of the brain.[95,98–113]

The typical sequence is as follows: First, a seizure disorder develops in the child, but it is usually well controlled with antiepileptic drugs. Aphasia then develops; its onset may be abrupt or insidious.[111] Unlike typically acquired childhood aphasia, receptive dysfunction usually is the dominant feature early in the course of the disorder.[98,114] Spontaneous verbal expression slowly becomes reduced, and the child may use stereotypies, perseverations, and paraphasias. In some cases the disorder progresses to the point where the child cannot even recognize sounds, so that total auditory agnosia develops. The child becomes indifferent to auditory stimulation and may not even recognize the sound of a telephone or barking dog, thus often appearing to be deaf or autistic. Reading, writing, and signing may be less impaired. Often an expressive aphasia develops later in the course of the disorder. In the original description of the syndrome, verbal auditory agnosia was the language disturbance,[105] but some patients may have expressive aphasia early in the course. The clinical course of the disorder fluctuates[109,112] and spontaneous remissions can occur.

As Landau and Kleffner[105] noted, not all patients have seizures. Seizures occur in approximately 70% of patients. In one-third of cases, a single seizure or status epilepticus occurs, usually early in the course of the syndrome. The seizures usually begin in children who are between 5 and 10 years of age. After age 10, only 20% of patients still have seizures. The patients usually have generalized tonic-clonic and atypical absence seizures. Complex partial seizures with automatisms are uncommon.

In addition to aphasia, the majority of patients have behavioral and psychomotor disturbances that may suggest autism. The neurologic examination findings, other than those from the mental status examination, are usually normal.

Electroencephalography

The EEG is nonspecific in this syndrome. Typical EEG findings are frequent and repetitive spikes, sharp waves, and spike-and-wave activity. Usually the discharges are bilateral and are located in the temporal region or the parietal-occipital region. Sleep usually activates the record and at times the abnormality is seen only in sleep recordings.[103,112] Often patients will have continuous spike-and-wave activity during sleep.

REFERENCES

1. Dreifuss FE. Proposal for revised clinical and electroencephalographic classification of epileptic seizures. *Epilepsia.* 1981;22:249–260.
2. Holmes GL. Partial seizures in children. *Pediatrics.* 1986;77:725–731.
3. Holmes GL. *Diagnosis and Management of Seizures in Children.* Philadelphia: WB Saunders; 1987:1–293.
4. Delgado–Escueta AV, Bascal EF, Treiman DM. Complex partial seizures on closed-circuit television and EEG: A study of 691 attacks in 79 patients. *Ann Neurol.* 1982;11:292–300.
5. Holmes GL. Partial complex seizures in children: An analysis of 69 seizures in 24 patients using EEG FM radiotelemetry and videotape recording. *Electroencephalogr Clin Neurophysiol.* 1984;57:13–20.
6. Holmes GL, McKeever M, Adamson M. Absence seizures in children: Clinical and electroencephalographic features. *Ann Neurol.* 1987;21:268–273.
7. Holmes GL. Breath-holding attacks in children. *Postgrad Med.* 1988;84:191–192, 196–198.
8. Schmidt D, Tsai JJ, Janz D. Generalized tonic-clonic seizures in patients with complex partial seizures: Natural history and prognosis relevance. *Epilepsia.* 1983;24:43–48.
9. Penry JK, Porter RJ, Dreifuss FE. Simultaneous recording of absence seizures with videotape and electroencephalography. *Brain.* 1975;98:427–440.
10. Holmes GL. The epilepsies. In: David RB, ed. *Pediatric Neurology for the Clinician.* East Norwalk, CT: Appleton & Lange; 1992:185.
11. Pearl PL, Holmes GL. Absence seizures. In: Dodson WE, Pollock JM, eds. *Pediatric Epilepsy.* New York: Demos Publications; 1993:157.
12. Porter RJ, Penry JK, Dreifuss FE. Responsiveness at the onset of spike-wave bursts. *Electroencephalogr Clin Neurophysiol.* 1973;34:239–245.
13. Egli M, Mothersill I, O'Kane M, et al. The axial spasm—The predominant type of drop seizure in patients with secondary generalized epilepsy. *Epilepsia.* 1985;26:401–415.
14. Gastaut H, Roger J, Ouahchi S, et al. An electroclinical study of generalized epileptic seizures of tonic expression. *Epilepsia.* 1963;4:15–44.
15. Holmes GL. Myoclonic, tonic, and atonic seizures in children. *J Epilepsy.* 1988;1:173–195.
16. Aicardi J. The problem of the Lennox syndrome. *Develop Med Child Neurol.* 1973;15:77–81.
17. Aicardi J. The Lennox-Gastaut syndrome. *Int Pediatr.* 1988;3:152–157.
18. Markand ON. Slow spike-wave activity in EEG and associated clinical features: often called "Lennox" or "Lennox–Gastaut" syndrome. *Neurology.* 1977;27:746–757.
19. Ikeno T, Shigematsu H, Miyakosi M, et al. An analytic study of epileptic falls. *Epilepsia.* 1985;26:612–621.
20. Schneider H, Vassella F, Karbowski K. The Lennox syndrome: A clinical study of 40 children. *Eur Neurol.* 1970;4:289–300.
21. Commission on Classification and Terminology of the International League against Epilepsy. Proposal for revised classification of epilepsies and epileptic syndromes. *Epilepsia.* 1989;30:389–399.
22. van Huffelen AC. A 16th-century description of benign focal epilepsy of childhood. *Arch Neurol.* 1989;46:445–447.
23. Beaumanoir A, Ballis T, Varfis G, et al. Benign epilepsy of childhood with rolandic spikes: A clinical, electroencephalographic, and telencephalographic study. *Epilepsia.* 1974;15:301–15.

24. Beaussart M. Benign epilepsy of children with rolandic (centro-temporal) paroxysmal foci: A clinical entity. Study of 221 cases. *Epilepsia.* 1972;13:795–811.
25. Beaussart M. L'epilepsie benigne de l'enfant avec paroxysmes E.E.G. intercritiques rolandiques ou E.P.R. *Pédiatrie.* 1975;309:249–263.
26. Beaussart M. Crises epileptiques apres guerison d'une (epilepsie a paroxysmes rolandiques). *Rév EEG Neurophysiol Clin.* 1981;11:489–492.
27. Beaussart M, Faou R. Evolution of epilepsy with rolandic paroxysmal foci: a study of 324 cases. *Epilepsia.* 1978;19:337–342.
28. Blom S, Brorson LO. Central spikes or sharp waves (rolandic spikes) in children's EEG and their clinical significance. *Acta Paediat Scand.* 1966;55:385–393.
29. Blom S, Heijbel J, Bergfors PG. Benign epilepsy of children with centro-temporal EEG foci: Prevalence and follow-up study of 40 patients. *Epilepsia.* 1972;13:609–619.
30. Dobrzynska L, Kamaraj-Mazurkiewica K. Benign childhood epilepsy with spike activity in the area of the precentral gyrus. *Neurol Neurochir Pol.* 1978;12:561–568.
31. Doose H, Baier WK. Benign partial epilepsy and related condition: Multifactorial pathogenesis with hereditary impairment of brain maturation. *Eur J Pediatr.* 1989;149:152–158.
32. Heijbel J, Blom S, Rasmuson M. Benign epilepsy of childhood with centrotemporal EEG foci: A genetic study. *Epilepsia.* 1975;16:285–293.
33. Holmes GL. Rolandic epilepsy: Clinical and electroencephalographic features. In: Degen R, Dreifuss FE, eds. *Benign Localized and Generalized Epilepsies of Early Childhood.* Amsterdam: Elsevier Science Publishers; 1992:29.
34. Kriz M, Grazdik M. Epilepsy with centrotemporal (rolandic) spikes: A peculiar seizure disorder of childhood. *Neurol Neurochir Pol.* 1978;12:413–419.
35. Loiseau P, Beaussart M. The seizures of benign childhood epilepsy with rolandic paroxysmal discharges. *Epilepsia.* 1973;14:381–389.
36. Nishiura N, Miyazaki T. Clinico-electroencephalographical study of focal epilepsy with special reference to "benign epilepsy of children with centro-temporal EEG foci" and its age dependency. *Folia Psychiatr Neurol Jpn.* 1976;30:253–261.
37. Lerman P. Benign partial epilepsy with centro-temporal spikes. In: Roger J, Dravet C, Bureau M, *et al.,* eds. *Epileptic Syndromes in Infancy, Childhood, and Adolescence.* London: John Libbey, Eurotext; 1985:150.
38. Lerman P, Kivity S. Benign focal epilepsy of childhood—A follow up study of 100 recovered patients. *Arch Neurol.* 1975;32:261–264.
39. Lombroso C. Sylvian seizures and midtemporal spike foci in children. *Arch Neurol.* 1967;17:52–59.
40. Fejerman N, Di Blasi AM. Status epilepticus of benign partial epilepsies in children: Report of two cases. *Epilepsia.* 1987;28:351–355.
41. Calamaria V, Sgrò V, Caraballo R, *et al.* Status epilepticus in benign rolandic epilepsy manifesting as anterior operculum syndrome. *Epilepsia.* 1991;32:329–334.
42. Roulet E, Deonna T, Despland PA. Prolonged intermittent drooling and oromotor dyspraxia in benign childhood epilepsy with centrotemporal spikes. *Epilepsia.* 1989;30:564–568.
43. Blom S, Heijbel J. Benign epilepsy of children with centro-temporal EEG foci: Discharge rate during sleep. *Epilepsia.* 1975;16:133–140.
44. Clemens B, Majoros E. Sleep studies in benign epilepsy of childhood with rolandic spikes. II. Analysis of discharge frequency and its relation to sleep dynamics. *Epilepsia.* 1987;28:24–27.
45. Clemens B, Oláh R. Sleep studies in benign epilepsy of childhood with rolandic spikes. I. Sleep pathology. *Epilepsia.*1987;28:20–23.
46. Dalla Bernardina B, Beghini G. Rolandic spikes in children with and without epilepsy (20 subjects polygraphically studied during sleep). *Epilepsia.* 1976;17:161–167.
47. Dalla Bernardina B, Pajno Ferrara F, Beghini G. Proceedings: Rolandic spike activation during sleep in children with and without epilepsy. *Electroencephalogr Clin Neurophysiol.* 1975;39:537.

48. Dalla Bernardina B, Tassinari CA. EEG of a nocturnal seizure in a patient with "benign epilepsy of childhood with rolandic spikes." *Epilepsia.* 1975;16:497–501.

49. Rose D, Duron B. Prognostic value of the interictal discharges during nocturnal sleep in children with rolandic spikes. *Rev Electroencephalogr Neurophysiol Clin.* 1984;14:217–226.

50. Gastaut H. A new type of epilepsy: Benign partial epilepsy childhood with occipital spike-waves. *Clin Electroencephalogr.* 1982;13:13–22.

51. Gastaut H. L'epilepsie benigne de l'enfant a pointe-ondes occipitales. *Rév EEG Neurophysiol Clin.* 1982;12:179–201.

52. Gastaut H. Benign epilepsy of childhood with occipital paroxysms. In: Roger J, Dravet C, Bureau M, *et al.,* eds. *Epileptic Syndromes in Infancy, Childhood, and Adolescence.* London: John Libbey, Eurotext; 1985:150.

53. Talwar D, Rask CA, Torres F. Clinical manifestations in children with occipital spike-wave paroxysms. *Epilepsia.* 1992;33:667–674.

54. Aicardi J. Epileptic syndromes in childhood. *Epilepsia.* 1988;29:Sl–S5.

55. Panayiotopoulos CP. Benign childhood epilepsy with occipital paroxysms: A 15-year prospective study. *Ann Neurol.* 1989;26:51–56.

56. Lerman P, Kivity S. The benign partial nonrolandic epilepsies. *J Clin Neurophysiol.* 1991;8:275–287.

57. Beaumanoir A. Infantile epilepsy with occipital focus and good prognosis. *Eur Neurol.* 1983;22:43–52.

58. Newton R, Aicardi J. Clinical findings in children with occipital spike-wave complexes suppressed by eye-opening. *Neurology.* 1983;33:1526–1529.

59. Kivity S, Lerman P. Benign partial epilepsy of childhood with occipital discharges. In: Manelis J, Bental E, Loeber JN, eds. *Advances in Epileptology: The XVIIth Epilepsy International Symposium.* New York: Raven Press; 1989:371.

60. Ludwig BI, Ajmone–Marsan C. Clinical ictal patterns in epileptic patients with occipital electroencephalographic foci. *Neurology.* 1975;25:463–471.

61. Struve FA. Lithium-specific pathological electroencephalographic changes: A successful replication of earlier investigative results. *Clin Electroencephalogr.* 1987;18:46–53.

62. Teraski T, Yamatgi Y, Otahara S. Electroclinical delineation of occipital lobe epilepsy in childhood. In: Andermann F, Lugaresi E, eds. *Migraine and Epilepsy.* London: Butterworth; 1987:125.

63. Gibbs EL, Gillen HW, Gibbs FA. Disappearance and migration of epileptic foci in childhood. *Am J Dis Child.* 1954;88:596–603.

64. Miles DK, Holmes GL. Benign neonatal seizures. *J Clin Neurophysiol.* 1990;7:369–379.

65. Plouin P. Benign neonatal convulsions (familial and non-familial). In: Roger J, Dravet C, Bureau M, *et al.,* eds. *Epileptic Syndromes in Infancy, Childhood, and Adolescence.* London: John Libbey, Eurotext; 1985:2.

66. Plouin P. Benign idiopathic neonatal convulsions (familial and non-familial). In: Roger J, Bureau M, Dravet C, *et al.,* eds. *Epileptic Syndromes in Infancy, Childhood, and Adolescence.* London: John Libbey, Eurotext; 1992:3.

67. Hirsch E, Velez A, Sellal F, *et al.* Electroclinical signs of benign neonatal familial convulsions. *Ann. Neurol.* 1993;34:835.

68. Navelet Y, D'Allest AM, Dehan M, *et al.* Are convulsions on the fifth day of life a distinct clinical and electrophysiological entity? *Rev Electroencephalogr Neurophysiol Clin.* 1977;7:366–370.

69. Dehan M, Quillerou D, Navelet Y, *et al.* Convulsions in the fifth day of life: A new syndrome? *Arch Fr Pediatr.* 1977;34:730–742.

70. Dravet C, Bureau M, Roger J. Benign myoclonic epilepsy in infants. In: Roger J, Bureau M, Dravet C, *et al.,* eds. *Epileptic Syndromes in Infancy, Childhood and Adolescence.* London: John Libbey; 1992:67.

71. Lombroso CT. Early myoclonic encephalopathy, early infantile epileptic encephalopathy, and benign and severe infantile myoclonic epilepsies: A critical review and personal contributions. *J Clin Neurophysiol.* 1990;7:380–408.

72. Janz D, Christian W. Impulsiv-petit mal. *J Neurol.* 1957;176:346–386.
73. Asconape J, Penry JK. Some clinical and EEG aspects of benign juvenile myoclonic epilepsy. *Epilepsia.* 1984;25:108-114.
74. Delgado–Escueta AV, Enrile–Bascal FE. Juvenile myoclonic epilepsy of Janz. *Neurology.* 1984;34:285–294.
75. Wolf P. Epilepsy with grand mal on awakening. In: Roger J, Bureau M, Dravet C, *et al.*, eds. *Epileptic Syndromes in Infancy, Childhood and Adolescence.* London: John Libbey; 1992:329.
76. Clancy RR. Sharp electroencephalographic transients in neonates with seizures. *Ann Neurol.* 1983;14:377–378.
77. Kellaway P, Hrachovy RA, Frost JD Jr, *et al.* Precise characterization and quantification of infantile spasms. *Ann Neurol.* 1979;6:214–218.
78. Lacy CR, Penry JK. *Infantile Spasms.* New York: Raven Press; 1976.
79. Lombroso CT. A prospective study of infantile spasms: Clinical and therapeutic considerations. *Epilepsia.* 1983;24:135–158.
80. Jeavons PM, Bower BD. *Infantile Spasms: A Review of the Literature and a Study of 112 Cases.* London: Heinemann; 1964.
81. Bellman M. Infantile spasms. In: Pedley TA, Meldrum BS, eds. *Recent Advances in Epilepsy.* Edinburgh, Scotland: Churchill Livingstone; 1983:113.
82. Gibbs EL, Fleming MM, Gibbs FA. Diagnosis and prognosis of hypsarrhythmia and infantile spasms. *Pediatrics.* 1954;13:66–73.
83. Watanabe K, Iwase K, Hara K. The evolution of EEG features in infantile spasms: A prospective study. *Dev Med Child Neurol.* 1973;15:584–596.
84. Hrachovy RA, Frost JD Jr, Kellaway P. Hypsarrhythmia: Variations on the theme. *Epilepsia.* 1984;25:317–325.
85. Friedman E, Pampiglione G. Prognostic implications of electroencephalographic findings of hypsarrhythmia in first year of life. *Br Med J.* 1971;4:323–325.
86. King DW, Dyken PR, Spinks IL, *et al.* Infantile spasms: Ictal phenomena. *Pediat Neurol.* 1985;1:213–218.
87. Chevrie JJ, Aicardi J. Childhood epileptic encephalopathy with slow spike-wave: A statistical study of 80 cases. *Epilepsia.* 1972;13:259–271.
88. Papini M, Pasquinelli A, Armellini M, *et al.* Alertness and incidence of seizures in patients with Lennox–Gastaut syndrome. *Epilepsia.* 1984;25:161–167.
89. Kurokowa T, Goya N, Fukuyama Y, *et al.* West syndrome and Lennox–Gastaut syndrome: A survey of natural history. *Pediatrics.* 1980;65:81–88.
90. Doose H. Myoclonic astatic epilepsy of early childhood. In: Roger J, Bureau M, Dravet C, *et al.*, eds. *Epileptic Syndromes in Infancy, Childhood, and Adolescence.* London: John Libbey; 1992:103.
91. Aicardi J. Early myoclonic encephalopathy (neonatal myoclonic encephalopathy). In: Roger J, Bureau M, Dravet C, *et al.*, eds. *Epileptic Syndromes in Infancy, Childhood, and Adolescence.* London: John Libbey; 1992:13.
92. Tassinari CA, Bureau M, Dravet C, *et al.* Epilepsy with continuous spikes and waves during slow sleep—Otherwise described as ESES (epilepsy with electrical status epilepticus during slow sleep). In: Roger J, Dravet C, Bureau M, *et al.*, eds. *Epileptic Syndromes in Infancy, Childhood, and Adolescence.* London: John Libbey, Eurotext; 1985:194.
93. Tassinari CA, Bureau M, Dravet C, *et al.* Electrical status epilepticus during sleep in children (ESES). In: Sterman MB, Shouse P. Passouant P, eds. *Sleep and Epilepsy.* London: Academic Press; 1982:465.
94. Morikawa T, Seino M, Osawa T, *et al.* Five children with continuous spike-wave discharges during sleep. In: Roger J, Dravet C, Bureau M, *et al.*, eds. *Epileptic Syndromes in Infancy, Childhood, and Adolescence.* London: John Libbey, Eurotext; 1985:205.

95. Hirsch E, Marescaux C, Maquet P, *et al.*, Landau–Kleffner syndrome: A clinical and EEG study of five cases. *Epilepsia*. 1990;31:756–767.
96. Patry G, Lyagoubi S, Tassinari A. Subclinical "electrical status epilepticus" induced by sleep in children. *Arch Neurol*. 1971;24:242–252.
97. Dravet C, Bureau M, Guerrini R, *et al.* Severe myoclonic epilepsy in infants. In: Roger J, Bureau M, Dravet C, *et al.*, eds. *Epileptic Syndromes in Infancy, Childhood, and Adolescence*. London: John Libbey; 1992:75.
98. Cole AJ, Andermann F, Taylor L, *et al.* The Landau–Kleffner syndrome of acquired epileptic aphasia: Unusual clinical outcome, surgical experience, and absence of encephalitis. *Neurology*. 1988;38:31–38.
99. Cooper J, Ferry P. Acquired auditory verbal agnosia and seizures in childhood. *J Speech Hear Disord*. 1978;43:176–184.
100. Deonna T, Beaumanoir A, Gaillard F, *et al.* Acquired aphasia in childhood with seizure disorder: A heterogeneous syndrome. *Neuropaediatrie*. 1977;8:263–273.
101. Deonna T, Fletcher P, Voumard C. Temporary regression during language acquisition: A linguistic analysis of a 2 1/2-year-old child with epileptic aphasia. *Dev Med Child Neurol*. 1982;24:156–163.
102. Deonna T, Peter C, Ziegler AL. Adult follow-up of the acquired aphasia–epilepsy syndrome in childhood. Report of 7 cases. *Neuropediatrics*. 1989;20:132–138.
103. Gascon G, Victor D, Lombroso CT. Language disorder, convulsive disorder, and electroencephalographic abnormalities. *Arch Neurol*. 1973;28:156–162.
104. Kellermann K. Recurrent aphasia with subclinical bioelectric status epilepticus during sleep. *Eur J Pediatr*. 1978;128:207–212.
105. Landau WM, Kleffner FR. Syndrome of acquired aphasia with convulsive disorder in children. *Neurology*. 1957;7:523–530.
106. Lerman P, Lerman-Sagie T, Kivity S. Effect of early corticosteroid therapy for Landau–Kleffner Syndrome. *Develop Med Child Neurol*. 1991;33:257–266.
107. Lou HC, Brandt S, Bruhn P. Aphasia and epilepsy in childhood. *Acta Neurol Scand*. 1977;56:46–54.
108. Marescaux C, Hirsch E, Finck S, *et al.* Landau-Kleffner syndrome: A pharmacologic study of five cases. *Epilepsia*. 1990;318:768–777.
109. Montovani JF, Landau WM. Acquired aphasia with convulsive disorder: Course and prognosis. *Neurology*. 1980;30:524–529.
110. Otero E, Cordova S, Diaz F, *et al.* Acquired epileptic aphasia (the Landau–Kleffner Syndrome) due to neurocystercercosis. *Epilepsia*. 1989;30:569–572.
111. Roulet E, Deonna T, Gaillard F, *et al.* Acquired aphasia, dementia, and behavior disorder with epilepsy and continuous spike and waves during sleep in a child. *Epilepsia*. 1991;32:495–503.
112. Sawhney IMS, Suresch N, Dhand UK, *et al.* Acquired aphasia with epilepsy—Landau–Kleffner Syndrome. *Epilepsia*.1988;29:283–287.
113. Shoumaker RD, Bennett DR, Bray PF, *et al.* Clinical and EEG manifestations of an unusual aphasic syndrome in children. *Neurology*. 1974;24:10–16.
114. Rapin I, Mattis S, Rowan AJ, *et al.* Verbal auditory agnosia in children. *Dev Med Child Neurol*. 1977;19:192–207.

CHAPTER 2

Radiographic Assessment of Patients
with Epilepsy

Gottfried Schlaug, M.D., Ph.D., and Mahesh Patel, M.D.

Neuroimaging studies have become increasingly important in the evaluation of patients with epilepsy. Computed tomography (CT) and conventional magnetic resonance imaging (MRI) allow identification of structural lesions, whereas functional imaging, including single photon emission computed tomography (SPECT), positron emission tomography (PET), and functional magnetic resonance imaging (fMRI), allow identification of localized disturbances of cerebral blood flow (CBF) and metabolism. Over the last decade, software and hardware improvements have led to a steady increase in the sensitivity and specificity of these methods and further refinement can be expected. Although conventional MRI has demonstrated high sensitivity and specificity in detecting structural lesions, functional neuroimaging methods have consistently shown disturbances of regional CBF (rCBF) or metabolism without structural lesions being detected by MRI. The significance and clinical value of these "functional lesions," without detectable evidence of a structural abnormality, require further investigation. Incorporating functional and structural imaging within one modality, such as with conventional and functional MRI, may increase the sensitivity and specificity of lesion detection and our understanding of the underlying pathology and pathophysiology of epileptic seizures.

SHOULD EVERY PATIENT WHO HAS A SEIZURE
HAVE AN IMAGING WORKUP?

Epilepsy is one of the most common neurologic disorders. It is estimated that about 7–8% of the population experience at least one epileptic seizure and that about 0.5–1% of the US population have epilepsy.[1] Epilepsy is the chronic condition (either genetic or acquired) that predisposes a person to recurrent epileptic seizures. In 15–30% of cases, epilepsy is refractory to medical intervention. Patients with medically refractory epilepsy often have structural brain abnormalities that are amenable to surgery, a treatment that is successful in controlling seizures in two-thirds of patients undergoing surgery.[2]

The Comprehensive Evaluation and Treatment of Epilepsy
Copyright © 1997 by Academic Press. All rights of reproduction in any form reserved.

Certain types of seizure disorders are likely to be associated with structural brain lesions. In adults, partial seizures are more likely to be associated with focal cerebral lesions than are primary generalized seizures. Partial seizures show either clinical or electrophysiologic evidence of onset from a localized area in the cerebral hemisphere. Many age-related epilepsies are associated with particular types of central nervous system lesions (e.g., tuberous sclerosis in patients with infantile spasms) or are known not to be associated with cerebral lesions (e.g., benign childhood epileptic syndromes). The dominant cause of epilepsy, in cases in which the cause is known or presumed, varies with the patient's age. During childhood, the most common cause of epilepsy is congenital abnormalities. In young adulthood, neurologic deficits since birth, brain tumors, trauma, and infection are important causative factors. Stroke is the leading cause of epilepsy in midlife and in the older years.

Every patient who experiences a seizure warrants an imaging evaluation to define or rule out underlying structural–functional pathologies. Conventional MRI with or without contrast should be the first approach. Repeated seizures may call for further evaluation by functional imaging, particularly if no lesion was detected in the first MRI study.

WHAT IMAGING METHODS ARE INDICATED AND WHAT SHOULD THE PHYSICIAN ORDER WHEN PERFORMING A WORKUP ON A PATIENT WITH SEIZURES?

The physician who is taking care of a patient who has had an epileptic seizure can select from several imaging methods, deciding which one is most appropriate. For example, MRI with contrast should be the first step for the adult patient who has had an epileptic seizure but who has no childhood or family history of seizures. The purpose of the study is to exclude a tumor or vascular lesion as the etiology of the seizure.

The patient with recurrent epileptic seizures, an epileptic syndrome, or an epilepsy disorder requires a more extensive evaluation, including a high-resolution MRI study to exclude hippocampal atrophy and focal cortical dysplasia. Probably either an interictal ^{18}F-2-deoxyglucose (FDG)-PET or an ictal SPECT study should also be performed. Functional studies are indicated in "nonlesional" MRI studies, particularly in extratemporal lobe epilepsy, to support electroencephalographic (EEG) findings of a focal onset and to guide semi-invasive and invasive electrophysiologic methods. Imaging strategies may differ between different epilepsy centers but, in general, patients with medically refractory epilepsy will need a more extensive imaging workup to locate accurately the epileptogenic focus for invasive electrophysiologic recordings and successful surgical intervention.

The standards used to determine the true sensitivity of an imaging method in detecting abnormalities have varied. Comparisons with EEG analysis, with pathologic findings in resected brain tissue, and with patient outcome after resective surgery have all been made. The last of these standards is considered by some to be the one against which all noninvasive neuroimaging should be judged. A summary of the most commonly employed methods follows.

SINGLE PHOTON EMISSION COMPUTED TOMOGRAPHY

SPECT is a radioactive method used primarily to assess CBF qualitatively or semiquantitatively by measuring the distribution of radionuclide tracer uptake and retention. The ideal radiopharmaceutical for SPECT imaging of CBF must fulfill the following criteria: It must freely diffuse into the brain through the intact blood-brain barrier; it must show complete first-pass extraction from the blood into the brain; it must distribute proportionally to CBF; it must remain fixed within the brain without redistribution and it must not undergo metabolism. None of the currently available tracers fulfills all these criteria. Therefore, it is difficult to quantify the rCBF with SPECT. The most commonly used SPECT tracers are Tc^{99m}–HMPAO (hexamethyl propylene amine oxime) and, Tc^{99m}–ECD (Tc^{99m}–ethyl cysteinate dimer). These tracers differ in their blood clearance, first-pass extraction, radioactive stability, and preparation ease. Because the first-pass extraction for both preparations is only moderate, the tracers certainly yield an underestimated CBF. Because temporal lobe blood flow has been shown to remain focally elevated immediately after the termination of a seizure, a SPECT with Tc^{99m}–HMPAO is considered ictal if the tracer is injected during the seizure or within 30 seconds of seizure cessation.

Often, little effort is made to ensure the true interictal nature of SPECT as well as PET scans. Yet, ensuring that these scans are interictal is important, particularly for patients whose seizures are poorly controlled medically. In only a few studies was an EEG routinely acquired while the patient underwent SPECT or PET scanning, but these studies are commonly referred to as ictal or interictal.

Interictal SPECT studies are less sensitive than ictal SPECT studies. Analysis of pooled results from the former has shown sensitivities ranging from 30–70%.[3,4] In comparison with other techniques (EEG, MRI, and PET), SPECT has always had lower sensitivities. Although an interictal SPECT study may be useful for comparison with an ictal or peri-ictal SPECT study, it is clearly inferior to a PET scan in the evaluation of focal epilepsies. On the other hand, ictal SPECT studies with radiolabeled perfusion tracers have shown a much higher sensitivity (up to 90% or higher) for temporal lobe seizures and 80% or higher for extratemporal lobe seizures.[4-6] Tc^{99m}–HMPAO or Tc^{99m}–ECD is trapped in the tissue, resulting in an increase in relative CBF. The high concentration in the epileptic focus and the long half-life of these SPECT tracers allow scanning of the patient's brain with some delay in the postictal period. Several studies have shown a high correlation between focal temporal hyperperfusion and mesial temporal sclerosis. Studies have also shown a high correlation between EEG localization and the ictal SPECT scan. Some studies have reported even higher sensitivities for ictal SPECT studies than for interictal FDG–PET studies. Furthermore, several ictal studies have demonstrated a network of abnormal regions that is possibly related to seizure propagation and ictal semiology.

SPECT is also used to image cell receptors. The two tracers most commonly used are I-123–iomazenil and I-123–dexetimide. I-123–iomazenil, a close analog of flumazenil, is a benzodiazepine antagonist with a high affinity for the central type of benzodiazepine receptors. The benzodiazepine receptor-binding density in epileptic foci is reduced by 15–35%.[22] I-123–dexetimide, which binds to muscarinic acetylcholine receptors, is also reduced in the epileptogenic focus.

Considering the high sensitivity of ictal SPECT and MRI studies independently, it has been suggested that ictal SPECT studies be reserved for MRI-negative cases or those in which conflict exists between the MRI study and the EEG. An interictal SPECT study alone is neither sensitive nor specific enough to be of value, although it can be extremely helpful as a comparison to an ictal study.

SPECT studies cost less than current PET studies, which is a significant advantage. Gamma cameras are cheaper, cyclotron-produced isotopes are not needed, and SPECT radiopharmaceuticals are more widely available. Another disadvantage of PET studies is that most are limited to interictal scans.

POSITRON EMISSION TOMOGRAPHY

PET permits measurement of the tissue distribution of a positron-emitting tracer (e.g., ^{18}F, ^{15}O, ^{11}C). A variety of radiopharmaceuticals, useful for the understanding of various metabolic, physiologic, and receptor processes, have been synthesized with these positron-emitting ligands. An on-site cyclotron is necessary to produce these isotopes because all of them have a short half-life. The clinical significance of PET studies is that these radioisotope tracers can be used to quantitatively measure regional cerebral glucose metabolism (rCMRGlc), regional cerebral oxygen metabolism (rCMRO$_2$), and rCBF, which are all indicators of synaptic activity of groups of neurons.[7,8] Glucose uptake and metabolism using FDG, and CBF using H$_2$$^{15}O$, are the two most common physiologic processes measured by PET. PET studies revealed for the first time that metabolism and blood flow were reduced in a region related to the EEG focus (Fig. 2.1). An epileptic seizure was associated with a focal metabolic increase in the interictally hypometabolic region.[9,10] FDG–PET studies have consistently shown a high sensitivity—approaching 90% and higher for temporal lobe epilepsy (TLE) and 50–80% for

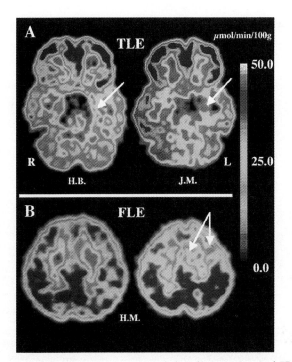

Figure 2.1 (A) Two patients with TLE by EEG and clinical criteria. Interictal FDG–PET images show a pronounced left mesial temporal hypometabolism extending into lateral temporal regions. (B) 7-year-old patient with SMA (supplementary motor area) epilepsy. Seizure-free after resection of posterior frontomesial (anterior to primary motor leg area) and lateral premotor epileptogenic zone. Interictal FDG–PET images show a pronounced hypometabolism in the left SMA and in the lateral premotor region to a smaller degree.

extratemporal lobe epilepsy—in detecting focal abnormalities.[11–18] Even in patients with normal MRI studies, FDG–PET showed focal abnormalities correlating with electroclinical localizing information.[13,15,16]

Similarly, there is a high correspondence between focus detection using semi-invasive EEG studies and regional FDG–PET abnormalities.[11] Temporal lobe hypometabolism was also a good predictor of seizure control after temporal lobectomy.[16] More sensitive and quantitative analysis methods revealed a network of abnormal cerebral regions rather than a single region.[14,16,17,19] Thus, FDG–PET, as well as ictal SPECT, may identify regions, remote to each other (Fig. 2.2), that are involved in seizure propagation and possibly ictal semiology (e.g., epileptogenic and symptomatogenic regions).

In one of the largest reviews on the sensitivities and specificities of PET, SPECT, and MRI in the presurgical evaluation of epilepsy, Spencer[4] reported a

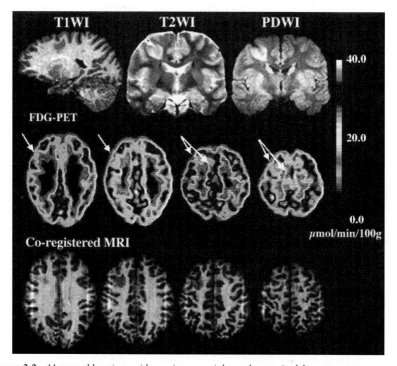

Figure 2.2   11-year-old patient with a seizure semiology characterized by a somatosensory aura involving both hands followed by a hypermotor seizure. Interictal FDG–PET demonstrates a pattern of hypometabolic areas, most pronounced in the dorsolateral frontal cortex (corresponding to a structural abnormality on MRI), but also in the left cingulate and frontomesial region (without underlying structural abnormality). T1WI = T1-weighted image, T2WI = T2-weighted image, PDWI = proton density weighted image (see also page 43). FDG–PET images in Figures 2-1 and 2-2 are shown with the permission of Dr. R. J. Seitz (Department of Neurology, University of Düsseldorf, Germany). The images were acquired while Dr. Schlaug was in Dr. Seitz's laboratory.

sensitivity and specificity of 84% and 86% for PET, 66% and 68% for interictal SPECT, and 55% and 78% for MRI, respectively. One should keep in mind that those data were collected in the years since 1982 and that technologic advances during that time have improved the diagnostic sensitivity and specificity of each of these modalities. The sensitivity of PET improved with scanning resolution and quantitative analysis methods from approximately 60% up to 90%.[12,15–17,20] PET sensitivity in predicting lateralization for the semi-invasive site or surgical outcome may be further improved if other areas of interictal hypometabolism, such as the thalamus, are also considered.

Radioactively marked receptor-ligands allow us to investigate further the epileptic focus. The opiate and benzodiazepine receptors are the two major classes of receptors examined with PET in patients with epilepsy. Opiates may mediate the postictal state and are involved in seizure termination.[21] Savic *et al.*[22] were able to show that the epileptic focus had a lower concentration of GABA-benzodiazepine receptors. This finding might implicate impairment of the GABA-benzodiazepine system in the seizure focus, leading to increased neuronal excitability and seizures.

COMPUTED TOMOGRAPHY

Several studies have shown that MRI has a higher sensitivity for all substrates of epilepsy than CT, mainly because of MRI's superior soft-tissue contrast, its multiplanar imaging capability, and the absence of beam-hardening artifacts.[23–25] Bronen *et al.*[25] reported that the rate of detection of histopathologically positive abnormalities was 95% with MRI and 32% with CT. MRI was found to be significantly superior to CT for localizing developmental disorders, hippocampal sclerosis, and neoplasms. The CT performance in assessing temporal lobe abnormalities was found to be particularly poor. CT is probably indicated only for patients with relative contraindications to MRI (e.g., pacemakers, noncompatible aneurysm clips, severe claustrophobia).

MAGNETIC RESONANCE IMAGING

MRI has been used since the early 1980s for structural imaging. Briefly, the MRI technique makes use of the following principles: (1) Magnetic nuclei align themselves in parallel with an externally applied magnetic field; (2) The orientation of the nuclear spins of these isotopes will change with respect to the static field if a second alternating magnetic field is applied at an appropriate radio frequency (RF). Changes in nuclear spin involve the absorption of energy by protons; this energy is subsequently emitted when the RF field is terminated and the nuclei assume equilibrium or relaxation. Two measures of the return of protons to their equilibrium are used in MRI: T1 is the time constant for the protons to return to the magnetized equilibrium with the main magnetic field (return to their aligned state); T2 is the time constant for loss of synchronization of the emitted signals in the plane perpendicular to the main magnetic field, which occurs as the spins of the nuclei lose coherence. T1 and T2 exhibit tissue specificity: Bone has a long T1 and a short T2, and liquid has a short T1 and a long T2. The sequencing of the applied RF pulses either emphasizes T1 or T2 in an image.

The role of MRI in the clinical management of patients with epilepsy is to identify a possible structural substrate of partial seizures and secondary generalized seizures. In addition, MRI can be used to identify potential surgical candidates and assist in surgical planning. MRI is sensitive in characterizing the morphologic substrates that underlie the electroclinical abnormalities noted in patients with epilepsy. The sensitivity of MRI has steadily increased because of imaging protocol optimization (e.g., coronal slices to evaluate hippocampal size as well as signal intensity, higher-field-strength magnets, and the development of new sequences with a higher sensitivity). Reports published in the early 1990s indicated a sensitivity of 50–80% for temporal lobe seizures and 40–60% for extratemporal lobe epilepsies. However, later reports indicated that a much higher yield can be achieved—up to 90% and higher for TLE.[25] Some studies, however, reflected a bias toward assessing patients with medically refractory epilepsy in whom macroscopic histopathologic abnormalities were likely.

Jack *et al.*[26] have reported the highest diagnostic sensitivity and specificity of MRI when using hippocampal volume measures (Fig 2.3). In one study that compared quantitative MRI and SPECT,[26] they reported an accuracy of 86%, which included the assessment of surgical outcome.

The histologic substrates detected by MRI can be divided into five major categories: tumors, disorders of neuronal migration and cortical organization, vascular malformations, mesial temporal sclerosis, and neocortical sclerosis attributable to brain injury (see Figs. 2.2, 2.4, 2.5, and 2.6).

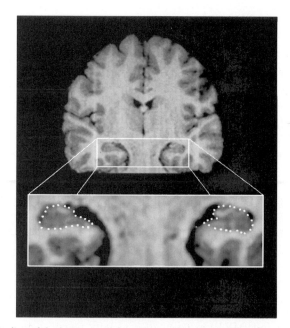

Figure 2.3 Outline of the hippocampal formation and morphometric analysis in an oblique MR image (perpendicular to the long hippocampal axis) of a healthy control subject.

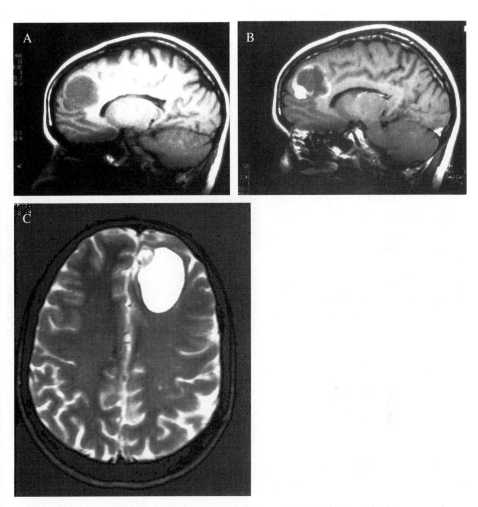

Figure 2.4   40-year-old woman with new onset of seizures. (A) Sagittal T1-weighted image reveals a 4-cm right frontal cystic lesion. (B) Sagittal T1-weighted postgadolinium image demonstrates peripheral enhancement with a more solid nodular enhancing component at the anteroinferior aspect. (C) Axial T2-weighted image reveals the predominantly cystic nature of the left frontal lesion, with a solid component at the anteromedial aspect. Biopsy confirmed a pilocystic astrocytoma.

Conventional MRI is employed primarily to obtain structural images of the brain. Newer methods, such as MR spectroscopy and functional MRI, have been developed and are already in clinical use to assess, with one modality, functional cerebral changes underlying structural abnormalities (see discussion later in this chapter).

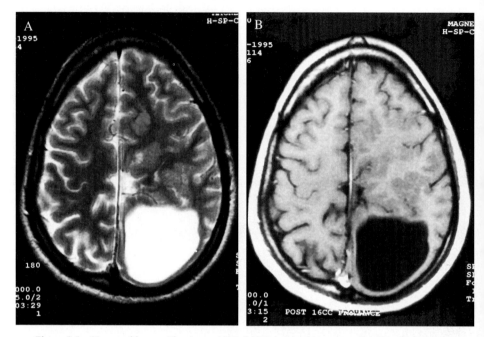

Figure 2.5   23-year-old man with seizures. (A) Axial T2-weighted image reveals a dilated left occipital horn consistent with colpocephaly, with heterotopic gray matter seen in the left frontal lobe as well as in the perirolandic region. (B) Axial T1-weighted image postgadolinium fails to demonstrate abnormal enhancement. This remains consistent with heterotopic gray matter.

WHAT TYPE OF LESION IS NEUROIMAGING MOST LIKELY TO SHOW?

Modern imaging techniques, particularly MRI, have been crucial in detecting formerly cryptic seizure-related lesions. Because of its noninvasiveness, high spatial resolution, and high tissue contrast, MRI is becoming the most sensitive and specific imaging technique for the identification of structural substrates underlying epileptic seizures, at least in TLE.[27] The following section will focus mainly on lesions identifiable with MRI. According to a sample of patients seen in an epilepsy surgery practice at the Mayo Clinic, 55% of epilepsy patients have mesial temporal sclerosis, 20% have a tumor, 15% have negative or nonspecific histologic findings, and fewer than 10% have a neuronal migration disorder, vascular malformation, or sclerosis from brain injury.[27]

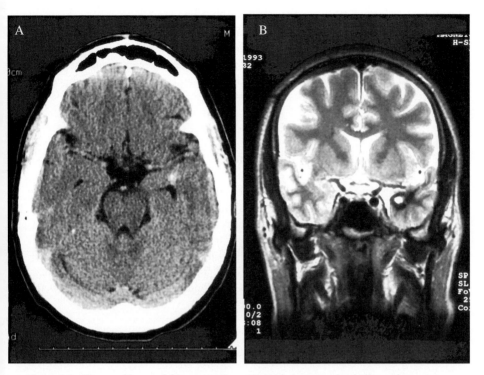

Figure 2.6   33-year-old man exhibits a new seizure. (A) Axial noncontrast head CT scan demonstrates a 7-mm calcification just anterior to the left temporal horn. No appreciable mass effect is seen. (B) A coronal T2-weighted image reveals a left temporal central hyperintense lesion with surrounding hypointensity consistent with hemosiderin. The findings are characteristic of a cavernous angioma.

MESIAL TEMPORAL SCLEROSIS

In mesial temporal sclerosis, cell loss and astrogliosis occur in the hippocampal formation, but also in the amygdala, parahippocampal gyrus, and entorhinal cortex. The MRI scan usually reflects atrophy (best seen and measured on a T1-weighted image) and signal change as an indication of increased tissue-free water (best seen on a T2-weighted image). A technique for measuring hippocampal volume (Fig. 2.3) was developed at the Mayo Clinic and has been implemented at various major epilepsy surgery centers.[26,28] The extent of loss of hippocampal volume correlates well with the degree of cell loss. Hippocampal atrophy is usually seen in more than 70% of cryptogenic TLE and has a high correspondence with electroclinical lateralization.[29,30] However, approximately 30% of patients with extratemporal epilepsy may also show hippocampal atrophy.[30] This could be because a chronic effect of extratemporal lobe seizures with propagation to the mesial temporal lobe or it could indicate a true dual pathology. Most commonly, such patients have mesial temporal sclerosis plus a tumor, cavernous hemangioma, or neuronal migration disorder. There is still controversy about the cause-and-effect relationship between seizures and tissue sclerosis: Is sclerosis the result of repetitive seizures or is it the source of seizures?

TUMORS

Patients with a primary diagnosis of epilepsy attributable to a brain tumor typically have a prolonged (many years) history of seizures and minor or no associated neurologic deficits. In contrast, patients with a primary diagnosis of brain tumor usually have neurologic signs and symptoms of recent onset and may have seizures secondary to their brain tumor. The following tumors are common among epilepsy patients and need to be differentiated: astrocytomas, oligodendrogliomas, mixed astrocytic-oligodendroglial tumors, gangliogliomas, dysembryoplastic neuroepithelial tumors, and hamartomas (see Fig. 2.4).

NEURONAL MIGRATION DISORDERS

The most common neuronal migration disorders associated with epilepsy are tuberous sclerosis, focal cortical dysplasia, polymicrogyria, and the nodular heterotopias.[27] In tuberous sclerosis, the defect is an abnormality in the radial neuron-glial unit; the cortical tuber component of this complex—composed of giant astrocytic and neuronal cells with abnormal organization—is most likely responsible for seizures.

The most obvious finding in focal cortical dysplasia is an abnormality of the cortical laminar organization, present either with or without polymicrogyria. The abnormal cortex is often centered on an abnormal cleft or sulcus of varied depth; the abnormal cleft may represent a rudimentary schizencephalic cleft.[27]

Two disorders of neuronal migration create the appearance of misplaced cortical matter. In diffuse subependymal nodular heterotopia, gray matter is found in an subependymal or subcortical location. Diffuse subependymal heterotopias have an X-linked inheritance pattern. Conglomerate masses of gray matter are called *focal subcortical nodular heterotopia.* Patients with this disorder often have neurologic deficits, developmental delay, and intellectual impairment.

Schizencephaly denotes an abnormal cleft that extends from the pial cerebral surface to the ependymal surface. The cleft is typically lined by dysplastic gray matter.[27] Laminar heterotopia, also referred to as *band heterotopia* or *double cortex syndrome,* is a laminar zone of gray matter bound on the inner and outer border by white matter; the overlying cortical mantle is usually abnormal.

Vascular Malformations

Cerebrovascular malformations include cavernous hemangioma, capillary telangiectasia, venous angioma, and arteriovenous malformation (AVM) (see Figs. 2.6 and 2.7). Hemorrhage and seizures are the most common initial manifestations in patients with an AVM. Occult vascular malformations are those that are not visualized on conventional arteriography (e.g., cavernous hemangioma, capillary telangiectasia, thrombosed AVM). MRI is more sensitive in detecting these occult vascular malformations. Sturge–Weber syndrome is characterized by facial leptomeningeal and ocular angiomatosis, mental retardation, epilepsy, and neurologic deficits that depend on the site of the leptomeningeal angioma. The main intracranial finding is a pial angioma.

Neocortical Sclerosis

Sclerosis, tissue loss, and astroglial proliferation can ensue from numerous types of brain insults, such as trauma, infection, inflammation, and infarction.[27] Any of these four mechanisms may produce an area of brain necrosis. The necrotic area is typically surrounded by an area of sclerosis. In cases of trauma, hemosiderin is often deposited in atrophic cortical tissue. Seizures are more likely to occur after a head injury if the dura is penetrated. Perinatal and neonatal vascular insults can produce cerebral infarctions that are associated with seizures. Seizures presumably originate from gliotic tissue at the periphery of such infarcted zones.[27] For unknown reasons, resective surgery does not produce as uniformly favorable results in neocortical sclerosis as it does in mesial temporal sclerosis.[27] Cerebral infarction is the most common cause of new-onset epilepsy in the elderly population.

Immune-Mediated Disorder (Rasmussen's Syndrome)

Rasmussen's encephalitis has been linked to an autoimmune response to subunit 3 of the glutamate neurotransmitter. The long-term prognosis is poor. Often patients have epilepsia partialis continua at the time of initial assessment. The disease may spread to involve an entire hemisphere and lead to severe neurologic and intellectual impairment.

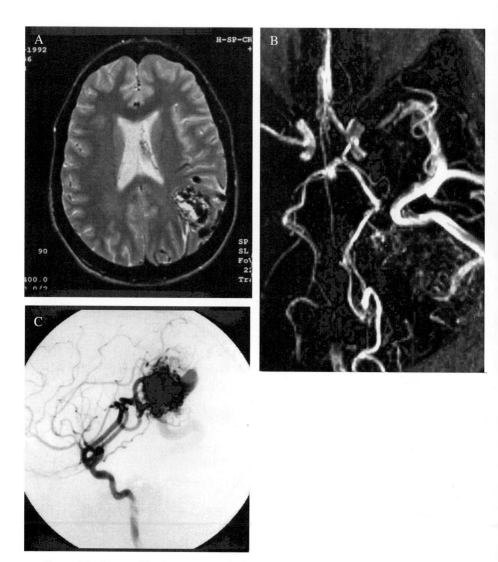

Figure 2.7 31-year-old pregnant woman with headaches and new onset seizures. (A) Axial T2-weighted image reveals left parietal serpiginous flow-voids characteristic of a nidus from an arteriovenous malformation. (B) Axial 3-dimensional time-of-flight MR angiogram demonstrates enlarged left middle cerebral artery branches supplying the malformation. (C) A selective left internal carotid artery digital subtraction angiogram confirms a left parietal arteriovenous malformation supplied by two angular branches of the middle cerebral artery, as well as a draining vein.

WHEN SHOULD THE PHYSICIAN ORDER A SPECT OR PET SCAN?

SPECT or PET is certainly indicated in patients with medically refractory epilepsies and in candidates for epilepsy surgery but may not be a priority in patients who have had a single epileptic seizure. It is important to recognize that a significant number of epilepsy patients can have a negative or nonfocal MRI evaluation. Functional studies have shown focal abnormalities even in this subset of patients.[4,13,15,17] Functional imaging methods have become more widely used, because epilepsy surgery has become an essential mode of treatment in medically refractory epilepsy patients and because these methods can provide information about localization of seizure onset and seizure propagation.[6,10,11,19,31,32]

Although the region of altered metabolism or blood flow appears to be much larger than the epileptogenic region as mapped by electrophysiologic methods, functional imaging can help to determine the focality of an epilepsy as well as guide semi-invasive and invasive electrophysiologic studies. Engel et al.[11] showed that there was a high correspondence between focal abnormalities determined with depth electrode recordings and those detected by FDG–PET. The role of PET, however, is not limited to its clinical benefits. Because PET can quantify cerebral metabolism, blood flow, oxygen extraction, and receptor kinetics, it plays an important role in understanding the pathophysiology of human epilepsy.

Although conventional MRI provides excellent anatomic information that is critical to the detection of neoplastic lesions, cortical dysplasias, and migrational disorders, it does not convey physiologic information about cerebral perfusion and metabolism. Functional and structural brain imaging have had a major impact on the presurgical evaluation of patients, particularly those with suspected TLE, but also those with extratemporal lobe epilepsy. It is believed that functional neuroimaging methods will play a more important role in defining the functional anatomy of the seizure focus and seizure propagation in addition to defining the underlying structural substrates seen with conventional MRI.

HOW SHOULD THE PHYSICIAN INTERPRET THE FINDINGS WHEN FUNCTIONAL IMAGING METHODS ARE USED?

Penfield[42] observed in 1939 that the ictal state in human beings is accompanied by an increase in CBF. Many years later, studies using animals demonstrated that seizures led to an increase in CBF. PET studies revealed for the first time that metabolism and blood flow in the human brain were reduced in a region related to the EEG focus. An epileptic seizure was associated with a focal metabolic increase in the interictally hypometabolic region.[9,10] Reports that demonstrate a temporal lobe hypometabolism in TLE patients approach sensitivities of 90% and more. There seems to be no clear correlation between the degree of hypometabolism and seizure frequency, duration of seizure disorder, presence of multiple seizure types, presence of secondarily generalized seizures, or frequency of interictal spiking.[33-35] It appears that cerebral metabolism in the temporal lobe more closely reflects the degree of general cerebral dysfunction or possibly loss of inhibitory input than the electrical activity within the abnormal neocortex.

The hypometabolic region can involve the mesial and lateral temporal lobe in patients with mesiotemporal onset or can even show remote areas of hypometabolism within the basal ganglia (putamen, thalamus) or the frontal and parietal cortex (Fig. 2.1).[18,19] Nevertheless, the correlation of the laterality and the general area of hypometabolism with the seizure focus according to surface and depth EEG is excellent.

The exact relationship between decreased FDG uptake and the pathology or pathophysiology of the seizure disorders is unknown. One hypothesis purports that a small hyperactive epileptic focus may reside within the hypometabolic focus usually seen. This hyperactive epileptic center will not be detected, in contrast to the far larger surrounding hypometabolism, as a consequence of the partial volume effect. Similar findings were seen in animal models of epilepsy in which the resolution of contact autoradiography allowed the visualization of a small central hypermetabolic focus and a surrounding hypometabolic region (for more details, see Witte et al.[10]). Neuronal inputs from surrounding brain regions might possibly function to inhibit chronically the spread of electrical activity out of the ictal brain region and might lead to interictal hypometabolism. Thus, the resolution of the PET scanner and partial volume effects may explain the local FDG–PET hypometabolism. Seizures appear to result in a prolonged increase in cerebral metabolism (possibly 24 h in duration) and may alter the metabolic activity in other brain regions for a long time. Because FDG–PET studies summate metabolic activity over 30–45 min, a seizure that occurs early in the study will reflect effects of the ictal and postictal state. Thus, one has to be careful in interpreting FDG–PET studies in patients with medically intractable seizures performed without simultaneous EEG recordings.

What is the relationship between CBF and metabolism? At rest, there is evidence of a close coupling between glucose uptake and blood flow. However, there is also evidence that CBF and metabolism may not be coupled in the epileptic focus and during a seizure. There also appears to be a higher interindividual variability in temporal lobe asymmetry of blood flow compared to glucose metabolism, a fact that could explain the lower sensitivity and specificity of SPECT to localize the epileptic focus in TLE as compared with FDG–PET.

Several FDG–PET and ictal SPECT studies have shown multiple regions with abnormal metabolism or blood flow remote to the presumed epileptogenic region.[6,14,15,17–19] This pattern of abnormal regions could indicate propagation pathways and could be related to the ictal behavior: for example, dystonic movements in TLE and focal motor manifestations in frontal lobe epilepsy with an epileptic focus in noneloquent cortex. In that respect, functional imaging studies are in a unique position to improve classification and anatomic localization of epileptic seizures by using signs and symptoms of the seizure semiology and relating them to anatomofunctional information.[36,37]

HOW CAN LESIONS BE DIFFERENTIATED BY A COMBINATION OF MAGNETIC RESONANCE IMAGING MODALITIES?

The majority of patients with symptomatic focal-onset epileptic syndromes are believed to have an abnormality detected by MRI that corresponds to a histopathologic abnormality.[27] The utility of CT in this context is limited because of its diminished sensitivity (other than its superior ability to detect calcification). Certain lesions, such as mesial temporal sclerosis, cortical dysplasias, and small cavernous angiomas, are not detectable by CT imaging; consequently, most of the discussion will be concentrated on differentiating properties by MRI criteria.

The fundamental sequences obtained include axial T1-weighted images, proton density–weighted images, T2-weighted images, gradient-echo susceptibility-weighted images, and postcontrast T1-weighted images that aid in the characterization of lesions. The most sensitive images for pathology involve the T2-weighted images that reveal a bright signal in the areas of abnormality, similar to cerebrospinal fluid (CSF). The proton density–weighted images continue to demonstrate abnormality, allowing their differentiation from CSF. Often T2 signal abnormalities can be seen out of proportion to the contrast-enhancing lesion, either indicating surrounding edema or reflecting the more extensive nature of the lesion.

The spectrum of lesions encountered include brain tumors, both primary and metastatic; neuronal migrational disorders, including focal cortical dysplasias and schizencephaly; vascular malformations; mesial temporal sclerosis; and sclerosis caused by brain injury. The latter category is the end result of any insult that causes loss of brain tissue (e.g., from trauma, infection). Each of these categories has a distinctive appearance on MRI, although clinical presentation and the patient's age are also important determinants of the likely diagnoses.

The primary brain tumors responsible for epilepsy are low-grade tumors rather than high-grade intra-axial supratentorial tumors that result in seizure presentation with a short, fulminant course. Similarly, metastatic lesions tend to be rare. These low-grade tumors are low-grade astrocytomas, oligodendrogliomas, dysembryopathic neuroepithelial tumors (DENTs), gangliogliomas, or hamartomas (see Fig. 2.4). These tumors are well-circumscribed, with little or no peritumoral edema, and may or may not have enhancement, and they tend to have a predisposition for the frontal and temporal lobes. The oligodendrogliomas calcify in 30–40% of cases, and spontaneous hemorrhage is frequent. Associated calvarial erosion has been noted in 17% of cases.[38] A significant number of these tumors fail to enhance. Mixed tumors with both astrocytic and oligodendral components are also seen in epilepsy patients. Gangliogliomas and ganglioneuromas are rare, low-grade, slow-growing tumors that arise from differentiated ganglion cells and mature neuroglia. Approximately 80% occur in patients younger than 30 years of age. These tumors appear as well-circumscribed lesions and are evenly divided between those with a solid and those with a cystic morphologic structure; the cystic ones may be multicystic. A variable enhancement pattern is seen. Punctate or flecklike calcification is seen in 30–40% of these tumors. The DENT consists of neuronal, oligodendroglial, and astrocytic elements with little atypia. These lesions have a predilection for the temporal lobe and are often cortically based; they typically occur in early childhood. MRI reveals them to be multicystic with areas of enhancement and perhaps of calcification. Because these lesions are sometimes found in association with areas of focal cortical dysplasia, they may be more appropriately classified between the categories of low-grade tumor or neuronal migrational disorder.

The disorders of neuronal migration typically arise from an in utero insult between the seventh and sixteenth gestational weeks. Focal cortical dysplasia represents a spectrum: Mild abnormalities appear only as a subtle area of thickened (greater than 4 mm) gray matter. The subjacent white matter may appear hyperintense on the T2-weighted images. Helpful in identifying this often subtle disorder are three-dimensional volume MRI acquisitions using gradient-echo technique with a 1.0–1.5-mm slice thickness using T1 weighting.

Schizencephaly is a result of an abnormal cleft lined with dysplastic gray matter (often with polymicrogyria consisting of small abnormal gyri). In Type I cases, the lips of the cleft are in apposition, whereas in Type II, the lips are open. In closed-lip schizencephaly, a small dimple may be seen on the ventricular surface on MRI. On MRI, heterotopias are clearly evident regions that follow gray matter in all sequences but that are in the wrong location. The nodular forms can be subependymal or subcortical, whereas the band form is bound on both the inner and outer surface by white matter. *Lissencephaly* refers to deficient sulcation and gyration along the surface of the brain. These abnormalities are subdivided into "agyria" with absent sulcation and "pachygyria" with broad, flat gyri. Unilateral hemimegaloencephaly refers to enlargement of all or part of one hemisphere, with associated dilatation of the ipsilateral ventricular system and increased ipsilateral white matter volume. The cortex organization is grossly abnormal. The affected portion of the brain is thought to be nonfunctional.

The vascular malformations include cavernous angiomas, capillary telangiectasias, venous angiomas, AVMs, and arteriovenous fistulas (see Figs. 2.6 and 2.7). The AVM is detectable on MRI by a nidus that contains serpiginous flow voids because of feeding arteries and draining veins. Cavernous angiomas are composed of dilated vascular spaces that are thought to ooze, resulting in surrounding hemosiderin. The gradient-echo susceptibility weighted images are most sensitive in demonstrating the hemosiderin-induced signal loss associated with these lesions. The lesion is often calcified, has a mulberry heterogeneous appearance within the center on all MRI pulse sequences, and may enhance centrally. The capillary telangiectasia often occurs in the pons and may have subtle enhancement. The venous angioma represents a "caput" of small veins that drains into a larger draining vein and is usually considered a normal variant because it provides the drainage pathway for the adjacent normal brain.

Mesial temporal sclerosis consists of cell loss and gliosis in the mesial temporal lobe and is considered the major cause of TLE in young adulthood. It is believed to be bilateral in as many as 80% of cases, although it is usually asymmetric. The MRI findings include atrophy and T2 hyperintensity. Atrophy is best determined by T1-weighted, thin-section coronal images obtained perpendicular to the hippocampal formation, and volumetric measurements are thought to be more sensitive than visual observation (Fig. 2.3). Associated findings include loss of the normal hippocampal architecture and unilateral atrophy of the mamillary body, columns of the fornix, amygdala, or parahippocampal white matter tracts. The associated finding of ipsilateral temporal horn dilatation is not regarded as reliable because it commonly occurs as a normal variant. T2 signal abnormality that extends outside the mesial temporal structures favors a low-grade glioma rather than mesial temporal sclerosis.

Neocortical sclerosis can occur from multiple etiologies and represents the final common pathway from trauma, infection, inflammatory processes, and infarction. All appear on MRI with hyperintensity on T2-weighted images and with associated atrophy. Cerebral infarcts are responsible for most new-onset epilepsy in elderly adults. These infarcts can usually be recognized by the involvement of vascular territories.

WHAT IS THE OPTIMAL RADIOGRAPHIC EVALUATION OF A PATIENT WITH EPILEPSY?

The MRI examination should include a sequence with a sufficient T2 contrast-to-noise ratio to identify subtle areas of increased signal intensity, such as in mesial temporal sclerosis. A fluid-attenuated inversion recovery (FLAIR) imaging sequence has been introduced to allow detection of subtle areas of signal abnormality without interference of CSF signal.[39] It was shown that the lesion-to-background contrast of small cortically based epileptogenic lesions was superior with FLAIR to standard T2-weighted sequences.[39] For patients with suspected TLE, these sequences should be obtained obliquely perpendicular to the principal axis of the hippocampal formation. It is important that the MRI protocol also include a pulse sequence with sufficient spatial resolution for detection of the most subtle alterations (e.g., a three-dimensional volumetric T1-weighted sequence). This high-resolution sequence will enhance the detection of hippocampal atrophy and focal cortical dysplasias.

Complementing MRI with functional imaging studies is important in patients being considered for epilepsy surgery; this combination may yield a higher positive predictive value for seizure relief. The combination of MRI, particularly with MRI morphometric evaluation of the hippocampal formation, and ictal SPECT studies in patients with suspected TLE may prove to be as useful as, or even achieve a higher sensitivity than, a combination of MRI and interictal FDG–PET. Functional studies will be needed to localize possible epileptogenic zones and, it is hoped, to define one day the epileptic focus, because Awad et al.[40] showed that the seizure focus in patients with suspected extratemporal lobe epilepsy was not within or contiguous to a structural lesion in one-third of their patients. Thus the combination of structural and functional imaging methods could provide adequate information for guiding semi-invasive and invasive procedures in extratemporal lobe epilepsies.

The differences in the sensitivities for each neuroimaging technique may mostly reflect the differences in the pathologic or pathophysiologic processes measured. MRI has an excellent spatial resolution and high tissue contrast and is the method of choice for identifying structural brain lesions. Because patients rarely proceed to surgery without the identification of a structural lesion or volumetric abnormality of the hippocampal formation (e.g., patients with temporal lobe epilepsy), MRI should be the first-choice, highest-priority imaging method in the workup of patients with medically refractory focal epilepsies. By acting as a combined measure of metabolism and anatomy, interictal FDG–PET has the highest sensitivity in "nonlesional" epilepsy cases. Studies indicate that ictal SPECT may be as sensitive as interictal FDG–PET in these cases.

MRI with contrast is not routinely indicated. Exceptions are adults with a recent onset of partial seizures or secondarily generalized seizures suggestive of neocortical origin, because a tumor is high on the differential diagnosis list. Magnetic resonance angiography may be of use in further delineating vascular malformations.

WHEN ARE FOLLOW-UP SCANS INDICATED?

Follow-up scans are indicated in cases of seizure exacerbation, reflected in either a change in seizure type or epilepsy syndrome or an increase in seizure frequency. A further indication is recurrent seizures after cortical resection or anterior temporal lobectomy. Although seizures can occur in the immediate postoperative period, continued seizures or a change in the seizure semiology or frequency warrants an imaging workup. Possible reasons for an increase in seizure frequency are incomplete lesion resection, postoperative scarring, or the presence of dual pathology. Dual pathology is seen mainly in patients with an extratemporal lobe type of epilepsy; these patients might exhibit seizures typical for TLE after removal of a neocortical lesion.

A further consideration is bitemporal lobe epilepsy. Autopsy studies have shown that bilateral mesial temporal sclerosis can occur in up to 80% of patients with mesial temporal sclerosis. If MRI-identified mesial temporal sclerosis is present along with an extratemporal lesion, careful electroclinical evaluation must be undertaken to determine which of the two abnormalities is responsible for the patient's recurrent seizures.

Any change in the neurologic examination results or in the patient's neurologic deficits warrants a repeat imaging workup. Also, repeated scans to monitor for potential tumor growth are necessary for patients who have identified nonresective tumors.

ARE THERE ANY NEW IMAGING METHODS OR TECHNIQUES FOR THE EVALUATION OF PATIENTS WITH EPILEPSY?

Magnetic resonance spectroscopy (MRS) utilizing hydrogen nuclei (^{1}H) and phosphorous nuclei (^{31}P) and fMRI utilizing MR parameters of blood flow and tissue perfusion may play an increasing role in the initial evaluation and subsequent management of patients with epilepsy. MRS has typically concentrated on ^{1}H imaging because of the increased signal.

For ^{1}H, MRS imaging (also called *chemical shift imaging*) allows simultaneous acquisition of spectra from all brain regions. The prime substance of interest is N-acetyl aspartate (NAA), which is predominantly neuronal in distribution and is not found in mature glial cells. In mesial temporal sclerosis, decreased NAA is seen because of neuronal loss with a 96% sensitivity. This technique may eventually diminish the need for invasive EEG monitoring. A limitation exists in spatial resolution of 1.7 cm^3 for MRS studies performed on a 2-Tesla magnet. Also, an increased lactate pool has been seen for up to several hours after a seizure within the epileptogenic region. This pool may also be of help in localization.

Use of ^{31}P imaging is limited by poor resolution, requiring a voxel size of 25 cm^3, but preliminary data have demonstrated a decrease in the phosphomonoesters. This technology requires the use of a special coil. An advantage of MRS is that it does not require a PET scanner with an on-site cyclotron, and it will likely be more useful in the future.

Functional MRI can be helpful not only in localizing epileptic foci but also in mapping, before surgery, primary sensorimotor regions and brain regions involved in the perception and production of language. Currently, these MRI methods rely on changes in the blood oxygen level–dependent (BOLD) contrast. The underlying premise is that increased CBF to a site of neuronal synaptic activity occurs with little change in oxygen extraction, resulting in an increased concentration of oxyhemoglobin and a decreased concentration of deoxyhemoglobin relative to adjacent areas. Thus the intrinsic contrast of deoxyhemoglobin is utilized, which causes signal loss on susceptibility-weighted images. Brain regions with increased perfusion and a decreased concentration of deoxyhemoglobin experience less signal loss. Discrete areas of cerebral signal changes in response to motion, cognition, and perception have been detected by this method. Functional MRI techniques have also been used to correlate focal magnetic resonance signal changes with subclinical epileptic discharges (demonstrated by EEG recordings) or constant focal motor activity, such as in epilepsia partialis continua.[31,32,41] These fMRI methods may allow identification of brain regions with blood flow changes related to either brief subclinical epileptic discharges or focal ictal motor activity (Fig. 2.8).

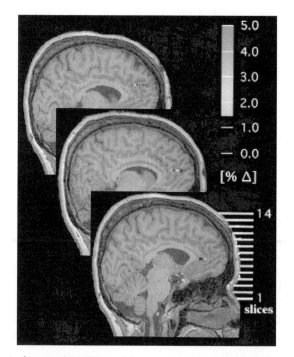

Figure 2.8 Foci of increased BOLD signal intensity time-locked to brief epileptic discharges in a 36-year-old patient with generalized spike-and-wave discharges; some discharges were limited to the right hemisphere or appeared to have right-sided onset with rapid generalization. The thresholded and spatially filtered percentage change maps are coregistered with T1-weighted MR images.

As more experience is gained in utilizing these techniques, and as higher field magnets become increasingly utilized, it is likely that fMRI techniques will contribute more significantly to the management of epilepsy patients.

REFERENCES

1. Hauser W, Hesdorffer D. *Epilepsy: Frequency, Causes, and Consequences.* New York: Demos Publications; 1990:378.
2. National Institutes of Health. Surgery for epilepsy: NIH Consensus Conference. *JAMA.* 1990;264:729–733.
3. Jibiki I, Yamaguchi N. Epilepsy and SPECT. *Neurosci Biobehav Rev.* 1994;18:281.
4. Spencer SS. The relative contributions of MRI, SPECT, and PET imaging in epilepsy. *Epilepsia.* 1994;35:S72.
5. Rowe CC, Berkovic SF, Sia STB, et al. Localization of epileptic foci with postictal single photon emission computed tomography. *Ann Neurol.* 1989;26:660–668.
6. Harvey AS, Hopkins IJ, Bowe JM, et al. Frontal lobe epilepsy: Clinical seizure characteristics and localization with ictal 99mTc–HMPAO SPECT. *Neurology.* 1993;43:1966–1980.
7. Borgström L, Chapman AG, Siesjö BK. Glucose consumption in the cerebral cortex of rat during bicuculline-induced status epilepticus. *J Neurochem.* 1976;27:971–973.
8. Kadekaro M, Crane AM, Sokoloff L. Differential effects of electrical stimulation of sciatic nerve on metabolic activity in spinal cord and dorsal root ganglion in the rat. *Proc Natl Acad Sci USA.* 1985;82:6010–6013.
9. Kuhl DE, Engel J Jr, Phelps ME, et al. Epileptic patterns of local cerebral metabolism and perfusion in humans determined by emission computed tomography of 18FDG and 13NH3. *Ann Neurol.* 1980;8:348–360.
10. Witte OW, Bruehl C, Schlaug G, et al. Dynamic changes of focal hypometabolism in relation to epileptic activity. *J Neurol Sci.* 1994;124:188–197.
11. Engel J Jr, Henry TR, Risinger MW, et al. Presurgical evaluation for partial epilepsy: Relative contributions of chronic depth-electrode recordings versus FDG–PET and scalp-sphenoidal ictal EEG. *Neurology.* 1990;40:1670–1677.
12. Theodore WH, Katz D, Kufta C, et al. Pathology of temporal lobe foci: Correlation with CT, MRI, and PET. *Neurology.* 1990;40:797–803.
13. Ryvlin P, Philippon B, Cinotti L, et al. Functional neuroimaging strategy in temporal lobe epilepsy: A comparative study of 18FDG–PET and 99mTc–HMPAO–SPECT. *Ann Neurol.* 1992; 31:650–656.
14. Swartz BE, Tomiyasu U, Delgado-Escueta AV, et al. Neuroimaging in temporal lobe epilepsy: Test sensitivity and relationships to pathology and postoperative outcome. *Epilepsia.* 1992;33:624–634.
15. Swartz BE, Khonsari A, Brown C, et al. Improved sensitivity of 18FDG-positron emission tomography scans in frontal and "frontal plus" epilepsy. *Epilepsia.* 1995;36:388–395.
16. Radtke RA, Hanson MW, Hoffman JM, et al. Temporal lobe hypometabolism on PET: Predictor of seizure control after temporal lobectomy. *Neurology.* 1993;43:1088–1092.
17. Schlaug G, Arnold S, Holthausen H, et al. Interictal cerebral hypometabolism reveals the epileptogenic and symptomatogenic zone in focal epilepsies involving the frontal lobe. *Neurology.* 1995;45:A313–A314.
18. Arnold S, Schlaug G, Niemann H, et al. Topography of interictal glucose hypometabolism in unilateral mesiotemporal epilepsy. *Neurology.* 1996;46:1422–1430.
19. Henry TR, Mazziotta JC, Engel J Jr, et al. Interictal metabolic anatomy of mesial temporal lobe epilepsy. *Arch Neurol.* 1993;50:582–589.

20. Theodore WH, Sato S, Kufta C, *et al.* Temporal lobectomy for uncontrolled seizures: The role of positron emission tomography. *Ann Neurol.* 1992;32:789–794.

21. Fisher RS, Frost JJ. Epilepsy. *J Nucl Med.* 1991;32:651–659.

22. Savic I, Roland P, Sedvall G, *et al.* In-vivo demonstration of reduced benzodiazepine receptor binding in human epileptic foci. *Lancet.* 1988;ii(8618):863–866.

23. Heinz ER, Heinz TR, Radtke R. Efficacy of MR vs CT in epilepsy. *Am J Neuroradiol* 1988;9:1123–1128.

24. Latack JT, Abou-Khalil BW, Siegel GJ, *et al.* Patients with partial seizures: Evaluation by MR, CT, and PET imaging. *Radiology.* 1986;159:159–163.

25. Bronen RA, Fulbright RK, Spencer DD, *et al.* Refractory epilepsy: Comparison of MR imaging, CT, and histopathologic findings in 117 patients. *Radiology.* 1996;201:97–105.

26. Jack CR Jr, Mullan BP, Sharbrough FW, et al. Intractable nonlesional epilepsy of temporal lobe origin: Lateralization by interictal SPECT versus MRI. *Neurology.* 1994;44:829–836.

27. Jack CR Jr. Magnetic resonance imaging in epilepsy. *Mayo Clin Proc.* 1996;71:695–711.

28. Jack CR Jr, Sharbrough FW, Cascino GD, *et al.* Magnetic resonance image-based hippocampal volumetry: Correlation with outcome after temporal lobectomy. *Ann Neurol.* 1992;31:138–146.

29. Cascino GD, Jack CR, Parisi JE, *et al.* MRI in the presurgical evaluation of patients with frontal lobe epilepsy and children with temporal lobe epilepsy: Pathologic correlation and prognostic importance. *Epilepsy Res.* 1992;11:51–59.

30. Adam C, Baulac M, Saint–Hilaire J-M, *et al.* Value of magnetic resonance imaging-based measurements of hippocampal formations in patients with partial epilepsy. *Arch Neurol.* 1994;51:130–138.

31. Detre JA, Sirvan JI, Alsop DC, *et al.* Localization of subclinical ictal activity by functional MRI: Correlation with invasive monitoring. *Ann Neurol.* 1995;38:618–624.

32. Warach S, Ives J, Schlaug G, *et al.* EEG triggered echo planar functional MRI for localization of epileptic discharges. *Neurology.* 1996;47:89–93.

33. Engel J Jr, Kuhl DE, Phelps ME, *et al.* Interictal cerebral glucose metabolism in partial epilepsy and its relation to EEG changes. *Ann Neurol.* 1982;12:510–517.

34. Engel J Jr, Brown W, Kuhl DE, *et al.* Pathological findings underlying focal temporal lobe hypometabolism in partial epilepsy. *Ann Neurol.* 1982;12:518–528.

35. Theodore WH, Newmark ME, Sato S, *et al.* 18F-fluorodeoxyglucose positron emission tomography in refractory complex partial seizures. *Ann Neurol.* 1983;14:429–437.

36. Lüders H, Awad I. Conceptual considerations. In: Lüders HO, ed. *Epilepsy Surgery.* New York: Raven Press; 1991:51–62.

37. Manford M, Fish DR, Shorvon SD. An analysis of clinical seizure patterns and their localizing value in frontal and temporal lobe epilepsies. *Brain.* 1996;119:17–40.

38. Kjos BO, Brant–Zawadzki M, Kuchardzyk W, *et al.* Cystic intracranial lesions: Magnetic resonance imaging. *Radiology* 1985;155:363–369.

39. Bergin PS, Fish DR, Shorvon DS, *et al.* Magnetic resonance imaging in partial epilepsy: Additional abnormalities shown with the fluid attenuated inversion recovery (FLAIR) pulse sequence. *J Neurol Neurosurg Psychiatry.* 1995;58:439–443.

40. Awad IA, Rosenfeld J, Ahl J, *et al.* Intractable epilepsy and structural lesions of the brain: Mapping, resection strategies, and seizure outcome. *Epilepsia.* 1991;32:179–186.

41. Jackson GD, Connelly A, Cross JH, *et al.* Functional magnetic resonance imaging of focal seizures. *Neurology.* 1994;44:850–856.

42. Penfield W, von Santha K, Cipriani A. Cerebral blood flow during induced epileptiform seizures in animals and man. *J Neurophysiol.* 1939;2:257.

CHAPTER 3

Treatment of Seizures

Steven C. Schachter, M.D.

WHAT ARE THE GOALS OF THERAPY?

The management of patients with epilepsy is both challenging and rewarding. The introduction of new antiepileptic drugs (AEDs) beginning in the mid-1990s and the increased emphasis on maximizing the quality of life for patients with epilepsy have led to a new set of goals for the treatment of seizures. These goals have evolved from complete control of seizures, whether or not side effects occurred, to enabling patients with epilepsy to lead lifestyles consistent with their capabilities.[1] Consequently, the introduction of new medications, the increased availability of epilepsy surgery (see Chapter 11), and the heightened awareness of quality-of-life issues have brought new hope to patients who have been unable to function up to their abilities because of seizures, medication side effects, or psychosocial difficulties.

The strategy for designing and implementing a treatment plan begins with an accurate diagnosis of the patient's seizure type(s) and a measurement of seizure frequency and severity. Referral to a neurologist may be appropriate to establish the diagnosis and to formulate a treatment plan, but subsequent follow-up is often managed by the primary care physician. In evaluating the effectiveness of treatment, the clinician takes into consideration any side effects of the medication and any psychosocial problems the patient may be experiencing. The treatment process is more likely to be successful when the clinician has a working knowledge of available AEDs, AED pharmacokinetics, drug–drug interactions, and AED side effects.

HOW DOES DIAGNOSIS OF THE PATIENT'S SEIZURE TYPE INFLUENCE THE CHOICE OF THERAPY?

The first step toward initiating therapy is to establish the patient's seizure type(s) within the framework of the seizure classification of the International League against Epilepsy[2] and, if possible, to establish the patient's epilepsy syndrome. Details about the classification of seizures are given in Chapter 1. The classifications of seizure type

The Comprehensive Evaluation and Treatment of Epilepsy
Copyright © 1997 by Academic Press. All rights of reproduction in any form reserved.

and epilepsy syndrome are made primarily on clinical grounds and may be supported by laboratory, neurophysiologic, and radiographic studies, as described elsewhere in this book. This determination has important implications for the selection of AEDs and requires that a thorough history be obtained from the patient and from observers, with close attention paid to descriptions of actual seizures. The patient may find it easier to describe any symptoms he or she has had during seizures by referring to published seizure descriptions.[3] If the patient is experiencing more than one type of seizure and can describe the different symptoms of each type, the clinician may be better able to categorize the patient's seizure types and epilepsy syndrome, as well as to plan the therapeutic approach more effectively.

It is often necessary for the clinician to ask pointed questions to uncover behaviors or environmental factors that may increase the possibility of a seizure. These so-called *seizure triggers,* such as sleep deprivation, alcohol intake, and stress, are potentially modifiable. Therefore, measures to limit exposure to these triggers may successfully augment AED therapy.

WHEN SHOULD TREATMENT BE STARTED?

The goal of AED therapy is to eliminate seizures without causing side effects. It follows, then, that AED therapy should be started when a patient appears to be at increased risk for recurrent seizures. Not all patients who have a single seizure are at risk for additional seizures; up to 10% of the general population may have a single seizure, but only about 0.5–1% of the general population are at risk for recurrent seizures. From a practical standpoint, AED treatment is usually started after the second seizure, because the appearance of the second seizure proves a propensity for seizure recurrence.

Factors that increase the risk of seizure recurrence include a history of brain insult (e.g., head injury with loss of consciousness), an identifiable brain lesion, focal abnormalities upon neurologic examination, a history of cognitive impairment, a partial seizure as the first seizure (with the exception of benign rolandic seizures), and an abnormal EEG (particularly epileptiform abnormalities). In selected cases, it may be reasonable to initiate AED therapy after the first seizure if the patient is considered at high risk for recurrence based on the factors just cited.

Table 3.1 presents the recommended initial treatment for the different types of seizures.

WHAT CAN BE DONE, AS TREATMENT IS INITIATED, TO MAXIMIZE THE LIKELIHOOD OF A SUCCESSFUL OUTCOME?

As soon as the patient begins AED therapy, the physician should establish a dialogue with the patient and the patient's family that will increase their understand-

Table 3.1

Recommended Treatment for Different Seizure Types

Seizure Type	Initial and First-Line Therapy	Second-Line or Adjunctive Therapy
Primary generalized tonic-clonic seizures	Carbamazepine Phenytoin Valproate	Phenobarbital Primidone
Partial seizures with or without secondary generalization	Carbamazepine Phenytoin Valproate	Felbamate[a] Gabapentin Lamotrigine Phenobarbital Primidone
Absence seizures	Ethosuximide Valproate	Trimethadione
Myoclonic seizures	Valproate	Clonazepam
Mixed seizures (myoclonic and tonic-clonic)	Felbamate[a] Valproate	Phenytoin Primidone

[a] Felbamate is not indicated as a first-line antiepileptic treatment. It is recommended for use only in those patients who respond inadequately to alternative treatments and whose epilepsy is so severe that a substantial risk of aplastic anemia or liver failure is deemed acceptable in light of the benefits conferred by its use.

ing of epilepsy and their ability to report important information. Because epilepsy affects each patient differently and each patient has a different capacity to understand various aspects of the disorder, the primary care provider should tailor the discussion on a personal basis to clarify the impact of the condition on the patient's quality of life and the expectations of the treatment plan.

The physician should also encourage the patient and family members to record the patient's seizures and medication dosages on a calendar. Seizure triggers, such as stress, sleep deprivation, and menses (when appropriate), should also be recorded. It is important to enlist the cooperation of the patient and family members or close friends in monitoring seizure frequency and severity, both of which can be recorded on the calendar. The calendar should be brought to the physician's office for review. This procedure helps to monitor and to encourage compliance and may demonstrate whether seizures do indeed correlate with factors such as stress or menses. Using a calendar also helps track the patient's response to AED therapy, including any symptoms that may represent side effects. The patient and family should be asked to note on the calendar the time of day that any symptoms occur.

Finally, the physician should stress the importance of taking the AED regularly and as prescribed. The patient should be given written instructions on how and when to take the AED, and the dosing regimen and any potential adverse effects or drug–drug interactions should be explained. If a patient is incapable of absorbing this information, it should be imparted to some other responsible person (e.g., a family member, friend, or case manager). Compliance with treatment is higher among patients who are well informed and who understand the expectations of the treatment plan and the potential benefits and risks of therapy. This understanding is particularly important with respect to medications that must be gradually increased during the initial phases of treatment. These AEDs include carbamazepine, valproate, lamotrigine, gabapentin, and felbamate. The patient should be encouraged to contact the physician before starting any other prescription or over-the-counter medication, because the serum levels of the AED could be affected. The patient should be warned not to suddenly stop taking an AED and should be sure to refill the prescription before the pills run out. Follow-up visits should be scheduled as necessary to monitor AED serum levels, blood counts, and liver and renal function and to address any concerns that the patient may have about possible side effects or taking the medication.

WHAT ARE THE RESULTS OF AED THERAPY?

Complete seizure control with minimal side effects can be achieved in approximately 70–80% of patients with single-drug therapy; combinations of AEDs enable an additional 10–15% of patients to achieve seizure control without significant side effects. If one AED is unsuccessful because of ineffectiveness or because of side effects, a second AED may be tried. In general, it is preferable to maintain a patient on a single AED. When it has been determined that the initial medication is ineffective, the second drug should be titrated to a therapeutic level or dosage before the old AED is tapered. As previously stated, combinations of AEDs may be necessary for some patients. Virtually all combinations of medications have been tried, although certain combinations should be avoided, such as any combination of phenobarbital, primidone, and diazepam—all three drugs are central nervous system (CNS) depressants.

Side effects are a major cause of medication intolerance and noncompliance. Table 3.2 lists the common and the rare side effects of the commonly used AEDs. The contraindications for each medication are given in the complete prescribing information for that drug.

The AEDs differ in how easily and rapidly a loading dose can be administered, as shown in Table 3.3, which also lists the likely mechanism of action for each AED.

Table 3.4 gives pharmacokinetic information, including frequency of dosing, number of days needed to achieve steady state, and frequency of initial monitoring (serum levels, liver and renal function, and complete blood counts). The number of days necessary to achieve steady state is particularly important in relation to the frequency of the patient's seizures. Patients with infrequent seizures can be more

Table 3.2

Common and Rare Side Effects of AEDs

AED	Brand	Systemic Side Effects	Neurotoxic Side Effects	Rare Idiosyncratic Reactions
Carbamazepine	Tegretol	Nausea, vomiting, diarrhea, hyponatremia, rash, pruritus, fluid retention	Drowsiness, dizziness, blurred or double vision, lethargy, headache	Agranulocytosis, Stevens–Johnson syndrome, aplastic anemia, hepatic failure, dermatitis/rash, serum sickness, pancreatitis
Ethosuximide	Zarontin	Nausea, vomiting	Sleep disturbance, drowsiness, hyperactivity	Agranulocytosis, Stevens–Johnson syndrome, aplastic anemia, dermatitis/rash, serum sickness
Felbamate[a]	Felbatol	Nausea, vomiting, anorexia, weight loss	Insomnia, dizziness, headache, ataxia	Aplastic anemia, liver failure: see package insert for details
Gabapentin	Neurontin	None known	Somnolence, dizziness, ataxia	Unknown
Lamotrigine	Lamictal	Rash, nausea	Dizziness, somnolence	Stevens–Johnson syndrome, hypersensitivity syndrome
Phenobarbital, Primidone	Mysoline	Nausea, rash	Alteration of sleep cycles, sedation, lethargy, behavioral changes, hyperactivity, ataxia, tolerance, dependence	Agranulocytosis, Stevens–Johnson syndrome, hepatic failure, dermatitis/rash, serum sickness
Phenytoin	Dilantin	Gingival hypertrophy, body hair increase, rash, lymphadenopathy	Confusion, slurred speech, double vision, ataxia, neuropathy (with long-term use)	Agranulocytosis, Stevens–Johnson syndrome, aplastic anemia, hepatic failure, dermatitis/rash, serum sickness
Valproate	Depakote	Weight gain, nausea, vomiting, hair loss, easy bruising	Tremor	Agranulocytosis, Stevens–Johnson syndrome, aplastic anemia, hepatic failure, dermatitis/rash, serum sickness, pancreatitis

[a] Felbamate is not indicated as a first-line antiepileptic treatment. It is recommended for use only in those patients who respond inadequately to alternative treatments and whose epilepsy is so severe that a substantial risk of aplastic anemia or liver failure is deemed acceptable in light of the benefits conferred by its use.

Table 3.3

Loading and Initial Dosing, Mechanism of Action of AEDs

AED	Brand	Iv Loading Dose	Oral Loading and Maintenance Dose	Mechanism of Action
Barbiturates	Mysoline	Phenobarbital: 90–120 mg every 10–15 min as needed to maximum of 1000 mg	1–5 mg/kg/day	Prolongs GABA-mediated chloride channel openings; decreases CNS excitability
Carbamazepine	Tegretol	N/A	Start at 2–3 mg/kg/day; increase dosage every 3–5 days to 10 mg/kg/day; dose may need to be increased further to 15–20 mg/kg/day after 2–3 months because of hepatic autoinduction	Blocks sodium-dependent action potentials; reduces neuronal calcium uptake
Ethosuximide	Zarontin	N/A	20–40 mg/kg/day in 1–3 divided doses	Modifies low-threshold or transient neuronal calcium currents
Felbamate	Felbatol	N/A	1200 mg/day in three divided doses; increase by 600–1200 mg/day every 2 weeks to recommended maximum of 3600 mg/day	Unknown
Gabapentin	Neurontin	N/A	300 mg first day, 300 mg bid second day, 300 mg tid third day; increased as needed to 1800 mg/day in three divided doses	Unknown
Lamotrigine	Lamictal	N/A	For patients taking an enzyme-inducing AED: 25 mg bid, titrated upward by 50-mg increments every 1–2 weeks as needed; for patients taking valproate: 25 mg every other day, with increases of 25–50 mg every 2 weeks as needed to a maximum of 300–500 mg/day; the maximum dosage used in US open-label drug trials is 700 mg/day	Inhibits voltage-dependent sodium channels, resulting in decreased release of the excitatory neurotransmitters glutamate and aspartate
Phenytoin	Dilantin	15–20 mg/kg (not more than 50 mg/min)	15 mg/kg in three divided doses over 9–12 hours; 5 mg/kg/day maintenance	Blocks sodium-dependent action potentials; reduces neuronal calcium uptake
Valproate	Depakote	N/A	15 mg/kg/day in three divided doses; increase by 5 to 10 mg/kg/day every week as needed	Reduces high-frequency neuronal firing and sodium-dependent action potentials; enhances GABA effects

N/A, not applicable.

Table 3.4

Pharmacokinetic Information for AEDs

AED	Percentage Bound to Plasma Protein	Elimination Half-Life (hours)	Time to Steady State (days)	Frequency of Dosing	Frequency of Initial Monitoring	Therapeutic Level (μg/ml)
Carbamazepine	70–80	11–17 (chronic therapy)	3–10	bid, tid, qid	3, 6, 9 weeks	4–12
Ethosuximide	0	40–50	6–12	qd, bid, tid	2–3 weeks	40–100
Felbamate	25	20–23	5–10	bid, tid	Every 2 weeks	32–137
Gabapentin	0	5–7; increases with decreased creatinine clearance (see prescribing information	2–3	tid	None	N/A
Lamotrigine	50–55	10–15 with enzyme-inducing AED; 40–60 with valproate	5–15	bid	None	N/A
Phenobarbital	40–60	30–50	16–21	qd	3–4 weeks	40–100
Phenytoin	90	15–30	5–15	qd or bid	2–3 weeks	10–20
Valproate	60–95 (decreases with serum levels over 100 μg/ml)	6–8	2–4	bid or tid	1–2 weeks	50–150

N/A, Not applicable.

safely begun on an AED with a slow loading or dose initiation schedule than patients with frequent seizures. The dosing information presented in Table 3.4 applies to adults; therefore, physicians who treat epilepsy in children should consult the prescribing information for correct dosing regimens of AEDs. In addition, modifications may be necessary in elderly patients, as discussed in Chapter 13.

IS NONCOMPLIANCE WITH AED THERAPY A SIGNIFICANT PROBLEM?

Up to half the patients with epilepsy may not take their medications as directed, and over half the patients seen in emergency rooms because of recurrent seizures are noncompliant. Patient-related factors that increase noncompliance are denial of the diagnosis of epilepsy, limited financial means to pay for AEDs, difficulty tolerating side effects, and frequent seizures or memory impairment. Iatrogenic factors include long intervals between visits to the physician and complicated medication regimens.

Noncompliance should be suspected if there is an unexpected increase in the number or severity of seizures, subtherapeutic or supratherapeutic AED serum levels, or a change in medical reimbursement systems. Noncompliance is the most common reason for incomplete seizure control or variable side effects. Clear communication with the patient provides the basis for an effective patient–physician partnership, and noncompliance often is a result of a communication failure.

Monitoring AED levels will help determine compliance, but variable levels can also occur when AEDs are stored in or near a humid environment, the patient takes generic medications from different manufacturers, or there is a significant change in the patient's weight.

WHAT ARE THE TYPICAL SIDE EFFECTS OF AEDs?

Within the first 6 months of treatment with a newly prescribed AED, systemic toxicity and neurotoxicity are as likely to contribute to AED failure as is lack of efficacy. Table 3.2 shows the common neurotoxic effects of AEDs; these include diplopia, nystagmus, dysarthria, ataxia, incoordination, tremor, sedation, mood alteration, dizziness, headache, and cognitive impairment. Sufficient time should be allowed during office visits to determine whether a patient is experiencing any side effects. Patients often complain of memory loss. Neuropsychologic testing, as described in Chapter 6, may help determine whether memory loss or trouble concentrating is medication-related.

For patients who have peak-level side effects from a particular AED, the usual strategy is to modify the medication regimen or treatment schedule to minimize side effects, such as by spreading out the daily dosage over several doses. The physician should attempt to correlate drug serum levels with the patient's side effects before abandoning a medication. Specifically, drug serum levels should be obtained when a patient is experiencing side effects, and these levels should be compared with those obtained when the patient is free of symptoms. Referring to the patient's seizure calendar may be helpful in planning the timing of drug levels, to prove a cause-and-effect relationship between peak levels and side effects. The serum levels that are associated with neurotoxicity vary from one patient to another and may occur within the so-called therapeutic range. Before the physician discontinues an AED because of side effects, an attempt should be made to adjust the timing or dose size of the AED taken during the day. For example, a patient may have only nocturnal seizures and may take equal doses of an AED twice a day. If the patient experiences side effects during the afternoon from the morning AED dose, the physician may succeed in eliminating those side effects without compromising seizure control by shifting part of the morning dose to the bedtime dose.

Total serum levels may be misleading. Free unbound serum levels of phenytoin and valproate should be checked in patients with low albumin levels or in patients who are taking multiple drugs that are tightly protein-bound. In such patients, free levels should be multiplied by 10 to approximate the desired total serum level. Further, serum levels may fluctuate even in compliant patients because of laboratory error, generic substitution for brand-name AEDs, and variable potency of pills (patients should avoid storing their pills in warm, humid places). Similarly, women with catamenial exacerbation of their seizures should have their serum AED levels checked in the premenstrual period and compared with midcycle levels, because AED levels may drop during the menses.

WHAT ARE THE ADVANTAGES OF MONOTHERAPY OVER POLYTHERAPY?

For most patients, treatment with a single AED enhances compliance, provides a wider therapeutic window, and is more cost effective than combination therapy; that is, there are usually fewer side effects, idiosyncratic reactions, and teratogenic effects and also no risk of AED–AED interactions.

Adding an AED to an existing AED (i.e., changing a patient from monotherapy to polytherapy) may result in increased AED side effects. For example, adding carbamazepine to phenytoin may increase mean total phenytoin serum levels by 35% and decrease phenytoin clearance by 37%. Other effects of adding one AED to another are outlined in Table 3.5.

Combinations of AEDs and other types of medications may also cause side effects or breakthrough seizures. Calcium-containing antacids may affect AED

Table 3.5

Common AED Drug–Drug Interactions

	Carbamazepine	Phenytoin	Valproate	Felbamate	Neurontin	Lamotrigine	Phenobarbital
AEDs that increase AED levels	Felbamate (increases carbamazepine epoxide) Lamotrigine (may increase carbamazepine epoxide) Valproate	Diazepam (these may increase free and/or total phenytoin levels) Ethosuximide Felbamate Valproate	Felbamate	Valproate	None	Valproate	Valproate
AEDs that decrease AED levels	Felbamate Phenobarbital Phenytoin Primidone	Carbamazepine	Carbamazepine	Carbamazepine Phenytoin	None	None	Carbamazepine

absorption. For instance, administering drugs that inhibit hepatic enzymes may increase levels of hepatically metabolized AEDs. As a result, propoxyphene, erythromycin, and verapamil often elevate carbamazepine levels. Cimetidine, which is now available over the counter, may also elevate levels of carbamazepine and phenytoin. Conversely, drugs that induce hepatic metabolism, such as rifampin and ethanol, may decrease AED levels. The common AED–non-AED interactions are listed in Table 3.6.

WHAT ARE THE ROLES OF AED LEVELS AND BLOOD TESTS?

Checking AED levels is useful for monitoring compliance, for following the results of AED dosage changes, and for establishing a patient's maximum tolerated serum level. Changes in dosages should be based on clinical grounds, such as seizure breakthrough or side effects, not because of the serum level. This rules applies particularly to lamotrigine, gabapentin, and felbamate, inasmuch as so-called therapeutic ranges have not been established for these AEDs.

Table 3.6

The Common AED Drug–Non-AED Drug Interactions

	Carbamazepine	Phenytoin	Valproate	Phenobarbital
Drugs that increase AED levels and/or enhance effects	Calcium channel blockers Cimetidine Erythromycin Fluoxetine Isoniazid Propoxyphene Valproate (may increase free level)	Aspirin Chloramphenicol Chlordiazepoxide Cimetidine Dicumarol Disulfiram Estrogens Halothane Isoniazid Methylphenidate Phenothiazines Phenylbutazone Sulfonamides Tolbutamide Trazadone	Aspirin Dicumarol	Amitriptyline Antihistamines Corticosteroids Imipramine MAO inhibitors Tranquilizers
Drugs that decrease AED levels	Doxycycline Haloperidol Oral contraceptives Theophylline Warfarin	Alcohol (chronic use) Isoniazid	None	None

WHEN CAN AEDs BE DISCONTINUED?

Even as they are beginning AED therapy, many patients ask how long they will need to stay on their treatment. Most, but not all, children and adults who are seizure free for 2 years while taking AEDs will remain so if they stop taking their medications. However, it is impossible to identify those prospective patients who will remain free from seizures after their AEDs are discontinued and those who will not. Factors that imply an increased risk for seizure recurrence include readily identifiable brain pathology (e.g., brain tumor, congenital anomaly, cerebral contusion), seizure onset after the age of 12, severe epilepsy before the initiation of AED therapy, specific epilepsy syndromes (particularly juvenile myoclonic epilepsy), abnormal EEGs (applies only to children with idiopathic epilepsy), and multiple seizure types occurring in the same patient.

The benefits of medication withdrawal are the avoidance of side effects (such as possible teratogenicity, behavioral and cognitive impairment, and cosmetic/soft tissue effects) and the removal of a visible reminder of the patient's diagnosis of epilepsy and, therefore, less chance that psychosocial issues will cause secondary problems.

The principal risk of discontinuing AED therapy is recurrent seizures. This risk poses a lesser problem for children than for adults, particularly adults who are gainfully employed, who drive, and whose lifestyle may be negatively affected by recurrent seizures. Therefore, the decision to taper AEDs must be made on a personal basis, with consideration given to the uncertainty of the risk of recurrence, the potential risk of continuing AEDs, and the risk of recurrent seizures after AEDs are discontinued.

When AEDs are withdrawn, special caution is warranted. Abrupt discontinuation of an AED may increase the risk of seizures and status epilepticus. Withdrawal from CNS depressants, such as phenobarbital and the benzodiazepines, should be accomplished over weeks to months in order to minimize the risk of withdrawal seizures.

IS AED TREATMENT DURING PREGNANCY SAFE? WHAT ARE THE SAFEST AEDs IN GENERAL?

A discussion of the teratogenicity of AEDs may be found elsewhere.[4] In general, women who take AEDs have double the risk of bearing a malformed infant as women who do not take AEDs. Features of the fetal anticonvulsant syndrome include limb abnormalities, craniofacial abnormalities, and growth and development abnormalities. Congenital malformations have been reported in association with all the older AEDs; clinical experience with the newer AEDs (felbamate, gabapentin, and lamotrigine) has not been extensive enough to determine risk. Unfortunately, there are no carefully controlled studies to identify which of the AEDs are safest for the fetus. Therefore, in general, the best approach is to select an AED on a case-by-case basis—an AED that has been proven in a particular patient to control seizures, especially generalized seizures—and to administer that AED at the minimum effective dosage. In every case, the physician must weigh the risk to benefit ratio. Valproate appears to carry a particular risk of neural tube defects.

When a pregnant woman takes multiple AEDs or has a personal or family history of birth defects or miscarriages due to birth defects, the risk to the fetus increases significantly. Any woman who is physically capable of becoming pregnant should be counseled on these issues and should be encouraged to take folic acid, 0.4 mg/day. Folic acid intake is particularly important before conception and should continue throughout pregnancy. Women with a previous pregnancy complicated by a fetal malformation, such as a neural tube defect, and women with a family history of birth defects should take 4 mg/day of folic acid and should probably avoid valproate and carbamazepine.

WHAT ARE THE OTHER ELEMENTS OF TREATMENT BESIDES MEDICAL THERAPY?

Pharmacotherapy is only one facet of a comprehensive approach to epilepsy management. Such factors as cognitive, physical, and psychosocial functioning may be as important to the patient's overall quality of life as seizure control. To have a positive impact on these nonpharmacologic aspects of epilepsy, the primary care physician may need to enlist the participation of various medical and social service professionals.

The psychosocial aspects of epilepsy are an important component of the disorder. Patients often have major concerns about health, independence, personal growth, relationships, well-being, and security. These issues are discussed more fully in Chapter 5 and can be appreciated and addressed only if the physician attempts to uncover the psychologic and social problems that adversely affect the patient's quality of life. This process begins with taking a complete psychosocial history, including information about any previous psychiatric illnesses or treatments, education, employment, driving, insurance, interpersonal relationships, and attitude toward having epilepsy. A number of questionnaires developed for this purpose supplement the psychosocial history and provide a quantifiable means of assessing and following patients as pharmacotherapeutic and psychosocial interventions are implemented.[5] Uncovering a source of psychosocial stress may lead to an effective strategy for reducing the impact of that stress on the patient, which in turn may help reduce seizure frequency. Patients with stress-induced seizures may be candidates for stress reduction, biofeedback, or relaxation training.

Support groups, individual or family counseling, legal assistance in cases of job discrimination or other legal problems, vocational training, and educational guidance are important adjuncts to medical therapy in selected patients. The primary care physician plays a key role in connecting the patient to the network of health care and psychosocial professionals when specific needs arise. Numerous resources are available, often through a local epilepsy association, to assist the patient. If there is no local epilepsy group, the patient should be encouraged to telephone the Epilepsy Foundation of America at 1-800-EFA-1000.

Negative preconceptions about epilepsy within certain ethnic groups may make some patients reluctant to seek treatment. The physician should be aware of and sensitive to these cultural differences. The acknowledgment of alternative forms of healing and spiritual healers may be meaningful to members of some ethnic groups and may have a place in the overall treatment plan of selected patients.

Finally, all patients with epilepsy and their family members and close friends should be familiar with first-aid techniques and safety considerations that lessen the risk of injury from seizures.[6]

CONCLUSION

The successful management of epilepsy is based on establishing an open dialogue with the patient and an accurate seizure diagnosis. Each patient must be closely followed for seizure frequency and severity, medication side effects, and psychosocial problems. The clinician should closely monitor the patient as his or her AEDs are adjusted and should make sure that the patient and family have access to appropriate resources, such as support groups, individual or family counseling, educational guidance, and stress reduction techniques.

As new AEDs are introduced, the range of options for patients increases. A rational approach to polypharmacy may emerge in the near future. Until then, cautious use of medications alone and in combination will minimize side effects and will enable the large majority of patients to achieve their potential within the limits of current therapy.

REFERENCES

1. Schachter SC. Advances in the assessment of refractory epilepsy. *Epilepsia.* 1993;34:S24–S30.
2. Commission on Classification and Terminology of the International League against Epilepsy: Proposal for revised classification of epilepsies and epileptic syndromes. *Epilepsia.* 1989;30:389–399.
3. Schachter SC. *Brainstorms: Epilepsy in Our Words.* New York: Raven Press; 1993:1–104.
4. Lindhout D, Omtzigt GC. Teratogenic effects of antiepileptic drugs: Implications for the management of epilepsy in women of childbearing age. *Epilepsia.* 1994;35:S19–S28.
5. Devinsky O. Clinical uses of the quality-of-life in epilepsy inventory. *Epilepsia.* 1993;34:S39–S44.
6. Schachter SC. *The Brainstorms Companion: Epilepsy In Our View.* New York: Raven Press; 1995: 1–134.

CHAPTER 4

Definition and Overview of Intractable Epilepsy

Orrin Devinsky, M.D.

WHEN IS EPILEPSY CONSIDERED INTRACTABLE?

Various terms are used to refer to seizures that are partially controlled, uncontrolled, or controlled only at the cost of disabling side effects. Since words define concepts and influence behavior, let us begin by considering dictionary definitions of *intractable* and *refractory*. The Oxford English Dictionary (OED) defines *intractable* as "not to be manipulated, wrought or brought into any desired condition; not easily treated or dealt with; resisting treatment or effort"; the OED defines *refractory* as "obstinate, not yielding to treatment." Both terms apply to seizures that persist despite antiepileptic drug (AED) therapy—seizures that are obstinate and that resist control. Although these terms focus on symptoms, in this case seizures, the picture is in reality more complex. In almost all patients, seizures can be brought under control or forced to yield, but the cost may be disabling side effects. Complete seizure control with a phenobarbital level of 75 μg/ml may be regarded as a success if one examines only the patient's seizure diary, but a miserable failure if one looks at the person.

Epilepsy is intractable when the patient has persistent seizures or medication side effects that interfere with quality of life. Intractability is not defined by a specific number or frequency of seizures or by the severity of seizures or side effects of AEDs. Although the term *intractable epilepsy* implies that the patient's seizures persist despite attempts to control them, there is no consensus on how long or vigorously a person's epilepsy must be treated before being labeled intractable.

With the dramatic increase in epilepsy surgery, intractable epilepsy has become strongly associated with surgical intervention. However, not all persons with intractable epilepsy are good candidates for epilepsy surgery. In some cases, intractability is because of misdiagnosis (i.e., the patient does not have epilepsy) or failure to try certain monotherapeutic regimens, such as valproate for juvenile myoclonic epilepsy. In other cases, a person's seizures are intractable to available medications but the patient is not an appropriate candidate for resective epilepsy surgery. Examples include patients with primary generalized epilepsy and multifocal partial epilepsy.

Intractable epilepsy is common, but experience in recognizing the disorder, and views on its implications, vary tremendously among physicians. Some physi-

The Comprehensive Evaluation and Treatment of Epilepsy
Copyright © 1997 by Academic Press. All rights of reproduction in any form reserved.

cians regard intractable epilepsy as simply a generic label for epilepsy in a person who they think deserves referral to an epilepsy center for enrollment in a monitoring study, for investigational drug therapy, or for surgery. Other physicians have only read about intractable epilepsy and have never observed it in their neurologic practices. Intractable epilepsy should be looked for and identified; it is a red flag—marking a patient whose AED therapy is not as effective or as well tolerated as the patient would like.

Practically speaking, a person can be said to have intractable epilepsy if his or her seizures or the side effects of treatment are unacceptable or significantly impair the quality of life. But how does one define unacceptable seizures or side effects and what constitutes significant impairment of quality of life? How many seizures or side effects are okay? Who should define intractable—the physician, the family, or the patient? The answers to these difficult questions are as individual as epilepsy is in different persons. In general, physicians decide who has intractable epilepsy. Unfortunately, many good candidates for investigational drugs or epilepsy surgery are not informed about these treatment alternatives.

HOW DO PHYSICIANS' AND PATIENTS' PERSPECTIVES ON INTRACTABLE EPILEPSY TEND TO DIFFER?

Important differences often exist between how physicians and patients view intractable epilepsy. The physician tends to be interested primarily in the patient's medical condition, whereas the patient tends to be interested primarily in quality of life. Quality of life should be defined from the patient's perspective, not the physician's. Many physicians consider medication changes or epilepsy surgery only for patients who have such frequent and severe seizures that they are unable to function, who frequently injure themselves, or who are experiencing obvious declines in cognitive function from seizures or polytherapy. Other physicians consider surgery only if there is evidence of a progressive lesion, such as a tumor. On the other end of the spectrum, some epileptologists consider patients with infrequent complex partial seizures to be good surgical candidates. Physicians focus on medical outcome—seizures and side effects. Patients are also concerned about seizures and side effects, but the seizures and side effects are perceived differently by the person who has them.

A CASE EXAMPLE

Consider a woman who has two tonic-clonic seizures a year and a complex partial seizure every other month. She takes high doses of carbamazepine, which produces diplopia one or two times a week for 1 to 3 hours, and she reports intermittent fatigue that she thinks is probably caused by her medication. From the neurologist's perspective, the patient's situation is acceptable. After all, her seizure frequency has been stable over the past 5 years; she is employed; she looks good, speaks well, and appears well. Of course, it would be better if she had no seizures, but her monotherapeutic regimen provides a reasonable balance between seizures and side effects. She's doing okay.

The patient's perspective of her disorder and her neurologist's are different. She finds the tonic-clonic seizures devastating. They can occur at work or on the street. Waking up confused with her coworkers surrounding her, losing control of her bladder during a seizure, having a seizure on the bus or street, being taken to an emergency room—all these experiences are embarrassing and disruptive. She must live with the constant anxiety of not knowing when the next seizure will occur. Will it happen tomorrow, 2 weeks from now, 4 months from now? Sometimes she gets a feeling that a seizure will occur soon so she restricts her activities that week. The woman's partial seizures also affect her adversely. They can cause problems when they occur during business meetings or important phone calls. She cannot drive a car. Her potential for career advancement is limited by her disorder. She must cope with the extra stress that her epilepsy imposes on her relationship with her boyfriend. She worries that after she gets married and becomes pregnant, her medication might harm the developing fetus. Will she be able to hold the baby, bathe the baby? The episodes of double vision she experiences are more than a minor nuisance: they last for about 2 hours and during that time she cannot function well so she avoids reading or using her computer. Trying to cope with spells of double vision makes her irritable and tired. The fatigue she feels is like having a touch of the flu 365 days a year. The zest that used to define her is missing or subdued. She has to push herself all the time to do things that she used to do without effort. Things are not okay!

THE IMPACT OF SOCIAL PROBLEMS

The psychosocial problems caused by chronic seizures often outweigh the medical ones. Driving restrictions; reduced social, educational, and employment opportunities; real and perceived stigmas; and fear of seizures pervade the existence of people with epilepsy. However, these problems usually receive minimal attention during routine medical office visits. With respect to driving, the physician may be unwilling to be the patient's advocate because of concern about protecting other drivers and pedestrians from potential seizure-caused accidents and because of concern about avoiding potential lawsuits should the patient have an accident while driving. Whether or not the physician is planning to refer a patient for investigational drug therapy or surgery, he or she should ask the patient how seizures and medications are affecting the patient's life. The impact of seizures on a person's life is impossible for the physician to measure fully.

Rare tonic-clonic seizures or occasional complex partial seizures can devastate quality of life for some persons, whereas others function without apparent problems and would not consider changing their medications or having surgery. Patients who take high doses of multiple AEDs may be tired, depressed, and dizzy throughout much of the day and may sleep more than 10 hours a night. Whether or not these patients have persistent seizures is secondary; the medications significantly disrupt their lives. Physicians may view the goal of therapy as eliminating the patient's seizures at any cost and the patient may passively cooperate with the physician's efforts, never considering that his or her own desires should determine "medical" decisions.

CONSIDERING ALTERNATIVES

The physician should offer patients whose seizures are not fully controlled with available medications *the chance to consider alternatives* such as investigational drugs or epilepsy surgery. Similarly, patients who are seizure free but who experience troublesome side effects may welcome a change in medications or, if the side effects are disabling, the possibility of a surgical procedure that would allow a reduction in the number or dosage of medications.

Referral of a patient to a comprehensive epilepsy center does not necessarily mean that the patient will undergo a monitoring study or that investigational drug therapy or epilepsy surgery will be recommended. In many cases, the patient will be reassured that no changes in the current regimen are needed. In other cases, a monitoring study may be recommended to confirm the diagnosis of epilepsy. Nonepileptic psychogenic seizures are a common cause of "intractable" epilepsy (see Chapter 9). If a patient is evaluated for possible surgery and is found to be a good candidate, a physician will review the workup results and surgical procedure with the patient so that he or she can choose whether or not to have surgery. Conversely, a patient who wishes to have surgery may be found to have multiple foci and therefore may be a poor candidate for surgery.

HOW DOES AED THERAPY AFFECT THE PROGNOSIS FOR PATIENTS WITH SPECIFIC EPILEPSY SYNDROMES?

The classification of epilepsy syndromes has provided a broader perspective from which to view the epilepsies than seizure type. Epilepsy syndromes are defined by a specific constellation of several factors, including the patient's age at onset, the patient's family history, seizure type and frequency, anatomic and pathophysiologic features, the patient's response to medication, medications of choice, and prognosis. Classifying epilepsy syndromes is more challenging and controversial than classifying seizure types. Our formulation of epilepsy syndromes continues to evolve. Some syndromes, such as febrile convulsions and juvenile myoclonic epilepsy, are well defined and widely accepted; others, such as dorsolateral frontal symptomatic epilepsies, are poorly defined and are difficult to distinguish without invasive electrode recordings.

Table 4.1 lists the degree of seizure control achieved with AEDs and the likelihood of remission for the major epilepsy syndromes. Although certain epilepsy syndromes are associated with good to excellent prognoses whereas others are not, some persons with intractable seizures have epilepsy syndromes that are generally responsive to AEDs. For example, childhood absence epilepsy is considered the easiest form of epilepsy to treat—less than 5% of patients have seizures that are intractable to currently approved AEDs.[1] Further, spontaneous remission of absence seizures often occurs. Despite these facts, one study of patients with absence epilepsy found that only 69% were free from absence seizures at the 7-year follow-up and 60% at the 9.5-year follow-up.[2,3] Studies in which patients' absence seizures were treated with either first-line drugs, ethosuximide, or valproate reported that complete control was achieved in 33–90% of patients.[4–8] Therefore, even among the

Table 4.1

Epilepsy Syndromes: Prognosis for Seizure Control and Remission

Syndrome	Seizure Control with AEDs	Remission of Epilepsy
Localization-related		
Benign rolandic	Excellent; AEDs may not be needed	>95%
Benign occipital	Excellent	90%
Mesial temporal	Variable; often intractable	Variable
Lateral temporal	Variable; often intractable	Variable
Frontal	Variable; often intractable	Variable
Primary generalized		
Benign neonatal convulsions	Excellent; AEDs may not be needed	>90%
Febrile	Usually not required; prophylactic benzodiazepines effective	>90%
West (infantile spasms)	Fair; may require ACTH	<50%
Lennox–Gastaut	Poor	<20%
Childhood absence (pyknolepsy)	Good	>70%
Juvenile myoclonic (impulsive petit mal)	Excellent	<5%
Tonic-clonic on awakening	Excellent	>50%
Progressive myoclonic	Poor	Rare

milder forms of epilepsy, intractability may be more common than is generally suspected.

The likelihood of remission is influenced by several factors, including not only the patient's specific epilepsy syndrome but also the results of neurologic examination and neuroimaging studies, any symptomatic causes, epileptiform activity reflected on an electroencephalogram (EEG), and degree of seizure control obtained with AEDs. Possible factors in intractable partial seizures include neuropsychiatric abnormalities, epilepsy of long duration, and psychosocial handicaps.[9]

Partial epilepsy is the most common seizure type in adults, but it is difficult to classify syndromically and prognostically. Although partial seizures are more likely to be intractable to pharmacotherapy than are primary generalized seizures, patients with partial epilepsy vary considerably in their response to medications and whether or not remission occurs at all. Long-term outcome is difficult to predict in the early stages for patients with partial epilepsy. After 1–2 years, a clearer picture emerges. If a patient's seizures remain uncontrolled after 1–2 years of treatment, despite accurate diagnosis and the use of two first-line medications, the chance of seizure remission or complete control is low.

HOW MANY MEDICATIONS SHOULD BE TRIED BEFORE A PATIENT IS EVALUATED FOR SURGERY?

No consensus exists about what constitutes an adequate trial of AEDs before surgery is considered. Overall, during the past decade there has been a marked reduction in the average duration between the onset of epilepsy and epilepsy surgery. In the past, patients lived with epilepsy for 10–30 years before they underwent surgery. Now, many persons undergo epilepsy surgery who have had epilepsy for only 1–5 years.

No absolute criteria exist, with respect to number of drugs, dosages, or drug-blood levels, that constitute an adequate trial of medication before surgery should be considered. In part, the decision depends on the individual case. For example, patients with structural lesions (e.g., cavernous angioma) may be considered for surgery relatively early, because these lesions tend to be intractable to medication and surgical success rates are high. When ictal behavioral features suggest a frontal focus and neuroimaging study results and EEGs are normal, the patient's epilepsy might be more aggressively treated with medications, because surgical success rates are lower in these cases. In general, our approach to therapy has been to institute a minimum of two monotherapeutic trials and at least one trial of a two-drug combination.

MONOTHERAPY

Because carbamazepine and phenytoin are considered first-line drugs for partial seizures, monotherapeutic trials with each drug are indicated for patients with partial epilepsy. For example, if a patient has persistent seizures and intolerable side effects when carbamazepine is added to primidone, the patient may still be well controlled on maximally tolerated doses of carbamazepine alone. In reviewing the patient's history of prior "intolerable side effects," it is critical to inquire whether the dosage was increased gradually until seizures were controlled or until unacceptable side effects developed. Many patients, in whom high intravenous doses of phenytoin or high doses of carbamazepine result in "disabling" or "intolerable" side effects, are able to tolerate those medications when therapy is initiated at low doses and the dosage is gradually titrated upward.

If a rash or another idiosyncratic side effect develops that mandates the discontinuation of a medication, a monotherapeutic trial of valproate or a barbiturate (phenobarbital or primidone) should be considered. If two monotherapeutic trials are ineffective, the chances of obtaining seizure control with additional medication trials are less than 15%.[10–13]

COMBINATION THERAPY

If two monotherapeutic trials are unsuccessful, the physician should consider trying a combination of two drugs (some epileptologists will consider surgery without a two-drug trial). Although some patients may have better seizure control with two AEDs, troublesome or disabling side effects are also more common. Many authorities suggest using drugs with different mechanisms of action. However, because the mechanisms of action of AEDs are not fully understood and drugs with similar but not identical mechanisms may act synergistically, such suggestions are premature. Other physicians recommend using drug combinations that do not cause significant pharmacokinetic or pharmacodynamic interactions (i.e., increased side effects). Unfortunately, data on the relative efficacy and tolerability of various two-drug regimens are scant. Carbamazepine in combination with phenytoin, a barbiturate, or valproate, and phenytoin in combination with a barbiturate or valproate are the most common two-drug regimens. Controlled studies comparing the efficacy and safety of different two-drug trials are needed. The number of possible two-drug combinations is growing rapidly because of the availability of many new AEDs, making clarification of this muddy water more difficult.

INVESTIGATIONAL DRUG THERAPY

For patients with persistent seizures, it is reasonable but certainly not mandatory to try an investigational drug before recommending epilepsy surgery. However, if trials of two first-line drugs and a combination of two drugs titrated slowly to the maximal tolerated doses are unsuccessful, the chances are slim (<10–15%) that a new drug will be highly effective. However, if the investigational drug improves seizure control and causes fewer side effects, that may be sufficient reason to use it and to decide against epilepsy surgery.

In rare cases, three-drug combinations or third-line (adjunctive) drugs, such as acetazolamide, methsuximide, ethotoin, or clorazepate, are effective in controlling otherwise refractory seizures. Control in such cases is usually temporary (especially with acetazolamide and benzodiazepines such as clorazepate), and in many instances three-drug combinations or benzodiazepines in combination with one or more other agents cause or exacerbate neurobehavioral and other side effects. In one study of 66 patients, those whose epilepsy was refractory to carbamazepine, phenytoin, phenobarbital, or primidone at maximally tolerated doses had only an 11% chance, at the end of the study, of achieving full seizure control (for periods of 1–6 months) when clorazepate, methsuximide, or valproate were added.[14] None of these three second-line drugs significantly reduced seizure frequency as compared with baseline in the overall patient group.[14] Further, of the seven (11%) patients who "responded" to second-line drugs, most had recurrent seizures after the study period ended, suggesting that the number who achieve long-term complete seizure control under these conditions is probably less than 5%.

HOW LONG SHOULD DRUG THERAPY BE TRIED BEFORE SURGERY IS CONSIDERED?

The length of time that drug therapy is tried before surgery is considered varies with each patient and center—no strict criteria can be applied across different patient groups. In most cases, patients' seizures are treated for at least 1–2 years before surgery is considered. However, the greater the seizure frequency, the more rapidly medications can be assessed. If seizures are frequent and disabling, surgery may be considered within 1 year after the onset of epilepsy. It is unfortunate that many patients are not referred for epilepsy surgery until their seizures have been uncontrolled for more than a decade. If the patient is a motivated, good candidate for epilepsy surgery, then the physician should not continue medication trials indefinitely, waiting for new drugs to be developed or approved. The longer that seizures remain uncontrolled, the less favorable (both in terms of seizure control and psychosocial benefits) the outcome after surgery.[15] If a patient's seizures are not fully controlled with AEDs after 2 years, chances are slim that they will ever be controlled by drugs. Early effective therapy may be important in preventing the evolution of chronic epilepsy.[16]

WHAT FACTORS CONTRIBUTE TO INCOMPLETE SEIZURE CONTROL OR DISABLING SIDE EFFECTS?

Persistent seizures or troublesome side effects have many causes. When intractable epilepsy is diagnosed, it implies poor seizure control because of biologic

Incomplete Seizure Control
  Misdiagnosis
    Nonepileptic physiologic events (e.g., cardiac)
    Nonepileptic conversion (psychogenic) seizures
    Nonepileptic, nonconversion paroxysmal psychiatric disorders (e.g., panic disorder,
      hallucinations)
    Undiagnosed progressive neurologic disorders (e.g., brain tumor)
    Noncompliance and partial compliance
    Incorrect epilepsy diagnosis (e.g., misdiagnosis of juvenile myoclonic epilepsy)
    Failure to use first-line AEDs
    Failure to use adequate doses of AEDs
    Use of an AED that can exacerbate seizures
  Polytherapy with hepatic microsomal enzyme-inducing drugs (lower drug levels)
  Lifestyle Factors
    Sleep deprivation
    Alcohol
    Stress
Disabling Side Effects
  Improper dosing (e.g., high-dose carbamazepine twice daily)
  Failure to adjust dosing based on symptoms (e.g., with nausea, taking carbamazepine or
    valproate after meals)
  Polytherapy
  Use of sedating drugs
  Chronic use of benzodiazepines

Figure 4.1 Factors contributing to incomplete seizure control or disabling side effects.

properties of the epilepsy. It also implies that the diagnosis is secure and the treatment has been rational and thorough. Regrettably, the label *intractable* is often applied in cases in which diagnostic or treatment errors have occurred or the patient has not cooperated with the treatment plan.

Many factors can cause incomplete seizure control or disabling side effects, as listed in Fig. 4.1.

WHEN SHOULD THE DIAGNOSIS OF NONEPILEPTIC SEIZURES BE CONSIDERED?

The use of video-EEG monitoring units has increased clinicians' ability to recognize nonepileptic seizures. The numbers vary with each treatment center, but about 10–30% of patients who are referred to these centers because of medically refractory seizures have nonepileptic episodes. The most common cause of nonepileptic seizures is conversion disorder (i.e., psychogenic factors). Medication toxicity, syncope, movement disorders, and other psychiatric disorders (e.g., panic or somatization disorder, dissociative disorders, factitious disorder) are among the many other causes.

The diagnosis of nonepileptic seizures should be considered for any patient who has not responded to several AED trials and whose seizures are atypical or have ambiguous clinical features. It is difficult to overemphasize the importance of maintaining a high index of suspicion because, in many cases, these patients' seizures have been misdiagnosed and incorrectly treated for decades. Furthermore, epileptic seizures coexist with nonepileptic seizures in approximately 20% of these patients, the reported frequency being between 10–60%.[15,17–19]

WHAT FACTORS CONTRIBUTE TO INCORRECT CLASSIFICATION OF SEIZURES?

Seizures are usually classified according to clinical characteristics and EEG findings. In many cases, seizure diagnosis is based on limited information about a single episode, even though witnesses' reports about specific features of the episode and its duration may be unreliable. Similarly, EEG interpretation can be problematic. In some cases, overinterpretation of an artifact or normal hyperventilation with an admixture of different frequencies can lead to "confirmation" of a clinical impression. In other cases, primary generalized epilepsies are associated with focal or unilaterally predominant discharges, or partial epilepsies are associated with bilaterally synchronous spike-and-wave discharges.

Incorrect classification of seizure type is not uncommon. For example, juvenile myoclonic epilepsy, which represents 4–10% of all epilepsies, frequently goes undiagnosed or misdiagnosed for a decade or more.[20,21] Often, patients who have been given the diagnosis of partial epilepsy actually have juvenile myoclonic epilepsy and so never receive valproate monotherapy.[22]

SEIZURE CHARACTERISTICS

The clinical manifestations and consequences of seizures vary, even for seizures of the same type. In considering the intractability of a patient's epilepsy, the physician must take into account the physical, psychologic, and neurologic effects of the person's seizures.

Seizures that cause impairment, or loss of consciousness, or loss of motor control pose the greatest threat to the patient's physical safety and independence. They limit driving privileges and various other activities. The degree to which seizures impair consciousness and motor control varies considerably. Further, whether or not a person is aware of seizure episodes when they are happening affects how disabling the seizures are. Sometimes, awareness is absent or incomplete. For example, a person who experiences both simple and complex partial seizures may find the former more disturbing and disabling than the latter since the person is aware during simple partial seizures but unaware during complex partial seizures.

Postictal symptoms can be major problems. Confusion, lethargy, irritability, agitation, and even aggressive outbursts (most often provoked by attempts at restraint) can lead to embarrassment, problems with social relations, and loss of employment. For persons with nocturnal tonic-clonic seizures, postictal symptoms may be the predominant disability. For some, clusters of tonic-clonic or complex partial seizures are followed by serious behavioral problems, such as psychosis or depression.

WHY DO PATIENTS SOMETIMES NOT COMPLY WITH TREATMENT?

Epilepsy is a chronic disorder with intermittent symptoms, the treatment of which is often associated with adverse effects. Therefore, problems with compliance are expected and frequently occur. Many patients whose seizures are well controlled will experiment with reducing or discontinuing their medication. Most patients who are receiving long-term pharmacotherapy occasionally forget one or more doses. In some cases, they frequently forget certain doses, such as the midday dose (because they are at work or busy) or the bedtime dose (because they fall asleep first).

Approximately 20% of patients with intractable complex partial seizures have compliance problems when they first visit an epilepsy center.[23] Some patients with refractory epilepsy question whether the medications they are taking are doing anything but causing side effects. Over a period of years, they have had their doses of AEDs increased and decreased and drugs added and removed, yet their seizures don't seem to change much. Common sense might argue that their seizure frequency and intensity are unrelated to their medications. It is important that patients understand why they take medications, why they must take them regularly, and why sudden cessation or even gradual withdrawal without the supervision of a physician can be dangerous.

HOW DO LIFESTYLE AND LIVING CONDITIONS AFFECT SEIZURE CONTROL?

For many people with epilepsy, it is possible to identify factors that may provoke seizures. In one study, patients reported that forgetting to take medication (84%), emotional state (58%), sleep loss (56%), menses (54%), physiologic state (32%), specific sensory stimuli (21%), alcohol consumption (20%), and illness (11%) were the most common factors that exacerbated their epilepsy.[24] For some persons, relaxation therapy or avoidance of stressors can help reduce seizure frequency, but these measures are rarely able to control seizures fully in someone whose epilepsy is intractable to medications. For patients who believe that alcohol use or withdrawal exacerbates their seizures, intake should be stopped or carefully restricted. Catamenial seizures remain a challenge because no treatment strategy is clearly effective in reducing them except hormonal therapy that renders the woman anovulatory.[25]

In some cases, identifying and remedying adverse living situations can improve seizure control. Sleep deprivation, stress, drug abuse, and poor nutrition, for example, may contribute to seizures.

WHAT SPECIAL RESOURCES DO COMPREHENSIVE EPILEPSY CENTERS OFFER?

Patients with refractory epilepsy should be considered for referral to a comprehensive epilepsy center. Reassessment by a different set of eyes and ears may shed new light on an old problem. In many cases, video-EEG monitoring helps clarify diagnostic and therapeutic questions, although patients are usually not referred for this procedure for seizure classification. But even when the diagnosis seems certain, monitoring may disclose that the patient's attacks are not seizures or that the patient has a different seizure type than was suspected. Correct classification of seizure type and epilepsy syndrome has important therapeutic and prognostic implications.

Monitoring studies are also a critical part of the phase I evaluation for epilepsy surgery. Lateralization and localization of the seizure focus using surface and sphenoidal electrodes is possible in many cases. In some instances, these data support localizing information from other diagnostic sources (e.g., unilateral hippocampal atrophy evident on magnetic resonance imaging, poor memory as revealed by the Wada test, in which the hemisphere contralateral to the presumed focus is injected) and permit epilepsy surgery without the use of invasive electrode recordings.

Epilepsy centers also offer a variety of other resources for patients with refractory seizures: neuropsychologic evaluation, psychologic counseling, psychiatric evaluation and treatment, social work evaluation and counseling, vocational rehabilitation, and the input of expert nurse clinicians, nurse practitioners, and patient support groups.

HOW DOES UNCONTROLLED EPILEPSY AFFECT THE PATIENT?

COGNITIVE AND BEHAVIORAL PROBLEMS

Seizures that persist despite pharmacotherapy or that are controlled only by medications or dosages that produce disabling side effects often have important consequences. These effects are difficult to measure. Further, in many cases, cognitive and behavioral problems develop that also impair function and quality of life. In some cases, these problems are progressive but may be halted or partially reversed by changes in the patient's AED regimen that reduce adverse effects or seizures or by epilepsy surgery. In many epilepsy patients with cognitive and behavioral problems (Fig. 4.2), it is difficult to define clearly the relevant pathogenetic mechanisms. Psychosocial problems (e.g., stigma, dependence, loss of control over events in one's life, educational and employment difficulties, life events such as death of a loved one or loss of job), AEDs, direct effects of epileptiform discharges or seizures, effects of chronic epilepsy, effects of the underlying neurologic disorder that caused the epilepsy, and genetic and other factors must be considered. Thus the challenge posed by cognitive and behavioral problems, which contribute greatly to the disability of epilepsy, is threefold: recognition, understanding of the pathophysiology, and treatment. We often fail at recognition in particular.

MEASUREMENT OF QUALITY OF LIFE

The ability to measure quality of life is an important step towards a more meaningful and global assessment of how epilepsy affects the individual. Comprehensive quality-of-life instruments for epilepsy are now available for researchers and clinicians.[26-28] The Quality of Life in Epilepsy Inventories (QOLIE) contain questions (QOLIE-10) and scales (QOLIE-89 and QOLIE-31) that examine different aspects of quality of life, including overall quality of life, health perceptions, energy and fatigue, social function, emotional well-being, cognitive function, physical function, pain, and role limitations caused by emotional, physical, or memory problems. Additional scales pertain to epilepsy: seizure-specific health perceptions, seizure worry, attention and concentration, memory, language, working and driving limitations, social support, and social isolation.

Obtaining quality-of-life measures for persons with epilepsy can help determine what care they need and can perhaps expand the definition of intractable epilepsy. Currently, intractable epilepsy is considered "severe" or "characterized by

Cognitive Disorders	Behavioral Disorders
Attention and vigilance	Anxiety
Short-term memory	Depression
Learning	Psychosis
Naming	Obsessive-compulsive behaviors
Reading	Aggression
Arithmetic skills	Dissociative states
Spatial analysis and constructional abilities	
Judgment and reasoning	

Figure 4.2 Cognitive and behavioral problems in patients with intractable epilepsy.

frequent, intense seizures." We may discover that patients with relatively infrequent seizures other than tonic-clonic are strongly affected by their epilepsy and that the disorder, even when under good control, can adversely affect the person's self-perception, security, independence, cognitive skills, social function, and emotional well-being. Should such a person—one who has well-controlled epilepsy but experiences disabling secondary effects—be considered a medical success or someone with intractable epilepsy? We must reconsider how we define our successes and failures.

REFERENCES

1. Penry JK. Diagnosis and treatment of absence seizures. *Cleve Clin Q.* 1984;51:284–286.
2. Sato S, Dreifuss FE, Penry JK. Prognostic factors in absence seizures. *Neurology.* 1976;26:788–796.
3. Sato S, Dreifuss FE, Penry JK, *et al.* Long-term follow-up of absence seizures. *Neurology.* 1983;33:1590–1595.
4. Suzuki M, Maruyama H, Ishibashi Y, *et al.* A double-blind comparative trial of sodium dipropylace-tate and ethosuximide in children, with special emphasis on pure petit mal epilepsy. *Med Prog (Jpn).* 1972;82:470–488.
5. Sato S, White BG, Penry JK, *et al.* Valproic acid versus ethosuximide in the treatment of absence seizures. *Neurology.* 1982;32:157–163.
6. Callaghan N, O'Hare J, O'Driscoll D, *et al.* Comparative study of ethosuximide and sodium valproate in the treatment of typical absence seizures (petit mal). *Dev Med Child Neurol.* 1982;24:830–836.
7. Covanis A, Gupta AK, Jeavons PM. Sodium valproate: monotherapy and polytherapy. *Epilepsia.* 1982;23:693–720.
8. Oller–Duarella L, Sanchez ME. Evolucion de las ausencias typicas. *Rev Neurol (Barcelone).* 1981;9:81–102.
9. Schmidt D. Medical intractability in partial epilepsies. In: Luders H, ed. *Epilepsy Surgery.* New York: Raven Press; 1991:83–90.
10. Mattson RH, Cramer JA, Collins JF, *et al.* Comparison of carbamazepine, phenobarbital, phenytoin, and primidone in partial and secondarily generalized tonic-clonic seizures. *N Engl J Med.* 1985;313:145–151.
11. Mattson RH. Drug treatment of uncontrolled seizures. In: Theodore WH, ed. *Surgical Treatment of Epilepsy.* New York: Elsevier; 1992:29–35.
12. Smith DB, Mattson RH, Cramer JA, *et al.* Results of a nationwide Veterans Administration cooperative study comparing efficacy and toxicity of carbamazepine, phenobarbital, phenytoin, and primidone. *Epilepsia.* 1987;28:S50–S58.
13. Schmidt D, Richter K. Alternative single anticonvulsant drug therapy for refractory epilepsy. *Ann Neurol.* 1986;237–257.
14. Dasheiff RM, McNamara D, Dickson LV. Efficacy of second line antiepileptic drugs in the treatment of patients with medically refractory complex partial seizures. *Epilepsia.* 1986;27:140–144.
15. Dreifuss FE. Goals of surgery for epilepsy. In: Engle J Jr, ed. *Surgical Treatment of the Epilepsies.* New York: Raven Press; 1987:31–49.
16. Reynolds EH. Early treatment and prognosis of epilepsy. *Epilepsia.* 1987;28:97–106.
17. Krumholz A. Psychogenic seizures: A clinical study with follow-up data. *Neurology.* 1983;33:498–502.
18. Lesser RP. Psychogenic seizures. *Neurology.* 1986;27:823–829.

19. Lempert T, Schmidt D. Natural history and outcome of psychogenic seizures: A clinical study in 50 patients. *J Neurol.* 1990;237:35–38.
20. Janz D. The natural history of primary generalized epilepsies with sporadic myoclonias of the impulsive petit mal type. In: Lugaresi E, Pazzaglia P, Tassinari CA, eds. *Evolution and Prognosis of Epilepsies.* Bologna, Italy: Auto Gaggi; 1973:55–61.
21. Obeid T, Panayitopoulos CP. Juvenile myoclonic epilepsy: A study in Saudi Arabia. *Epilepsia.* 1988;29:280–282.
22. Vazquez B, Thacker K, Luciano D, *et al.* Juvenile myoclonic epilepsy: Misdiagnosis as partial epilepsy and coexisting psychiatric disorders. *Epilepsy.* 1992;33(suppl 3):115.
23. Schmidt D. Single drug therapy for intractable epilepsy. *J Neurol.* 1983;229:221–226.
24. Mattson RH. Emotional effects on seizure occurrence. In: Smith D, Treiman D, Trimble M, eds. *Advances in Neurology,* vol 55. New York: Raven Press; 1991:453–460.
25. Mattson RH, Cramer JA, Caldwell BV, *et al.* Treatment of seizures with medroxyprogesterone acetate: Preliminary report. *Neurology.* 1984;34:1255–1258.
26. Devinsky O, Vickrey BG, Cramer JA, *et al.* Development of the quality of life in epilepsy inventory. *Epilepsia.* 1995;36:1089–1104.
27. Vickrey BG, Hays RD, Graber J, *et al.* A health related quality of life instrument for patients evaluated for epilepsy surgery. *Med Care.* 1992;30:299–319.
28. Devinsky O, Baker G, Cramer J. Health-related quality of life scales to assess epilepsy. In: Engel J Jr, Pedley TA, eds. *Comprehensive Textbook of Epilepsy.* New York: Raven Press (in press).

CHAPTER 5

Psychosocial Aspects of Epilepsy

Patricia O. Shafer, R.N., M.N.,
and Eileen Salmanson, M.S.W, L.I.C.S.W.

WHAT IS THE PATIENT'S PERSPECTIVE ON EPILEPSY?

Interest in the psychosocial aspects of epilepsy and how they may affect the patient's quality of life is growing. Listening to persons with epilepsy and their family members is necessary to appreciate the inherent limitations, changes, and losses that may occur. Listen to what it feels like to have a seizure in public, to feel "different," to be dependent, or to take medicines daily. Listen to how it feels to arrive at the physician's office with a list of questions, only to leave with half of them unanswered or explanations not understood!

Seizures pose special problems for patients, their intimate partners, and their families. The ultimate challenge for patients and their loved ones is coping with the hidden nature and unpredictability of the disorder. Others may not appreciate or understand memory problems, cognitive problems, or the sudden anxiety, panic, or mood swings that may accompany seizures. These symptoms may be invisible to others yet can be devastating to persons with epilepsy. Seizures can often be more of a threat than an active condition. Unlike heart, lung, or liver disease, epilepsy has no consistent pattern; the disability can be transient, changeable, and, at times, unknown.[1]

The majority of persons with epilepsy have good seizure control and receive their medical care from primary care providers or general neurologists. Yet, control of seizures does not necessarily mean the absence of psychosocial difficulties. Surveys have shown that the majority of respondents were still having seizures, yet half perceived that their seizures were well controlled.[2] In addition, when members of a state epilepsy association were queried, the majority indicated that they had no specific problems when asked global questions about epilepsy. When asked specific questions, however, the majority "strongly agreed" or "somewhat agreed" that their epilepsy caused problems in such areas as transportation, housing, finances, employment, or relationships.[3] These results reaffirm the importance of listening to the patient's perspective, understanding the patient's definition of control, and asking specific questions about psychosocial concerns. This chapter will discuss

The Comprehensive Evaluation and Treatment of Epilepsy
Copyright © 1997 by Academic Press. All rights of reproduction in any form reserved.

some of the psychosocial aspects of epilepsy and the treatment strategies that clinicians may find useful in assisting patients to manage the disorder and its impact on their daily lives.

WHAT IS THE SPECTRUM OF EPILEPSY?

Epilepsy is now considered to be a disorder with onset from childhood to old age, the incidence being highest during these extremes of life.[4] The disorder is usually categorized by seizure type, severity, or epileptic syndrome. Although these categories may be helpful in understanding the medical aspects, they do not describe the disorder fully.

Epilepsy can also be described along a spectrum of categories ranging from the "uncomplicated" to "compromised" or "devastated."[5,6] The person with epilepsy may move from one category to another at different times throughout life because of changes in seizures, medications, developmental levels, or because of psychosocial factors. For example, the person may have, at one point in life, an uncomplicated course with well-controlled seizures, no medication side effects, and no significant psychosocial issues. The person may then switch jobs, a change that leads to sleep deprivation and more frequent seizures. Or the person may need to stop driving, a change that creates stress because of inaccessible transportation and financial hardship. The frequency and severity of the person's seizures may still be considered mild medically; the person's life, however, may still be compromised by the consequences of their seizures. Care should be directed at suggesting lifestyle modifications to decrease seizure triggers, providing resources to cope with new transportation and financial concerns, and helping the person manage stress. A person whose epilepsy is considered "devastating" is usually one with refractory seizures and significant psychosocial problems affecting the quality of life. These operational categories can be used easily in clinical practice to reflect the special needs and problems of people with seizures (Table 5.1).

WHAT FACTORS AFFECT A PERSON'S COPING AND ADJUSTMENT TO SEIZURES?

Coping can be thought of as balancing the demands on daily life with available resources.[7] The demands of epilepsy may be thought of as the impact of the disorder on daily life, whereas resources include the person's internal coping abilities and external supports from other people, systems, or society. Certain areas of the brain are necessary for effective coping, such as temporolimbic and hypothalamic structures. Because epilepsy and its treatment may affect these areas and their functions, one may postulate that the development and maintenance

Table 5.1

The Spectrum of Epilepsy

Operational Category	Descriptors
Uncomplicated	Seizures controlled Medicines: minimal side effects No concomitant neurologic problems Rare psychosocial and/or functional problems, usually short-lived Supports: good Treatment: usually primary care providers
Compromised	Seizures controlled; occasional "breakthrough" seizures Medicines: variable side effects No serious neurologic problems or deficits Psychosocial and/or functional problems affecting quality of life Supports: variable Treatment: medical reevaluation warranted, increased support and periodic psychosocial and educational interventions needed
Devastated	Seizures uncontrolled Medicines: polytherapy; side effects often present but tolerated Concomitant neurologic problems or deficits Psychosocial and/or functional problems affecting quality of life Supports: limited or strained Treatment: comprehensive epilepsy team for seizures, psychosocial problems, and education; frequent reevaluation needed; surgical and other alternative therapy options considered

Adapted from: Santilli N. The spectrum of epilepsy. *Clin Nurs Pract Epilepsy*. 1993;1:4–7.[6]

of effective coping strategies is directly or indirectly affected in some people with epilepsy.

External resources, such as family, friends, finances, or community supports, supply the necessary social support that is so crucial in coping with a chronic illness. When the demands exceed available resources or when resources are limited, the person's health and coping must be reevaluated. The extent or severity of demands, which may vary, may be influenced by societal reactions, feelings, and attitudes of the individual and family and by seizure and behavior variables. Many other factors can affect a person's adaptation and coping abilities, such as their knowledge and beliefs, perceived self-efficacy, goals and priorities for management, age, and developmental level.

SOCIETAL REACTIONS

Many myths and misperceptions about epilepsy persist today. The word *epilepsy* (*epilepsius*) means "a taking hold," connoting that the victim is carried off by some mysterious, supernatural power. An array of mystical medicines have been used to treat epilepsy. Some people regarded epilepsy as sacred, whereas others perceived it as a devil-like illness.[8] These primitive thoughts and misconceptions have been passed down through history. Many have been shed, but others continue to exist. A survey revealed that 66% of the general public ($N = 1000$) still believe that a person's tongue must be secured to prevent the person from swallowing it during a seizure.[9] Society still values the ability of people to conform, to display self-control, and to know when something is going to happen. Unfortunately, having seizures conflicts with these values. During seizures, people may display abnormal behaviors, which do not conform with socially accepted norms. Seizures signify a loss of control and changes occur in the body, mind, or emotions during seizures and in many facets of life between seizures. Most important, the unpredictability of seizures and the hidden nature of the disorder conflict with society's need for predictability.[10]

A patient describes what the unpredictability of seizures is like for her: "Put a gun to your head. Slowly pull the trigger. Click. 'What's that Mommy? Oh, another seizure.' Suppose you never knew the gun was loaded, whether every time that little click, that tiny discharge in your brain goes click, if you'll even come out alive" (p. 301).[11]

INDIVIDUAL REACTIONS

Societal values and reactions may affect the patient's view and love of self, but so, too, can the patient's feelings and reactions. It is normal for the person initially to experience a wide range of feelings such as denial, anger, frustration, shame, embarrassment, or even fear. These reactions may be transient and resolve as the person learns how to cope with the changes in his or her life. Yet these feelings may recur over time as the patient experiences changes over time. If these feelings are chronic or left untreated, the person may also have other emotional or behavioral responses, such as decreased self-esteem and confidence, loss of self-identity, social isolation, dependency, or impaired social skills. The patient may feel angry or rejected sometimes, leading to maladaptive, aggressive, or demanding behavior, including the blaming of others for the person's own problems.

FAMILY REACTIONS

Parental and sibling reactions are vital to the development of healthy self-esteem in the person with epilepsy. Initially, parents may deny the existence of seizures in a child with epilepsy. The longer a person is seizure-free, the more likely family members or the person will continue to deny the disorder.[12] People may manifest this denial by forgetting to take or dispense medications, because medications are the visible reminder of their epilepsy and that the person is "different." If seizures persist, denial usually disappears, often being replaced by anxiety, fear, or worry.

Out of worry and concern, parents often excuse the child with epilepsy from responsibilities or chores that the other children are asked to do, a practice that may foster resentment on the part of the siblings. Parents may also prevent their child from participating in such activities as climbing trees, swimming, or riding bikes, for fear that these activities might precipitate seizures or lead to injuries. These concerns are understandable, but safety precautions can be taken to avoid injury, such as having the child wear a helmet or having the child play with a friend instead of alone.

Guilt is another common and understandable parental reaction. Parents may blame themselves for their child's epilepsy or for their imperfect child, leading to overprotection. The child may respond by displaying learned helplessness or by adopting the "sick role," contributing to the parents' tendency to excuse the child from normal responsibilities. Guilt feelings can also lead to the opposite reaction. The person with seizures or his or her family may deny that anything has to be confronted or grieved for, or that there is any way to create some order, safety, or predictability in their lives.

Seizures can disrupt family relationships. Parents may disagree about how to treat the child, or the stress of coping with the child's seizures may distance the parents from each other. The child may sense these disruptions within the family and may become anxious or depressed, or may blame himself or herself for these problems or for the perceived loss of parental love. Siblings may feel neglected and jealous of the child with epilepsy, who may receive more attention than the other children. Siblings may also be embarrassed by the child's seizures. Unfortunately, the child with epilepsy may be left with feelings of rejection.

GRIEVING PROCESS

Health care providers must appreciate the fact that persons with epilepsy and their families need to grieve for actual or perceived losses and limitations. Being unable to control, stop, or predict seizures in spite of medical treatment may adversely affect the patient's feelings of productivity, independence, trust, and love. The patient's perceived loss of control can lead to feelings of being misunderstood or feared, as the following quote demonstrates:

> While my first seizures were more terrifying than subsequent seizures because I had no idea what was happening to me, having seizures does not become any easier with familiarity. If anything, each one is a frustrating setback: a reminder that my epilepsy is not under control, an indication that my medication dosage is not sufficient, a signal

that I must start over my "countdown" until the day I may drive again, another reason
for my family to worry about me. (p. 96)[13]

Some people with epilepsy, like those with other chronic disorders, may
engage in self-destructive behaviors, such as alcohol or drug abuse, to ease the
pain they feel because of chronic losses and limitations. In some women with
epilepsy, eating disorders may develop as they desperately attempt to gain control
of their own bodies.

Mood disorders, such as depression, are important for all health care professionals to evaluate. The incidence of suicide is four times higher in people with
epilepsy than in the general population.[11] Anxiety disorders, thought disorders,
hypomania, or bipolar disorder can coexist with epilepsy. The cause and frequency
of these disorders is still a matter of controversy, but the possibility of a disturbance
in brain function related to the epilepsy should not be overlooked. Some mood
disorders, however, occur as a reaction to having epilepsy and may be diagnosed
as adjustment disorders. It is important for persons with seizures to remember that
everyone becomes angry sometimes and has mood swings for one reason or another.
Attributing all their feelings or behavior to epilepsy can negatively affect their self-
esteem and sense of identity. They may come to view themselves as tolerated in
spite of their seizures, rather than loved and accepted with their seizure disorder.

The first step in the grieving process is for patients to accept the reality of
their losses and limitations. Inherent in that task is experiencing the pain of those
losses. Some people will try to cut the grieving process short and move on or
avoid it altogether. Or, they may isolate themselves so that they will not feel the
pain of their limitations or the fear of seizures. Family members also may be
uncomfortable with the grieving process. However, unresolved pain or anger can
easily return at a later date, exhibiting themselves in somatic or behavioral problems.

Grieving can be a lengthy process. People may become increasingly aware
of their losses over a period of months or years. Some may resent having to make
accommodations or modify their activities after receiving a diagnosis of epilepsy
or after having their seizures recur. Others may assume a helpless posture or refuse
to make necessary changes in their lifestyle or environment. They may feel as if
they are being held prisoner in a situation they cannot resolve. As a person works
through the grief, however, he or she is able to reinvest their emotional energy
into other relationships and activities.[14]

WHAT PSYCHOSOCIAL INTERVENTIONS ARE APPROPRIATE FOR PATIENTS WHOSE EPILEPSY HAS NOT BEEN CONFIRMED?

Many persons who have had one or more seizures struggle with their feelings
about epilepsy even though they may not yet know whether they truly have the

disorder. They may ask, "Do I have epilepsy? Will I need medication? May I drive? Am I the same person?" These are common questions, yet the answers will vary for each person, depending upon the number of seizures, the nature of the seizure(s), and the circumstances involved. If people question whether or not they have epilepsy, it is important to discuss their attitudes and beliefs about epilepsy and mental health issues, and what impact the diagnosis may have on their lives.

Although a single seizure is usually not diagnosed as epilepsy, a person who has had a seizure will have many of the same initial feelings and concerns as one whose epilepsy has been diagnosed. In particular, fears about seizures and of physical harm have been noted in parents and children with first seizures.[15,16] Thus, regardless of whether the person has a single seizure or many seizures, attention should be paid to the person's and the family's initial reactions, feelings, and concerns. For example, experiencing a first seizure can be particularly difficult for women who are planning to have children. Some may wish to put their plans to become pregnant on hold until the medical picture is clearer. Other patients may cope better by not embracing the idea of having epilepsy until it is clearly diagnosed. Some patients may have more difficulty coping or obtaining access to care if the terms *seizure* and *epilepsy* are not defined appropriately. Education and support tailored to the specific patient's and family's coping styles, supports, and needs are helpful.

Nonepileptic events may coexist with seizures in many patients with epilepsy. The clinician needs to explain carefully to patients the difference between epileptic and nonepileptic events. If patients are told that they are not having "real seizures," they may feel angry, distrustful, or invalidated. But the events are real regardless of the cause and must be addressed. Some patients will be relieved to learn that they may not have epilepsy. Others may be confused or disappointed that there is no medical reason that can be identified for the events. Many patients who have nonepileptic events may also have been abused physically, mentally, or sexually in the past. Or they may have experienced a traumatic event or loss. Exploring these traumatic events with patients in a psychotherapeutic setting may provide emotional relief and may reduce the frequency of the nonepileptic events.

WHAT SEIZURE VARIABLES MAY AFFECT THE PATIENTS' PSYCHOSOCIAL ADJUSTMENT?

The type, severity, and frequency of a person's seizures may affect the person's susceptibility to psychosocial problems. Although generalized tonic-clonic seizures usually raise the most fears and worries, partial seizures are usually harder to diagnose, treat, and manage. Persons with partial seizures are often given incorrect diagnoses, such as substance abuse, mental illness or retardation, or behavioral problems. Partial seizures, particularly simple partial seizures, are also often scarier for the person experiencing the seizure because of preserved awareness, perceptual distortions, experiential phenomena, or memory disturbances that may occur. These subjective perceptions about the seizure experience have been found to be more strongly related to psychologic and social adjustment than to the actual seizure type or frequency.[17]

The frequency of a person's seizures may play a role in the development or manifestation of psychosocial problems by affecting the patient's coping behaviors. Epileptiform discharges in temporolimbic structures may predispose the person to changes in behavior, either ictal or interictal. Cognitive changes may occur as a result of epileptiform discharges in areas of the brain responsible for various cognitive functions. Medication side effects, postictal disinhibition, or underlying neurologic problems may also affect a person's cognitive abilities.

The patient's emotional behavior may be affected if temporolimbic structures are involved during or between seizures. These structures are important to functions such as motivation, basic drives and instincts, and the generation and expression of feelings, memory, and learning. Memory disturbances in people with partial seizures may be related to epileptiform discharges or to the adverse effects of medications. Negative feelings, such as anxiety, fear, or a sense of impending doom, or even positive emotions can be manifestations of a seizure.

Fears of death and brain damage are common in people with epilepsy.[18] They also fear getting injured and the worsening of their seizures over time. Status epilepticus is a life-threatening condition that is especially alarming to patients. Many persons who have epilepsy never experience an episode of status, whereas others have these episodes frequently. The clinician should explore the patient's history of status and discuss the feelings and thoughts that having this condition may raise. Again, misunderstandings about seizures and fear of death may affect the person's psychologic and social adjustment more than the seizure type or frequency.[19]

WHAT IMPACT DO SEIZURES HAVE ON PATIENTS' DAILY LIVES?

The severity of a person's epilepsy depends partly on how the patient and family subjectively experience the patient's seizures. A patient-based seizure severity scale, which incorporates the patient's perspective on seizures, has been developed as an outcome measure for treatment.[19] The patient's definition of control is also necessary to determine, which may vary from the provider's or family's perspective. Many persons with epilepsy focus on control of their seizures, whereas others hope to control not only their epilepsy but all its consequences as well. The clinician should explore these different objectives early in the treatment period so that appropriate goals can be set.

The psychosocial and functional problems that people with epilepsy may encounter can be grouped into three main categories using a model of enforced dependency.[20] These categories are personal care and safety, mobility, and social relationships and community living (Fig. 5.1). For each category, the effect of seizures, medications, psychosocial concerns, and resources needs to be explored, as does the degree of dependency present.

PARENTING CONCERNS

Persons with epilepsy face additional demands when they are parents. Careful planning and extra support are essential for effective family functioning. Concerns in pregnancy may range from the effect of seizures and medications on the fetus to postpartum worries about breast feeding and safety. Safety remains a concern throughout life for parents with epilepsy, particularly those with uncontrolled seizures. Other parenting issues, such as involving a child in caring for a parent during or after a seizure or explaining seizures to a child, need to be addressed with all families.

Personal Care and Safety
General safety
First aid for seizures
Fears and feelings about seizures
Activities of daily living
Lifestyle modifications for seizure
  control and safety
Sleep, rest, and nutritional status
Home management
Financial ability to provide for self and
  family
Access to health care
Mobility
Physical deficits (permanent or
  temporary) affecting walking, sitting,
  stair climbing, traveling, exercising
Effects of medications on movement,
  coordination, balance, vision
Potential for injury and need for safety
  precautions
Ability to drive
Availability of accessible alternative
  transportation
Recreational opportunities

Social Relationships and Community Living
View of self and others
Cognitive or emotional problems affecting
  behavior
Perceived stigma
Education
Employment
Social skills
Social opportunities
Sexuality
Relationships
Housing or independent living
Community involvement

Figure 5.1 Psychosocial and functional aspects of epilepsy.

SEXUALITY AND COUPLES ISSUES

Couples may find that epilepsy in one partner interferes with sex, intimacy, and sexuality. For example, having a seizure disorder may make a person feel unattractive and undesirable because of an altered self-image. Certain antiepileptic medications may cause cosmetic problems, such as coarsened skin, darkened facial hair, or periodontal disease, that may contribute to those negative feelings. Normal behavior during sexual activities, including abnormal breathing, altered facial expression, or stiffening of the body, may mimic seizure activity, causing patients or their partners to distance themselves or avoid sexual activity. Persons with epilepsy often worry about the possibility that they will have a seizure during sex. It is essential to address the impact of epilepsy on relationships and intimacy in counseling.

WHAT TREATMENT OPTIONS EXIST FOR PSYCHOSOCIAL PROBLEMS?

HEALTH EDUCATION

Health education enables people with seizures to take charge of managing their epilepsy and their lives. Health care providers recommend treatment alternatives, yet it is up to the person with epilepsy and his or her family to use these recommendations. Encouraging the patient and family to take an active role in treatment is the first step in the educational process and can enhance treatment success. Mutual goals and expectations should be identified, and factors that may inhibit treatment assessed. Including other health care team members, such as the nurse, social worker, or psychologist, in the exploration of psychosocial variables and the patient and family's ability to manage the epilepsy is an essential part of any educational program.

Individual or group education should be offered to everyone who has epilepsy, to help patients cope with their disorder regardless of seizure control. Key content areas to include in general epilepsy education for people at different developmental phases are found in Table 5.2.

If attempts at achieving seizure control are not successful, patients and providers need to reevaluate their efforts to see if the seizures and psychosocial problems are truly refractory. Nursing and social work evaluations may be helpful to look at other factors that can affect seizure control. When questioning seizure control or treatment, however, providers must be careful not to invalidate a person's diagnosis or feelings.

Medication Management

Many factors affect the efficacy of pharmacotherapy, most of which are not under the control of providers. Appropriate drug selection, dosage, and duration of use is vital to successful therapy, but patient-controlled variables probably have a greater impact on seizure control. For example, if a person is unable to remember to take pills or to manage a complex regimen, compliance with drug therapy will be erratic and thus drug efficacy compromised. If a person is unable to afford medication or even to get to a pharmacy, financial and transportation problems must be resolved before treatment is considered a failure. Figure 5.2 lists some factors that affect the success of pharmacotherapy. These points should be assessed routinely for all people with seizures, particularly those whose seizures are in the compromised or devastated category.

Lifestyle Modifications

Triggers or precipitants of seizures, although one of the least understood aspects of epilepsy, are often easy to manage. Providers tend to regard noncompliance with therapy as the primary precipitant of seizures, followed by sleep deprivation, alcohol or drug use, and intercurrent illness. Patients, however, often cite such lifestyle variables as inactivity, exercise, irregular eating patterns, the eating of certain foods, hormonal changes, or stress, either alone or in combination, as key seizure triggers. Some providers avoid addressing the subject of triggers out of concern that patients or families will become overprotective or fearful. However, avoiding this topic encourages passivity and dependence on medications and providers. Helping patients and families to identify seizure triggers can enhance their feelings of control and responsibility. Discussing patients' lifestyles and environments with them may reveal adjustments that need to be made to minimize the risk of injury. A safety management plan may be devised that incorporates strategies for patients to prevent injury, to minimize triggers, and to enhance feelings of control.

Health care professionals can offer practical, supportive help to people in managing their epilepsy in a variety of ways. The clinician can help the patient to focus on personal strengths rather than weaknesses and then to develop a plan to enhance those strengths or to change perceived weaknesses into strengths. Easily obtainable goals and small, concrete steps can be identified. Using seizure diaries to measure the amount of change that has occurred will provide feedback to the patient and clinician and will reinforce success. These strategies may be particularly helpful for a person or family who wish to focus on the lifestyle variables that may be affecting seizure control. Although seemingly simplistic, this approach is easily replicated in any clinical situation.

Table 5.2

Educational Needs of Persons with Epilepsy at Various Stages of Development

Patient with Newly Diagnosed Epilepsy (Any Age)	Preschool Child	School-Aged Child
Who to Include in Education	1. Parents or guardians	1. Juvenile with epilepsy
1. Person with epilepsy	2. Child with epilepsy	2. Parents/guardians
2. Immediate family, including siblings or children	3. Siblings	3. Teacher
3. Extended family, especially grandparents	4. Babysitter	4. Classmates
	5. Extended family, especially grandparents	
	6. Preschool/nursery school teacher	
Topics to Be Included	1. Limit setting; what is realistic? (a) discipline; (b) safe activities	1. Review: (a) what is epilepsy? (b) taking medication; (c) making safe choices
1. What is epilepsy?	2. Explaining epilepsy to the child	2. Support systems for learning needs
2. What will this mean in my life?	3. Taking and monitoring medications	3. Instruction on how to explain to the teacher, coach, etc.: (a) first aid; (b) safety features; (c) seizure diary; (d) medication monitoring
3. Taking and monitoring medications	4. Explaining epilepsy to relatives and friends	
4. Safe living and first aid	5. Instructions on how to explain to friends and babysitters: (a) first aid; (b) making safe choices for activities; (c) seizure diary; (d) medications	4. How to tell classmates about epilepsy and first aid
5. Seizure diary		
6. Wearing/carrying medical alert		
7. Support networks available to the person and his/her family (e.g., EFA and affiliates/state agencies)		

Adolescent	College Student	Adult
Who to Include in Education	1. Person with epilepsy	1. Person with epilepsy
1. Adolescent with epilepsy	2. Roommate	2. Employer/employees
2. Parents/guardians	3. Friends	3. Friends/significant others
3. Friends	4. Dorm counselor	4. Vocational rehabilitation counselors
4. Teachers, especially the driver, education teacher, gym teacher, coaches	5. College infirmary staff	
	6. Dean of students	

Topics to Be Included

1. Talking to friends about epilepsy	1. Living on your own: (a) telling others; (b) proper eating and sleeping habits	1. Employment: (a) limitations and options; (b) prejudices, perceived stigma
2. Medical insurance	2. Taking and monitoring medication	2. Job applications and interviews: how to handle them
3. Driver's license (including driver's education teacher)	3. Support networks in college community for learning needs, self-help/support groups; EFA affiliate	3. Employment resources
4. Car insurance	4. Dating: (a) how to handle a seizure while on a date; (b) sex and seizures; (c) anticonvulsants and birth control pills	4. Talking to fellow employees about epilepsy and first aid
5. Dating: (a) how to handle a seizure while on a date; (b) sex and seizures; (c) anticonvulsants and birth control pills		5. Insurance
6. Drinking and recreational drugs		

Adult Considering Marriage	Adult with Children	Elderly Person

Who to Include in Education

1. Person with epilepsy	1. Person with epilepsy	1. Person with epilepsy
2. Prospective spouse	2. Spouse	2. Caretakers
3. In-laws	3. Children	3. Other professionals providing routine care
	4. Neighbors	
	5. Children's friends	

Topics to Be Included

1. Informing spouse	1. Parenting: how to provide safe child care	1. Safe living and first aid, with special emphasis on coordination, balance, and prevention of falls and injury
2. Sex and seizures	2. Maintaining parental responsibilities	2. Medications: (a) taking and monitoring; (b) coordination of all prescribed drugs
3. Informing in-laws	3. How and when to explain seizures to children	3. Seizure diary
4. Pregnancy, including heredity concerns	4. Safe living and first aid	
5. Parenting	5. Informing neighbors and public servants	

Adapted from: Santilli N. The patient's perspective on epilepsy. In: Lesser RP, ed. *The Diagnosis and Management of Seizure Disorders*. New York: Demos; 1991:135–150.[21]

Adequate trial of appropriate drug and dose
Acceptability of side effects
Complexity of dosing regimen
Number of pills per day
Presence of cognitive or behavioral deficits
Fears, fantasies, misbeliefs, or inadequate knowledge about medication regimens
Cost of medicines and insurance coverage
Ability to get to pharmacy
Amount of change required to take medicines as prescribed

Figure 5.2   Aspects of medication management to assess.

COUNSELING

Many persons with epilepsy, especially those with compromising or devastating courses, benefit from counseling. Helpful counseling modalities include individual and family psychotherapy using psychoanalytic or cognitive behavioral restructuring approaches. Clinical social workers or psychologists are usually the health care providers that address the psychosocial issues and help individuals, couples, and families make sense of this misunderstood condition. Social work intervention with couples provides a forum, often for the first time, to address the impact of seizures on relationships and family functioning. Helping patients and their spouses or partners feel supported, informed, and involved can lead to more adaptive coping strategies.

Relationships and Family Dynamics

Every couple and family has a certain lifestyle and structure and a change in that structure can be threatening. The unknown can elicit all kinds of fears. Assessment of individual roles within the family is necessary to understand the family dynamics. A patient's role may range from the "underachiever"—demonstrating dependence, learned helplessness, and adoption of the sick role—to the "superachiever"—demonstrating extreme independence and an unwillingness to allow seizures to stand in the way. Most people fall between these two extremes.

Underachievers often have learned the role in their own families of origin or, if the seizures develop later in life, have been unable to compensate for losses and limitations. Feelings of hopelessness and loneliness predominate, and they engage in minimal daily activities. Spouses or significant others may feel overburdened with family obligations as the "quintessential caretakers." Spouses may become overprotective of the person with epilepsy for fear of injury or seizures, yet they may also feel desperate because of their emotional and physical burden. Their goal in therapy is often to find some relief and respite for themselves.

Independent *superachievers* often deny any losses or limitations in their lives. They avoid being a burden at any cost. This behavior can lead to healthy coping, such as moving closer to public transportation and gainful employment. In its extreme, however, it may lead to detrimental behavior, such as engaging in excessive exercise, becoming exhausted, or ignoring personal needs. In this situation, spouses may feel left out of medical treatment and may be difficult to engage in therapy. They may assume a passive role in the family and wonder if they are needed.

Treatment Implications

Motivation is the single most important variable in family counseling. The social worker's goals are to foster a sense of security and trust and to help families tolerate discomfort. Areas to address include, but are not limited to, education about epilepsy, family structure and roles, communication, and cognitive and behavioral techniques for sexual concerns.

People may fear what they don't understand and family members often lack the necessary knowledge to cope with epilepsy. Clinicians who provide epilepsy education should involve family members in teaching. Therapists may then provide follow-up education to help lessen fears, identify concerns, and enhance coping strategies.

Making known one's needs and experiences can be a difficult task in a family system. Understanding each person's role and how it works in the context of the family can increase awareness and understanding between family members. Are one's needs being met? Are one's needs and experiences changing as the family progresses through different life cycles? Addressing these changes and communication barriers can improve relationships and family functioning.

TREATMENT OF SEXUALITY PROBLEMS

Sexual issues are important to address in couples therapy, because sexual behavior represents the ultimate bonding of partners. Cognitive and behavioral techniques can be particularly helpful. Simple strategies to enhance communication and intimacy are often the best, such as encouraging couples to set specific times to talk to each other or make tapes for each other to enhance listening. Alternatively, sharing written thoughts and feelings can be beneficial. Listening to music together can foster a connected feeling, can induce relaxation, and can reduce stress. Couples may need to be encouraged to explore creative therapeutic strategies such as massaging and stroking, allowing patients and their partners to feel cared for and attractive. Referring patients for treatment of medical concerns, such as impotence or lack of sexual drive, are necessary additions to psychotherapy.

STRESS MANAGEMENT

Many persons with epilepsy report that stress can precipitate seizures or diminish quality of life. They feel stress from the seizures themselves, the treatment regimen, or the effect of the disorder on daily life. An epilepsy stressor inventory has been developed to identify concerns related to seizures that are perceived as stressful to patients or families.[22] Many people respond readily to talking about their feelings and to receiving validation and practical guidance on stress management techniques. Others may benefit from structured stress management approaches, either individually or in groups. Alternatives such as relaxation exercises or tapes, meditation, biofeedback, yoga, or massage may be helpful for some people.

SUPPORT GROUPS

Support groups are a useful treatment approach for many people. Groups may be offered by institutions with specialized epilepsy services or they may be community-based epilepsy groups. Support groups provide a sense of commonality and a chance to help others that cannot be found in individual counseling. They can be a good adjunct to individual and family counseling. Learning about epilepsy and sharing concerns with others may lessen patients' fears and help them develop useful coping strategies. However, the most important benefit of support groups is the sense of empowerment, support, and validation that people experience as they share successes and losses.

WHAT PSYCHOSOCIAL ISSUES NEED TO BE ADDRESSED BEFORE AND AFTER EPILEPSY SURGERY?

PRESURGICAL PREPARATION

Surgical approaches to the treatment of epilepsy are not new. Since the Egyptians drilled holes in peoples' skulls to let out the bad spirits, surgeons have tried to develop a method of localizing the source of seizures within the brain. During the long, arduous presurgical workup, it is not uncommon for patients to experience heightened anxiety and emotionality. Committing to a presurgical workup may involve compromising other life commitments and considerable time away from family, friends, and employment. There is no guarantee that surgery will take place or that it will be successful. But for many, it is a last hope for leading a more productive and satisfying life.

Patients and couples need a setting to explore psychosocial issues associated with surgery. Often the wish for a complete cure can mask significant psychosocial problems that may not be changed by surgery alone. Bringing these issues to the foreground during the surgical workup helps the clinician assess readiness for surgery and identifies needs for further education, support, and rehabilitation.

Discussing stresses, fears, and fantasies about surgery can be a great relief to patients and spouses. They can then focus their energies on setting realistic expectations and preparing for life after surgery.

BENEFITS OF SURGERY

The effect of surgery on a patient's quality of life is less clear than the medical effects on patients' lives. Medical benefits can be measured by changes in seizure frequency, severity, or type, as well as by medication usage. Psychosocial benefits are more difficult to quantify, yet several tools to assess quality of life have been developed. Comprehensive psychiatric and psychosocial assessments can be good predictors of postoperative emotional and psychosocial functioning. Findings have suggested that a complete cessation of seizures is closely associated with major improvements in emotional and behavioral functioning.[23]

REHABILITATION AFTER SURGERY

Patients with epilepsy and their families must be counseled that the surgical procedure is only the "halfway mark" in the process. Rehabilitation must begin immediately after surgery, starting with physical recuperation and incorporating psychosocial rehabilitation of both the patient *and* family. The rehabilitation process should include self-management strategies for enhancing seizure control, activity, and safety; emotional adjustment to life without seizures or to life with continued seizures; promoting and coping with changes in independence and mobility; impact on socialization and relationships; vocational rehabilitation; and independent living and community reentry.

WHAT COMMUNITY RESOURCES AND SUPPORTS ARE AVAILABLE TO PERSONS WITH EPILEPSY AND THEIR FAMILIES?

EMPLOYMENT

One of the major problems affecting people with epilepsy is unemployment or underemployment. Potential employment problems include actual or perceived discrimination against the person with epilepsy; the perceived stigma of epilepsy; misunderstandings about epilepsy in the workplace; safety concerns; lack of job skills, experience, or education on the part of the person with epilepsy; and learning disabilities or other cognitive problems that may interfere with the person's ability to obtain a job or to perform a job well. The person with epilepsy needs to consider carefully his or her strengths and weaknesses when exploring employment options and to obtain vocational counseling from people who are knowledgeable about epilepsy.

Local epilepsy associations and the Epilepsy Foundation of America (EFA) offer health care providers, employers, and people with epilepsy specific information on employment. Individual and group counseling and job-seeking support may also be available through local or state groups. In addition, the Department of Vocational Rehabilitation in most states is a good source of employment assistance. The Americans with Disabilities Act (ADA) prohibits discrimination based solely on a disability. Employers are required to base hiring decisions on a person's ability to perform a job and to provide reasonable accommodations for people with disabilities. People with epilepsy should be informed about the ADA and its implications for their own employment. Educational materials on the ADA and epilepsy are available from the EFA.

HEALTH CARE ACCESS

Health care has increasingly become a problem for people with chronic disabilities, particularly those with preexisting conditions. People with epilepsy may experience problems obtaining or maintaining adequate health care. Counseling and advocacy resources are recommended to help people with epilepsy obtain access to care, medication coverage, and referral to epilepsy specialists when they have compromising or devastating forms of the disorder. People with epilepsy and their families should get involved in a public policy network to become aware of the issues and to advocate for their own needs.

INDEPENDENT LIVING

Resources for independent living or housing are often a concern for people with epilepsy, particularly those with uncontrolled seizures. There may be times when seizures prohibit persons with epilepsy from living alone yet it is not appropriate or possible for them to live with family members. In those situations, supported living arrangements may be desired. Resources for independent living options vary in each state. They can be found by contacting the state Department of Vocational Rehabilitation, Developmental Disability Councils, head injury programs, local epilepsy associations, or the EFA. The requirements for independent living programs vary; unfortunately, many times people with seizures are excluded from these options. Providers may help obtain housing resources by advocating for patients and educating the community.

DRIVING

Driving regulations for persons with epilepsy vary from state to state. In most states, people who have seizures are required to be seizure-free for 3–12 months before being permitted to drive. Some states still require mandatory reporting of people with seizures by physicians and other providers; however, the majority support self-report of seizures by individuals. Clinicians must educate people with epilepsy and their families about the legal restrictions, public safety concerns, and financial impact of driving with seizures. In addition, alternatives to driving and the accessibility of public transportation should be explored with each patient.

EPILEPSY FOUNDATION OF AMERICA

The EFA is a national voluntary agency for everyone who is concerned with epilepsy. EFA has a network of affiliate associations throughout the United States serving people with epilepsy at local and state levels. Services include, but are not limited to, public information and education; professional education and research; legal and advocacy information; employment, self-help, and support networks; and school alert programs. Further information about EFA or its affiliates can be obtained by calling EFA at 1-800-EFA-1000.

CONCLUSION

The majority of people with epilepsy achieve control of their seizures with medications and lead a satisfactory life. Some, however, experience a wide range of psychosocial difficulties irrespective of seizure type or frequency. It is important for providers to recognize that psychosocial problems may exist, that treatment options are available, and that treatment is necessary to prevent chronic disability. Comprehensive assessment of the psychologic and social functioning of patients and families will help identify problems and facilitate referrals to appropriate professionals or community resources. The real challenge for health care providers lies in learning to listen to patients and families and to appreciate the demands of living with epilepsy and its consequences.

REFERENCES

1. Lechtenberg R. *Epilepsy and the Family*. Cambridge, MA: Harvard University Press; 1984:1–30.
2. *Living with Epilepsy: A Quality of Life Survey*. New York: The Roper Organization; 1992:7.

3. Schachter SC, Shafer PO, Murphy W. The personal impact of seizures: Correlation with seizure frequency, employment, cost of medical care, and satisfaction with physician care. *J Epilepsy.* 1993;6:224–227.

4. Hauser WA. Seizure disorders: The changes with age. *Epilepsia.* 1992;33:S6–S14.

5. Marshall RH, Cupoli JM. Epilepsy and education: The pediatrician's expanding role. *Adv Pediatr.* 1986;33:159–180.

6. Santilli N. The spectrum of epilepsy. *Clin Nurs Pract Epilepsy.* 1993;1:4–7.

7. Carnevali D, Patrick M. *Nursing Management for the Elderly.* Philadelphia: J.B. Lippincott; 1979:7–11.

8. Nuland SB. The sacred disease. *Discover.* 1991; February: 88–90.

9. *Myths and Misperceptions about Epilepsy.* Greenwich, CT: NFO Research; 1995:25.

10. Ozuna J. Psychosocial aspects of epilepsy. *J Neurosurg Nurs.* 1979;11:242–246.

11. Spiers PA, Schomer DC, Blume HW, Mesulam MM. Temporolimbic epilepsy and behavior. In: Mesulam MM, ed. *Principles of Behavioral Neurology.* Philadelphia: F.A. Davis; 1985:289–326.

12. Lessman S. Accepting epilepsy: social and emotional issues for patients and their families. In: Black R, Hermann B, Shope J, eds. *Nursing Management of Epilepsy.* Rockville, MD: Aspen Systems; 1982:73–82.

13. Schachter SC. *Brainstorms: Epilepsy in Our Words.* New York: Raven Press; 1993:96.

14. Worden JW. Bereavement. *Semin Oncol.* 1985;12:472–475.

15. Austin JK. Concerns and fears of children with seizures. *Clin Nurs Pract Epilepsy.* 1993;1:4–7.

16. Austin JK, Oruche UM, Dunn, DW, *et al.* New onset childhood seizures: Parents' concerns and needs. *Clin Nurs Pract Epilepsy.* 1995;2:8–10.

17. Smith DF, Baker GA, Davey M, *et al.* Seizure frequency, patient-perceived seizure severity, and the psychosocial consequences of intractable epilepsy. *Epilepsy Res.* 1991;9:231–241.

18. Mittan RJ. Patients' fears of death and brain damage from seizures. *Merritt Putnam Q.* 1989;5:3–19.

19. Baker GA, Smith DF, Dewey M, *et al.* The development of a seizure severity scale as an outcome measure in epilepsy. *Epilepsy Res.* 1991;8:245–251.

20. Benoliel JQ, McCorkle R, Young K. Development of a social dependency scale. *Res Nurs Health.* 1980;3:3–10.

21. Santilli N. The patient's perspective on epilepsy. In: Lesser RP, ed. *The Diagnosis and Management of Seizure Disorders.* New York: Demos; 1991:135–150.

22. Snyder J. Revised epilepsy stressor inventory. *J Neurosci Nurs.* 1993;23:9–13.

23. Hermann BP, Wyler AR, Somes G. Preoperative psychological adjustment and surgical outcome are determinants of psychosocial status after anterior temporal lobectomy. *J Neurol Psychiatry.* 1992;55:491–495.

CHAPTER 6

Neuropsychological Assessment and Application to Temporal Lobe Epilepsy

Peter J. Hayashi, Ph.D., and Margaret O'Connor, Ph.D.

In this chapter, we discuss the neuropsychological evaluation of patients with epilepsy, and, in particular, temporal lobe epilepsy (TLE). Basic principles of neuropsychological assessment, neuropsychological aspects of TLE, and specialized neuropsychological procedures in surgical patients are reviewed. The evaluation of cognition is emphasized because other neuropsychological issues, such as quality of life, psychiatric issues, and psychosocial adjustment, are discussed elsewhere in this book.

WHAT IS NEUROPSYCHOLOGY?

Neuropsychology is a discipline that focuses on the complex relationship between the brain and behavior. Through close observation of patients and the administration of standardized tests, neuropsychologists describe and quantify the cognitive and behavioral manifestations of brain dysfunction. Modern neuropsychology was shaped by two major influences: a statistically oriented approach with roots in American psychology and a clinical–theoretical approach emphasizing careful observations of single cases, best exemplified by the Russian neuropsychologist A. R. Luria. The influences of these competing approaches remain evident: Current methods can be arranged on a continuum based on the degree to which quantitative (statistical) versus qualitative (clinical–observational) data are emphasized.

The neuropsychological methods used in the Comprehensive Epilepsy Center at Beth Israel Deaconess Medical Center are based on the Boston process approach developed by Kaplan.[1] This method focuses on the *process* whereby a person solves a given problem in addition to whether or not the problem is solved correctly. A core set of tests is administered to each patient, and supplemental tasks are used to evaluate clinical hypotheses developed during the evaluation. In this manner, the cognitive status of the patient is defined with increasing precision throughout the evaluation. Standardized tests are adapted to provide additional qualitative information while retaining the standardized procedures necessary for

The Comprehensive Evaluation and Treatment of Epilepsy
Copyright © 1997 by Academic Press. All rights of reproduction in any form reserved.

normative comparison. Both qualitative and quantitative information are thus obtained. A more detailed description of the Boston process approach can be found in Milberg *et al.*[1]

WHAT IS THE ROLE OF NEUROPSYCHOLOGY IN THE CARE OF PATIENTS WITH EPILEPSY?

Neuropsychological assessment can be useful in the diagnosis of epilepsy, in the functional assessment of patients, and in intervention. Neuropsychologists are closely involved in the care of patients for whom surgical intervention for the treatment of refractory seizures is being considered, but neuropsychological services can be an important part of the care of nonsurgical patients as well.

Historically, lesion localization has been a major use of neuropsychological investigation, and it remains an important role for neuropsychologists in the care of epilepsy patients. Additional treatment concerns include the assessment of medication effects, educational and occupational guidance, intervention for cognitive problems, and referral for additional services. Functional concerns, such as the patient's ability to manage independently, can be addressed through neuropsychological testing. Eligibility for state and federal services and disability benefits is often based on neuropsychological data. Neuropsychological data are also used to assist in the differentiation of nonelectrical (psychogenic) seizures from electrically based seizures, although clear demonstrations of efficacy are lacking.[2]

Neuropsychologists provide additional services for patients who are considering surgical resection for the treatment of intractable epilepsy. Through the intracarotid amobarbital test (IAP), neuropsychologists can determine which patients are at risk for memory and language problems as a result of surgery, which is information that permits improved patient selection and the identification of patients who require cortical mapping studies. Intraoperative cortical mapping permits the cortical representation of language, sensory, and motor functions to be discerned. This information enables the surgeon to tailor the resection and thus improves surgical outcome. These procedures (the IAP and intraoperative cortical mapping) are discussed in detail later in this chapter.

HOW DOES TEMPORAL LOBE EPILEPSY AFFECT COGNITIVE STATUS?

Changes in cognition during epileptic seizures are widely appreciated and are a defining characteristic of complex partial seizures. Interictal (between seizure) changes in cognition, behavior, and personality also occur, but there is considerable controversy about the nature, frequency, and causes of these changes. Memory difficulties are the most common cognitive complaint of patients with epilepsy.[3] Other common cognitive complaints include attention problems,[4] reduced speed of mentation,[5] language disturbances,[6] and poor academic–occupational performance.[7]

A number of seizure variables have been shown to be related to cognitive functioning in TLE. The laterality of the seizure focus, for example, is a major influence. There is considerable evidence that left temporal seizure foci are associated with verbal memory deficits and language dysfunction. Right temporal seizure disorders more often produce nonverbal memory deficits.[6,8] The role of other seizure variables (e.g., age of onset, etiology) and demographic factors (e.g., sex, handedness) have yet to be clarified. Although many of these variables are known to correlate with cognitive functioning, the critical multivariate analyses necessary to determine the variables' unique contributions have rarely been performed.[9] Two of the more frequently cited factors are seizure etiology and early age of onset. Seizures of known etiology are associated with poorer neuropsychological performance than idiopathic epilepsy (see Tartar[10] for a review), and early age of onset is associated with poorer performance.[11]

HOW DOES TEMPORAL LOBE EPILEPSY AFFECT EMOTIONAL AND PSYCHOLOGICAL STATUS?

Emotional and psychosocial disturbances have often been linked with epilepsy, but the exact nature of the relationship is the subject of much debate. A number of investigators have examined the incidence of psychopathology in relation to the presence of epilepsy, particularly TLE. Bear and Fedio[12] proposed that patients with TLE were prone to specific clusters of behaviors as a consequence of enhanced neuronal connections between cortical and limbic brain regions. This "TLE personality syndrome" included increased philosophical concerns, deepened emotionality, unusual sexual proclivities (or lack of sexual interest), hypergraphia (excessive writing), and interpersonal dependency or "viscosity."[12] A later neurophysiologic study, which demonstrated that patients with TLE have increased galvanic skin responses (GSRs) to visual stimuli, was seen as further evidence that persons who have epilepsy are prone to heightened emotionality.[13] Further distinctions between patients with left and right TLE were emphasized; patients with left TLE were seen as more ideative (i.e., religious, philosophic, and paranoid), whereas patients with right TLE were seen as more emotional. A study by Perini[14] partially upheld this typology, emphasizing increased depression and paranoia in patients with left TLE and increased emotionality in association with right TLE. However, a number of other researchers have vehemently disagreed with the Bear–Fedio personality syndrome, arguing that patients with TLE do *not* differ substantively from patients with other types of neurologic illness or from patients with other types of epilepsy (see Ref. 15 for a review). Furthermore, the psychosocial impact of TLE must be considered, because it is well known that many patients with TLE experience social isolation and stigmatization, which may lead to unusual emotional reactions.[16]

WHAT DOES COMPREHENSIVE NEUROPSYCHOLOGICAL EVALUATION ENTAIL?

Before patients undergo psychometric evaluation, they receive a thorough clinical interview, during which the examiner gathers information relevant to the complex interplay of factors that influence the patient's psychological and cognitive status. This interview includes a review of seizure characteristics, cognitive problems, emotional status, prior medical history, family history, and psychosocial adaptation. Early development and education are reviewed, because this information is necessary to interpret current findings and may indicate the presence of a long-standing lesion. Ideally, information is also obtained from family members or other informants, because often patients cannot report seizure phenomena or provide information about interictal cognitive or behavioral changes.

Neuropsychological investigation is guided by the nature of the pathology, cognitive complaints, and treatment objectives. Cognition must be sampled in sufficient breadth so that all major cognitive domains and cortical areas are tested. The evaluation of cognitive processes is organized according to major domains of attention, memory, language, visuospatial abilities, executive functions, problem solving and reasoning, and sensorimotor functions. Although these categories reflect clinical abstractions rather than fundamental principles of brain organization, the model is a clinically useful means of structuring assessment and possesses anatomic correlation. Domains are sampled widely and in sufficient detail to allow for convergent and discriminate comparisons. The method yields a profile of cognitive and behavioral strengths and weaknesses and points to any underlying neuropathology.

WHAT ARE SPECIFIC CONSIDERATIONS IN THE NEUROPSYCHOLOGICAL EVALUATION OF PATIENTS WITH TLE?

Neuropsychological assessment in our clinic is based on a flexible, hypothesis-driven approach. Assessments thus vary in emphasis and test selection. However, there are important general considerations in both the test selection and interpretation of test results.

With regard to test selection:

1. Memory evaluation is emphasized because of the epileptogenic nature of temporal lobe structures and the importance of anterior and medial temporal lobe structures in memory.

2. Functions associated with frontal brain regions (attention, judgment, reasoning, set maintenance and set-shifting abilities, and capacity for temporal order) are assessed in detail because of the possibility of frontal lobe seizures and the frequency with which temporal lobe seizures interfere with these functions.

3. Identification of lateralized dysfunction is stressed throughout the evaluation. Although localized dysfunction is occasionally noted, more often strongly localized dysfunction is absent but lateralized dysfunction can be seen across domains.

4. Psychosocial and psychological functioning are important to assess because of the frequency of psychosocial/psychological problems in patients with TLE and the possible direct relationships between epilepsy and psychological function.

With regard to the interpretation of results:

1. Early brain injury can result in atypical cortical organization, particularly with regard to language. Early left hemisphere damage may cause a shift of language to the nondominant hemisphere or atypical organization within the left hemisphere.[17] Functions associated with the right hemisphere (such as visuoperceptual abilities) may be impaired in patients with right hemisphere language, presumably because of a "crowding" effect.[18]

2. Impairment in functions associated with structures distant from the seizure focus are regularly encountered, as indicated by studies showing improvement in verbal memory (presumably mediated by the left hemisphere) after successful right temporal lobectomy.[19]

3. Neuropsychological tests require multiple cognitive operations; deficient performance on a single test is rarely of localizing value.

4. The neuropsychological presentation of epilepsy varies considerably from one patient to the next.

5. Current methods of assessing nondominant hemisphere integrity are relatively insensitive[20]; patients whose electroencephalogram (EEG) and neuropsychological data lack congruence are more likely to have right hemisphere foci.[21]

6. It is necessary to consider medication effects. Antiepileptic drugs (AEDs) have been associated with impairments in attention, memory, information processing, and motor speed.[22] These effects appear to be dose-dependent, and polypharmacy has been shown to raise the risk of cognitive impairment.[23] However, the assessment of cognitive effects of AEDs has been impeded by serious methodologic problems,[24] and earlier studies indicating potent cognitive effects may have been misleading. Later studies addressing some of the methodologic problems[22] indicate

that the effects are less severe than previously indicated, with the exception of phenobarbital, which has significant negative effects on attention, concentration, speed of mentation, and learning.[25] Except for phenobarbital, differences in the cognitive effects of AEDs appear subtle.[22]

These considerations highlight the need for comprehensive evaluation utilizing multiple convergent methods of assessment (particularly in critical areas such as memory) and interpretation of neuropsychological findings within the context of developmental, psychosocial, and other medical information.

WHAT NEUROPSYCHOLOGICAL TESTS ARE USED IN THE EVALUATION OF PATIENTS WITH EPILEPSY?

Some neuropsychologists argue for the use of epilepsy-specific tests; however, the majority of practitioners employ traditional neuropsychological tests of broader applicability.[26] Our approach emphasizes flexible, individualized assessment structured around a core of standardized instruments. Comprehensive discussions of these tests can be found in Lezak[20] and Spreen and Strauss.[27] The evaluation usually includes additional tests to investigate specific hypotheses.

GENERAL INTELLECTUAL FUNCTIONS

Tests of intelligence such as the Wechsler Adult Intelligence Scale–Revised (WAIS–R)[28] are almost always included in the neuropsychological evaluation of patients with epilepsy. The Wechsler scales have a long history in neuropsychology, are well-normed, provide a measure of overall level of adaptation, and can be used to place other specific tests in context. The WAIS–R is not a sensitive measure of lateralized dysfunction or surgery-related changes in TLE.[29,30] However, several subtests are of considerable value. For instance, the Block Design subtest is an excellent measure of constructional abilities and also provides rich qualitative data concerning problem-solving abilities. Selection of WAIS–R subtests reflects both specific questions raised during the evaluation and the examiner's preferences.

ATTENTION

Higher cognitive functions such as memory and problem solving require the patient to select and attend to relevant environmental stimuli. The person must be able to sustain concentration in the face of potentially distracting stimuli, to attend to multiple sources of information simultaneously, and to monitor the environment as well as his or her behavior. This group of variables has been referred to as the *attentional matrix*.[31] Impairment in these areas leads to a variety of clinical conditions, including states of inattentiveness, distractibility, impulsiveness, and perseveration. Attentional deficits can be due to discrete lesions, diffuse neuronal dysfunction, or both. Tests used in our clinic to assess aspects of the attentional matrix include the Digit Span and Visual Span subtests of the Wechsler Memory Scale–Revised (WMS-R),[32] Stroop Color-Word Interference Test,[27] Trail-Making Tests,[33] Controlled Oral Word Association Test,[34] Paced Auditory Serial Addition Test,[35] and Go–No Go paradigms.[36]

MEMORY

Memory evaluation of the patient with TLE is emphasized because of the critical role of temporal lobe structures in learning and memory. New learning is assessed both immediately after stimulus exposure and after a delay. Delayed recall is a more sensitive measure of temporal lobe dysfunction.[8,37] Assessments are made across modalities (auditory–visual) and material (verbal–nonverbal). When the opportunity arises, patients are tested postictally, because postictal recognition is a sensitive measure of lateralized deficit.[38]

Verbal memory is assessed by having the patient recall prose passages such as those in the Logical Memory subtest from the WMS-R[32] and supraspan word lists such as the Rey Auditory Verbal Learning Test[39] or the California Verbal Learning Test.[40] List learning appears to be more sensitive to hippocampal dysfunction than prose passage recall,[41] but both types of assessment are typically included to provide convergent validity. Complaints of memory dysfunction correlate more strongly with prose passage than word list learning performance.[42] Assessment of nonverbal memory includes the Visual Reproduction subtest of the WMS-R and the Rey or Taylor Complex Figure recall.[43,44] Recognition memory can be tested with the Warrington Recognition Memory Test.[45] This test allows comparison of visual–verbal and visual–nonverbal memory and is frequently used in epilepsy centers.[26] However, its validity as a measure of lateralized temporal lobe dysfunction in epilepsy and its sensitivity to epilepsy-related changes have yet to be demonstrated.

LANGUAGE

The comprehensiveness of the language assessment is dictated by clinical factors (e.g., a planned left hemisphere resection), historical information (e.g., a developmental learning disability), or educational and occupational concerns. Language assessments vary widely in degree of comprehensiveness and in test selection. Brief assessments of naming and vocabulary skills and screening level measures of other language functions may be performed in patients with demonstrated right TLE and left hemisphere language. At the other end of the spectrum, detailed language evaluations are indicated in patients with demonstrated language dysfunction related to the seizure disorder.

Confrontation naming, the ability to name objects on presentation, is the single most important language function in the neuropsychological assessment of patients with epilepsy because word-finding complaints are common in TLE[6] and because surgical resection can result in an aphasic syndrome characterized by word-finding problems.[46] The Boston Naming Test,[47] a test of visual naming, is the most commonly used language measure in surgical centers.[26] The test is sensitive to left hemisphere seizure disorders and to postsurgical changes.[48] Additional subtests of the Boston Diagnostic Aphasia Examination[49] or the Multilingual Aphasia Examination[34] are used when indicated. Vocabulary skills correlate well with general mental abilities, are relatively resistant to the effects of acquired brain dysfunction, and can serve as a measure of overall language integrity.[20] Vocabulary skills can be assessed in auditory or visual modalities. Various forms of the Token Test originally devised by De Renzi and Vignoli[50] provide a sensitive measure of auditory comprehension.[51] Measures of academic skills can be assessed with the Wide Range Achievement Test–Revised or similar instruments.[52,53] Dichotic listening techniques, in which information is presented to both ears simultaneously, have been used to study language lateralization. Kimura[54] found that dichotic listening performance correlated with language laterality, with superior recall of the information presented to the ear contralateral to the language-dominant hemisphere occurring. However, consistent demonstration of validity has been lacking, and procedures vary across centers.[26]

VISUOSPATIAL PERCEPTION AND CONSTRUCTIONS

Visuospatial tasks are used especially in evaluation of the right hemisphere. Tasks commonly used to assess visual perceptual abilities include the Judgment of Line Orientation Test,[55] the Facial Recognition Test,[56] the Hooper Visual Organization Test,[57] and visual cancellation tests.[36] The majority of the visuospatial tests have limited anatomic specificity: They are particularly susceptible to right posterior lesions, but lesions in other areas can interfere with performance. Single findings are difficult to interpret, and concurrence among related tests is important in the interpretation of deficient performance.

Visual construction tasks, which require perceptual, motor, and problem-solving abilities, can be disrupted by lesions in a variety of areas. Qualitative data such as location of error, type of error, and strategy are often more informative than quantitative data in determining lesion localization. Constructional ability is assessed in both copy and spontaneous drawing conditions. Often there is a dissociation between these abilities. The patient is asked to reproduce simple two-dimensional line drawings (e.g., a clock) as well as three-dimensional figures (e.g., a cube) and more complex stimuli (e.g., the Rey Osterreith figure). Spontaneous drawing is measured by asking the patient to produce figures on command (e.g., a clock or a daisy). The WAIS–R Block Design and Object Assembly subtests also provide information about constructional skills.

PROBLEM-SOLVING AND EXECUTIVE FUNCTIONS

In addition to their dominant role in attention, the frontal lobes are intimately involved in problem-solving and executive functions. Executive functions concern the person's ability to understand, monitor, and control behavior and to act in a responsible, appropriate manner. These behaviors cannot always be directly measured. It is therefore often necessary to rely on clinical observation and data from reliable informants.

Problem-solving and reasoning skills require a high degree of integrated cognitive activity, including attention, memory, and executive systems. Thus, they are vulnerable to a variety of lesions. Isolated problem-solving and reasoning deficits are indicative of damage, usually of the bilateral frontal systems. The Wisconsin Card Sorting Test[58] is the most frequently used single instrument to measure problem-solving skills.[26] Other aspects of problem-solving abilities are measured by the Similarities and Comprehension subtests of the WAIS–R,[32] the Short Category Test,[59] and the Raven Matrices,[60,61] which emphasizes nonverbal deductive reasoning.

MOTOR FUNCTIONS

The assessment of motor functions is an important part of the determination of lateralized dysfunction. Handedness is assessed using preference measures, such as the Edinburgh Handedness Inventory,[62] and performance measures. Commonly used performance tests include measures of speed (e.g., the Finger Tapping Test),[33] strength (hand dynamometer), and dexterity, which is often assessed using one of the various pegboard tests (e.g., the Grooved Pegboard Test).[63] Interpretation of performance should be based on patterns across multiple measures. The significance of left-handedness must be viewed within the context of family history.

AFFECTIVE FUNCTIONING AND PERSONALITY

Objective methods of assessing psychological adaptation, such as the Washington Psychosocial Seizure Inventory,[64] are widely used in epilepsy centers,[26] and their use is strongly recommended. Psychometric assessment of psychological functioning is most often performed using the Minnesota Multiphasic Personality Inventory (MMPI)[65] or its revised version, the MMPI-2.[66] Concerns have been raised about the appropriateness of the test for populations with neurologic problems.[67] Cautious interpretation and the need for convergent data are highly suggested. Differentiation of pseudoseizure patients from those with epilepsy on the basis of MMPI scores has been reported,[68,69] but replication efforts have been unsuccessful.[70,71] It is likely that patients with nonelectrical seizures are a diverse population with heterogeneous MMPI profiles.

WHAT ROLE DOES NEUROPSYCHOLOGY PLAY IN THE CARE OF PATIENTS WHO ARE UNDERGOING SURGICAL RESECTION?

For surgical patients, neuropsychological data may indicate lateralized or localized dysfunction, implicating that region as the seizure focus. This information may agree with EEG findings or, in the case of a discrepancy, suggest a need for further study. These data also provide a baseline against which postsurgical changes are measured. Neuropsychological data have utility, albeit limited, in predicting neuropsychological functions after surgery.[72] More important neuropsychological information on surgical outcome is obtained through the IAP, or Wada test, which consists of selective anesthetization of each cerebral hemisphere to determine its functional capacities.[73,74] The test allows determination of language laterality and improves prediction of the likelihood of postsurgical amnesia. In patients who are undergoing resection of areas likely to be involved in language functions (typically left temporal resection), areas critical to language functions can be identified through intraoperative cortical mapping.

WHAT IS THE INTRACAROTID AMOBARBITAL TEST?

For patients who will undergo surgical resection, identification of cerebral dominance for language is critical in minimizing the effects of surgery on language. The IAP was developed as a means of determining language laterality. If a patient has aphasia, amnesia, or both after sodium amytal has been injected, that suggests that the inactivated hemisphere is critical for normal speech or memory functions and that the contralateral hemisphere, by itself, is incapable of supporting these processes. Information obtained from the IAP influences decisions about the need for cortical mapping at the time of surgery as well as the extent of surgical resection.[75]

Consequently, the IAP has become an integral part of the neuropsychological evaluation of patients who are considering surgical intervention as treatment for refractory seizures. Despite widespread consensus about the clinical importance of the IAP, considerable controversy surrounds fundamental aspects of IAP design and the relevance of the test to the evaluation of specific neuropsychological processes.[76,77]

HOW IS THE INTRACAROTID AMOBARBITAL TEST ADMINISTERED?

Although the version of the IAP used at each epilepsy center varies, fundamental aspects of the test are the same at all sites. The IAP is a brief exam, typically lasting 5–10 min. It is therefore imperative that the neuropsychologist work efficiently and that the patient cooperate as fully as possible. The procedure is extensively reviewed the day before the IAP to ensure optimal performance and to gauge the patient's baseline performance on specific tasks. Immediately before the exam, the patient undergoes cerebral angiography to detect atypical vasculature. A catheter is guided radiographically into the internal carotid artery, which feeds the middle and anterior cerebral arteries, which in turn supply the lateral and mesial areas of the frontal and anterior temporal lobes. The expectation is that functions typically associated with these brain regions will be disrupted by the infusion of medication. Once the amytal is injected, the patient is observed for drug effect, which may be manifested, seconds later, by contralateral hemiplegia, facial droop, ipsilateral pupil dilation, eye gaze deviation, speech dysfunction, EEG slowing, and a number of other behavioral changes. Evaluation of language, memory, perception, and other processes then begins. Often the contralateral hemisphere is injected either the same day (approximately 45 min after completion of the first exam) or on a different day; sometimes one injection is deemed sufficient.

Language is divided into constituent processes, which are examined separately during anesthetization. These include measures of spontaneous speech, recitation of an overlearned series, naming, repetition, word comprehension, and reading. Not all language processes are disrupted simultaneously, and some (e.g., word comprehension) seem relatively impervious to the effects of the amytal injection.[78] Estimates of language dominance vary considerably. Loring et al.[76] conducted a comprehensive review of 10 different IAP studies involving large samples of patients with epilepsy. Exclusive left hemisphere dominance was reported in 57–90% of patients, whereas right hemisphere dominance was seen in 2–23% and bilateral dominance (i.e., involvement of both hemispheres in language) in 5–36%. Snyder et al.[77] attributed variations in estimates of language dominance to several factors, including the use of different criteria for determining language dominance (in particular, the practice of inferring right hemisphere dominance from preservation of low-level language skills), differences in the doses of amytal (60–200 mg), and differences in the stimuli used to assess language.

Memory testing during the IAP varies tremendously across epilepsy centers. In some programs, stimuli are presented before the amytal is injected and retrieval is assessed while the medication is effective, providing a measure of retrograde amnesia (i.e., amnesia for events that occurred before injection). Anterograde memory (i.e., new learning) is often evaluated by presenting stimuli after injection at a time when medication effects are most pronounced; recall and or recognition of this material is then tested when the effects of medication have worn off. Many types of stimuli are used for memory testing, including words, sentences, nursery rhymes, geometric figures, faces, and real objects. Factors that influence memory performance include laterality of seizure focus, timing of presentation relative to injection of amytal, nature of the stimuli (i.e., verbal vs nonverbal) in relation to the side of injection, and density of hippocampal structures on the side opposite the injection.

Researchers have consistently demonstrated that bilateral temporal lobe damage is necessary for the occurrence of amnesia.[79–81] Based on these observations, Milner et al.[82,83] proposed that amnesia during the IAP was evidence of a preexisting lesion in the contralateral hemisphere. Over time, the use of the IAP as a predictor of risk for postoperative amnesia has become a standard part of the IAP protocol. A number of investigators have shown that memory performance during the IAP predicts postsurgical memory abilities. In particular, volumetric analyses highlight an association between IAP memory deficits and magnetic resonance imaging evidence of contralateral hippocampal cell loss.[84,85] Other studies have shown material-specific memory problems during the IAP so that greater verbal memory deficits are noted after left hemisphere injection, whereas nonverbal memory problems emerge during right hemisphere injection.[86] In addition, memory deficits during the IAP are viewed as an effective way to identify seizure focus. Amnesia upon injection suggests that the contralateral hemisphere is dysfunctional.[87]

In all likelihood, the IAP will be replaced by newer and less cumbersome imaging technologies in the future. However, the current and historical relevance of this procedure should not be underestimated. For several decades IAP findings have influenced decisions about surgical intervention for the treatment of epilepsy by enhancing the identification of seizure focus and by predicting surgical outcome from both cognitive and medical perspectives. IAP investigations have greatly enriched our understanding of a variety of neuropsychological processes relevant to issues of cerebral dominance and brain–behavior relationships in general.

WHAT IS CORTICAL MAPPING?

Successful surgical intervention for the treatment of epilepsy involves the removal of epileptogenic tissue while sparing cortical brain regions critical to motor and cognitive functions. These separate and sometimes competing goals are partially achieved by means of careful evaluation of patients in the presurgical phase. At the time of surgery, the neurosurgeon has a wealth of information on each patient's cerebral functions through neurophysiologic, neuropsychological, and imaging studies. Nonetheless, surgeons in many epilepsy surgery centers rely on one more test—intraoperative cortical stimulation—as a way of delineating the boundaries of resectable brain tissue.

Cortical mapping procedures were introduced by Penfield[88,89] and were further refined by Ojemann *et al.,* who conducted numerous validation studies. Individually tailored brain maps are derived by administering small electrical currents to a variety of brain regions while the patient is awake. Localization of motor and cognitive functions is inferred by either the production or disruption of behaviors known to be associated with specific brain regions. Cortical mapping provides a way of tailoring the boundaries of the resection to each patient's brain. This procedure is particularly important because in patients with long-standing epilepsy, language and other cognitive functions are often located in anomalous brain areas; heterogeneity in the representation of these functions suggests that traditional brain models are not relevant to patients with chronic epilepsy.[90,91]

At the Beth Israel Deaconess Comprehensive Epilepsy Center, cortical stimulation studies proceed as follows: The night before surgery, the procedure is thoroughly reviewed and baseline functional skills are assessed with specific tasks to be used during intraoperative mapping. Surgery proceeds with the craniotomy, during which a fast-acting anesthetic is used. The patient is subsequently awakened and cortical stimulation commences. The surgeon administers small electrical pulses to designated brain areas in order to elicit behavioral change. The neuropsychologist is in direct contact with the patient and is not aware of the particular region being stimulated. Typically, sensory and motor functions are tested first. During the sensory part of the exam, the patient is asked whether he or she feels any unusual sensations. Often patients report feeling pain related to the craniotomy that is not of immediate consequence. The neuropsychologist probes for more discrete sensations (e.g., buzzing or tingling sensations in the face, mouth, or hand). Stimulation of prerolandic areas may result in a variety of motor changes, such as clonic movements of the mouth and hand. Alterations in behavior are described in detail for the surgeon, who labels the brain areas associated with evoked activity.

Language functions are assessed using a variety of tasks. Frequently patients are asked to recite overlearned series (e.g., the ABCs, months of the year) or to name items presented rapidly. Disrupted speech, speech hesitations, and perseverations are viewed as evidence of language localization. Naming has been described as discretely organized, whereas other language processes, such as reading, may be associated with a wider cortical network.[92] Memory is evaluated in some epilepsy centers, although this is not a routine part of the exam at the Comprehensive Epilepsy Center. Memory investigation entails the application of stimulation during encoding, consolidation, or retrieval of new information. Disruption in a specific stage of memory suggests an association with the stimulated neural region.

Clinical research studies using cortical stimulation procedures have produced some interesting and provocative findings. A consistent theme is the variable localization of functions in patients with epilepsy. Motor and sensory functions may not correspond to traditional zones (i.e., the postcentral and precentral gyri) and have been elicited in widely distributed regions.[93,94] Language studies have shown that many patients have two or more critical language zones,[95,96] the location of which may vary with sex,[91] verbal intelligence, and date of onset of seizures. Studies with bilingual patients reveal discrete language sites for different languages.[95] The clinical significance of cortical stimulation studies is underscored by a number of studies from Ojemann's laboratory. Patients who underwent cortical resections that came within 2 cm of identified language zones demonstrated transient aphasia postsurgically. Tumor patients who, by necessity, underwent resections that came within 5–7 mm of language sites were left with permanent aphasia.[97] Other research has shown that language functions are significantly altered as a result of temporal lobe resection when mapping is not used.[98]

WHAT NEUROPSYCHOLOGICAL CHANGES ARE ASSOCIATED WITH SURGERY FOR SEIZURES?

Language and memory deficits are the most common neuropsychological changes after temporal lobectomy. The presence and severity of those changes vary according to surgical and neuropsychological factors. Use of the IAP and cortical mapping reduces but does not altogether eliminate cognitive changes after temporal lobe resection.

Language dysfunction has been associated with left, but not right, temporal resection except in patients with right hemisphere or bilaterally represented language functions. However, there is controversy concerning the risk of language impairment after temporal lobectomy: some studies indicate that standard anterior temporal lobectomies with conservative resection do not produce significant language dysfunction,[99] whereas other studies suggest a significant risk.[48] Word-finding difficulty (dysnomia) is the most common clinically significant language disturbance after lobectomy,[100] and the risk of dysnomia appears to be greater in patients with late-onset seizures,[48] presumably because of diminished or absent cortical reorganization of language. As described earlier, the use of cortical mapping improves language outcome.[98]

With the use of the IAP, the risk of global amnesia after surgery is minimal, but material-specific memory deficits are relatively common and appear to be long-lasting. Diminished verbal learning capacities after left temporal lobe surgery have often been reported.[101] Declines in nonverbal memory after right temporal lobectomy are less frequently observed.[30] Improvement in memory functions associated with the hemisphere contralateral to resection has been reported.[19]

Memory outcome has been associated with several factors. Memory outcome after surgery is related to the degree of seizure control: Less decline in verbal memory has been noted in patients with good seizure control,[102] and improvements in memory functions associated with the hemisphere contralateral to resection have been seen only in seizure-free patients.[19] Patients with higher preoperative verbal memory scores show a greater decline postoperatively.[103] The age of onset of epilepsy may influence the pattern of memory changes, early-onset left temporal seizures being associated with a risk of decline in nonverbal memory.[30]

Although anterograde amnesia has been extensively studied, effects on retrograde amnesia have received little attention. Barr et al.[104] found evidence of impairment of retrograde amnesia in patients who underwent left temporal lobectomies but not in those who underwent right temporal lobectomies, and the investigators cited anecdotal evidence of retrograde amnesia in other patients. This finding has not been replicated.

HOW DOES SURGERY FOR THE TREATMENT OF EPILEPSY AFFECT THE PATIENT'S EMOTIONAL–PSYCHOLOGICAL STATE?

Most of the neuropsychological literature on the psychological impact of epilepsy surgery has focused on generic changes in various aspects of daily life, such as dependency on others, work performance, family relationships, and personal satisfaction. Extent of improvement correlates positively with amount of family support, lack of premorbid psychopathology, extent of seizure control, and lack of cognitive side effects from surgery.[105] Other studies have focused more directly on alterations in personality functions. Fedio and Martin[106] found that surgery resulted in attenuation of the behavioral features of the TLE personality syndrome. Patients who underwent left temporal lobectomy were less ideational than their presurgical counterparts, whereas patients who underwent right temporal lobectomy were less emotional than patients with right TLE. More subtle aspects of emotional processing have been examined in neurophysiologic studies, in which resection of right temporal lobe structures has been associated with hypoarousal on GSR, whereas left temporal lobe surgery has been associated with mild hyperarousal.[107] Other studies have shown hypoarousal in both right and left temporal lobe resection groups in response to emotional slides.[106]

CONCLUSION

The neuropsychological aspects of TLE differ from those of other seizure disorders in important ways, but many of the principles and procedures discussed in this chapter are applicable to the care of patients with other seizure disorders as well. It is our position that neuropsychological evaluation can and should play a significant role in the care of patients with epilepsy and that outcome is improved when neuropsychological services are utilized appropriately. Neuropsychological evaluation can be stressful for patients, particularly those who are already suffering the stigma and adaptive challenge of epilepsy. But when evaluation is done sensitively and framed within the larger picture of patients' strengths and adaptive abilities, most patients respond favorably. Indeed, many persons with epilepsy find that the resulting neuropsychological description of their cognitive deficits serves as a strong validation of problems they have complained about in the past but that have been dismissed, left untreated, or both.

REFERENCES

1. Milberg WP, Hebben N, Kaplan E. The Boston process approach to neuropsychological assessment. In: Grant I, Adams KM, eds. *Neuropsychiatric Disorders.* New York: Oxford University Press; 1986:65–86.
2. Hermann BP, Connell BE. In: Bennett TL, ed. *The Neuropsychology of Epilepsy.* New York: Plenum Press; 1992:59–70.
3. McGlone J, Wands K. Self-report of memory function in patients with TLE and temporal lobectomy. *Cortex.* 1991;27:19–28.
4. Loiseau P, Signoret JL, Strube E. Attention problems in adult epileptic patients. *Acta Neurol Scand.* 1984;69(suppl 99):31—34.
5. Bruhn P, Parsons O. Reaction time variability in epileptic and brain-damaged patients. *Cortex.* 1977;13:373–384.
6. Mayeux R, Brandt J, Rosen J, et al. Interictal memory and language impairment in TLE. *Neurology.* 1980;30:120–125.
7. Dodrill CB. Cognitive and psychosocial effects of epilepsy on adults. In: Wylie E, ed. *The Treatment of Epilepsy: Principles and Practice.* Philadelphia: Lea & Febiger; 1993:1133–1139.
8. Delaney RC, Rosen AJ, Mattson RH, et al. Memory function in focal epilepsy: A comparison of non-surgical, unilateral temporal lobe, and frontal lobe samples. *Cortex.* 1980;16:103–117.
9. Dodrill CB. Interictal cognitive aspects of epilepsy. *Epilepsia.* 1992;6:S7–S10.
10. Tartar R. Intellectual and adaptive function in epilepsy: A review of fifty years of research. *J Nerv Ment Dis.* 1972;33:763–770.
11. Bourgeois BMP, Prensky AL, Palkes HS, et al. Intelligence in epilepsy: A prospective study in children. *Ann Neurol.* 1983;14:438–444.
12. Bear DM, Fedio P. Quantitative analysis of interictal behavior in TLE. *Arch Neurol.* 1977; 34:454–467.
13. Bear D, Schenk L, Benson H. Increased autonomic response to emotional stimuli in patients with TLE. *Am J Psychiatry.* 1981;138:843–845.
14. Perini GI. Emotions and personality in complex partial seizures. *Psychother Psychosom.* 1986;45(3): 141–148.
15. Dodrill CB, Batzel LW. Interictal behavioral features of patients with epilepsy. *Epilepsia.* 1986;27:S64–S76.
16. Beit–Jones M, Kapust L. TLE: Social and psychological considerations. *Soc Work Health Care.* 1986;11:17–33.

17. Rausch R, Walsh GO. Right hemisphere language dominance in right handed epileptic patient. *Arch Neurol.* 1984;41:1077–1080.

18. Satz P, Strauss E, Hunter M, *et al*. Re-examination of the crowding hypothesis: Effects of age of onset. *Neuropsychology.* 1994;8:255–262.

19. Novelly R, Augustine EA, Mattson RH, *et al*. Selective memory improvement and impairment in temporal lobectomy for epilepsy. *Ann Neurol.* 1984;15:64–67.

20. Lezak M. *Neuropsychological Assessment, 3rd ed.* New York: Oxford University Press; 1994.

21. Williamson PD, French JA, Thadani VM, *et al*. Characteristics of medial TLE, II: Interictal and ictal scalp electroencephalography, neuropsychological testing, neuroimaging surgical results, and pathology. *Ann Neurol.* 1993;34:781–787.

22. Meador KJ, Loring DW, Huh K, *et al*. Comparative cognitive effects of anticonvulsants. *Neurology.* 1990;40:391–394.

23. Thompson PJ. Antiepileptic drugs and memory. *Epilepsia.* 1992;33:S37–S40.

24. Dodrill CB. Problems in the assessment of cognitive effects of antiepileptic drugs. *Epilepsia.* 1992;33:S29–S32.

25. Dodrill CB. Effects of antiepileptic drugs on abilities. *J Clin Psychiatry.* 1988;49(suppl):31–34.

26. Jones–Gotman M, Smith ML, Zatorre RJ. Neuropsychological testing for localizing and lateralizing the epileptogenic region. In: Engel J Jr, ed. *Surgical Treatment of the Epilepsies, 2nd ed.* New York: Raven Press; 1993:245–261.

27. Spreen O, Strauss E. *A Compendium of Neuropsychological Tests.* New York: Oxford University Press; 1991.

28. Wechsler D. *Wechsler Adult Intelligence–Revised.* New York: Psychological Corporation; 1981.

29. Bornstein RA. Verbal IQ–performance IQ discrepancies on the Wechsler Adult Intelligence Scale–Revised in patients with unilateral or bilateral cerebral dysfunction. *J Consult Clin Psychol.* 1983;51:779–780.

30. Saykin AJ, Gur RC, Sussman NM, *et al*. Memory deficits before and after temporal lobectomy: Effect of laterality and age of onset. *Brain Cogn.* 1989;9:191–200.

31. Mesulam M-M. Attention, confusional states, and neglect. In: Mesulam M-M, ed. *Principles of Behavioral Neurology.* Philadelphia: F.A. Davis; 1985.

32. Wechsler D. *Wechsler Memory Scale–Revised.* New York: Psychological Corporation; 1987.

33. Reitan RM, Wolfson D. *The Halstead–Reitan Neuropsychological Test Battery.* Tucson: Neuropsychology Press; 1985.

34. Benton AL, Hamsher KDES. *Multilingual Aphasia Examination.* Iowa City: AIA Associates; 1983.

35. Gronwall DMA. Paced auditory serial-addition task: A measure of recovery from concussion. *Percept Motor Skills.* 1977;44:367–373.

36. Weintraub S, Mesulam M-M. Mental state assessment of young and elderly adults in behavioral neurology. In: Mesulam M-M, ed. *Principles of Behavioral Neurology.* Philadelphia: F.A. Davis; 1985:71–123.

37. Làdavas E, Umiltà C, Provinciali L. Hemisphere-dependent cognitive performance in epileptic patients. *Epilepsia.* 1979;20:493–502.

38. Andrewes DB, Puce A, Bladin PF. Post-ictal recognition memory predicts laterality of temporal lobe seizure focus: Comparison with post-operative data. *Neuropsychologia.* 1990;28:957–967.

39. Rey A. L'examen clinique en psychologie. Paris: Presses Universitaires de France; 1964.

40. Delis DC, Kramer, JH, Kaplan E, et al. *California Verbal Learning Test: Adult Version.* San Antonio: Psychological Corporation; 1987.

41. Rausch R, Babb TL. Hippocampal neuron loss and memory scores before and after temporal lobe surgery for epilepsy. *Arch Neurol.* 1993;50:812–817.

42. Cavanaugh JC, Poon LW. Metamemorial predictors of memory performance in young and older adults. *Psychol Aging.* 1989;4;365–368.

43. Rey A. L'examen psychologique dans les cas d'encephalopathic traumatique. *Arch Psychol.* 1941;28:286–340.

44. Taylor LB. Localization of cerebral lesions by psychological testing. *Clin Neurosurg.* 1969; 16:269–287.

45. Warrington EK. *Recognition Memory Test.* Windsor, England: NFER–Nelson; 1984.

46. Hermann BP, Wyler AR, Somes G, *et al.* Dysnomia after left anterior temporal lobectomy without functional mapping: Frequency and correlates. *Neurosurgery.* 1994;35:52–56.

47. Kaplan E, Goodglass H, Weintraub S. *The Boston Naming Test, 2nd ed.* Philadelphia: Lea & Febiger; 1983.

48. Stafiniak P, Saykin AJ, Sperling MR, *et al.* Acute naming deficits following dominant temporal lobectomy: Prediction by age at first risk for seizures. *Neurology.* 1990;40:1509–1512.

49. Goodglass H, Kaplan E. *The Assessment of Aphasia and Related Disorders, 2nd ed.* Philadelphia: Lea & Febiger; 1978.

50. De Renzi E, Vignoli L. The Token Test: A sensitive test to detect receptive disturbances in aphasics. *Brain.* 1962;85:665–678.

51. Boller F. Dennis M. *Auditory Comprehension: Clinical and Experimental Studies with the Token Test.* New York: Academic Press; 1979.

52. Reid N. Wide Range Achievement Test (WRAT–R). 1984 Edition. *J Counseling Dev.* 1986; 64:538–539.

53. Reynolds D. Wide Range Achievement Test (WRAT–R). 1984 Edition. *J Counseling Dev.* 1986;64:540–541.

54. Kimura D. Cerebral dominance and the perception of verbal stimuli. *Can J Psychol.* 1961; 5:166–171.

55. Benton AL, Hannay HJ, Varney NR. Visual perception of line direction in patients with unilateral brain disease. *Neurology.* 1975;25:907–910.

56. Benton AL, Van Allen MW. Impairment in facial recognition in patients with cerebral disease. *Cortex.* 1986;4:344–358.

57. Hooper HE. Hooper Visual Organization Test (VOT). Los Angeles: Western Psychological Services; 1983.

58. Berg EA. A simple objective technique for measuring flexibility in thinking. *J Gen Psychol.* 1948; 39:15–22.

59. Wetzel L, Boll TJ. *Short Category Test: Booklet Format.* Los Angeles: Western Psychological Services; 1987.

60. Raven JC. *Progressive Matrices: A Perceptual Test of Intelligence: Individual Form.* London: H.K. Lewis; 1938.

61. Raven JD. *Colored Progressive Matrices Sets A, Ab, B.* London: H.K. Lewis; 1947.

62. Williams SM. Handedness inventories: Edinburgh versus Annett. *Neuropsychology.* 1991;5:43–48.

63. Matthews CG, Kløve H. *Instruction Manual for the Adult Neuropsychology Test Battery.* Madison: University of Wisconsin Medical School; 1964.

64. Dodrill CB, Batzel LW, Quiesser HR, *et al.* An objective method for assessment of psychological and social problems among epileptics. *Epilepsia.* 1980;21:123–135.

65. Graham JR. *The MMPI: A Practical Guide.* New York: Oxford University Press; 1977.

66. Butcher JN, Dahlstrom WG, Graham JR. *MMPI–2: Minnesota Multiphasic Personality Inventory–2. Manual for Administration and Scoring.* Minneapolis: University of Minnesota Press; 1989.

67. Dikmen S, Hermann BP, Wilensky AJ, *et al.* Validity of the Minnesota Multiphasic Personality Inventory (MMPI) to psychopathology in patients with epilepsy. *J Nerv Ment Dis.* 1983; 171:114–122.

68. Shaw DJ, Matthews CG. Differential MMPI performance of brain damaged vs pseudoneurologic groups. *J Clin Psychol.* 1965;21:405–408.

69. Wilkus RJ, Dodrill CB, Thompson PM. Intensive EEG monitoring and psychological studies of patients with pseudoepileptic seizures. *Epilepsia*. 1984;25:100–107.

70. Vanderzant CW, Giordani B, Berent S, *et al*. Personality of patients with pseudoseizures. *Neurology*. 1986;36:664–668.

71. Heinrichs TF, Tucker DM, Farha J, *et al*. MMPI indices in the identification of patients evidencing pseudoseizures. *Epilepsia*. 1988;29:184–187.

72. Dodrill CB, Hermann BP, Rausch R, *et al*. Neuropsychological testing for assessing prognosis following surgery for epilepsy. In: Engel J Jr, ed. *Surgical Treatment of the Epilepsies*. New York: Raven Press; 1993:263–312.

73. Wada J. A new method for the determination of the side of cerebral speech dominance: A preliminary report on the intracarotid injection of sodium amytal in man. *Igaku Seibutsugaku*. 1949;14:221–222.

74. Wada J, Rasmussen T. Intracarotid injection of sodium amytal for the lateralization of cerebral dominance: Experimental and clinical observations. *J Neurosurg*. 1960;17:266–282.

75. Petersen RC, Sharbrough FW, Jack CR. Intracarotid amobarbital testing. In: Wyllie E, ed. *The Treatment of Epilepsy: Principles and Practice*. Philadelphia: Lea & Febiger; 1993.

76. Loring DW, Meador KJ, Lee GP, *et al*. *Amobarbital Effects and Lateralized Brain Function*. New York: Springer-Verlag; 1992.

77. Snyder PJ, Novelly RA, Harris LJ. Mixed speech dominance in the intracarotid sodium amytal procedure: Validity and criteria issues. *J Clin Exp Neuropsychol*. 1990;12:629–643.

78. Hart J, Lesser RP, Fischer RS, *et al*. Dominant side intracarotid amobarbital spares comprehension of word meaning. *Arch Neurol*. 1991;48:55–58.

79. Milner B. Amnesia following operation on the temporal lobes. In: Whitty CWM, Zangwill OL, eds. *Amnesia*. London: Butterworth; 1966:109–133.

80. Parkin AJ, Leng RC. *Neuropsychology of the Amnesic Syndrome*. East Sussex, England: Lawrence Erlbaum Associates; 1993.

81. Scoville WB, Milner B. Loss of recent memory after bilateral hippocampal lesions. *J Neurol Neurosurg Psychiatry*. 1957;20:11–12.

82. Milner B, 1972. Disorders of learning and memory after temporal lobe lesions in man. *Clin Neurosurg*. 1972;19:421–446.

83. Milner B, Branch C, Rasmussen T. Study of short term memory after intracarotid injection of sodium amytal. *Trans Amer Neurol Assoc*. 1962;87:224–226.

84. Rausch R, Babb TL, Engel J, *et al*. Memory following intracarotid amobarbital injection contralateral to hippocampal damage. *Arch Neurol*. 1989;46:783–788.

85. Sass KJ. The neural substrate of memory impairment demonstrated by the intracarotid amobarbital procedure. *Arch Neurol*. 1991;48:48–52.

86. Perrine K, Gershengorn J, Brown ER, *et al*. Material specific memory in the intracarotid amobarbital procedure. *Neurology*. 1993;43:706–711.

87. Loring DW, Murro MD, Meador KM, *et al*. Wada memory testing and hippocampal volume measurements in the evaluation for temporal lobectomy. *Neurology*. 1993;43:1789–1793.

88. Penfield W, Jasper H. *Epilepsy and the Functional Anatomy of the Human brain*. Boston: Little Brown; 1954.

89. Penfield W, Roberts L. *Speech and Brain Mechanisms*. Princeton: Princeton University Press; 1959.

90. Devinsky O, Perrine K, Llinas DJ, *et al*. Anterior temporal language areas in patients with early onset TLE. *Ann Neurol*. 1993;34:727–732.

91. Ojemann GA. Functional mapping of cortical language areas. In: Devinsky O, Aleksander B, Dogali M, (eds.) *Electrical and Magnetic Stimulation of the Brain and Spinal Cord*. New York: Raven Press; 1993:155–163.

92. Ojemann GA. Brain organization for language from the perspective of electrical stimulation mapping. *Behav Brain Res* 1983;6:189–230.

93. Uematsu S, Lesser R, Fisher RS, *et al.* Motor and sensory cortex in humans: Topography studied with chronic subdural stimulation. *Neurosurgery.* 1992;31:59–71.

94. Lesser R. Extraoperative cortical functional localization in patients with epilepsy. *J Clin Neurophys.* 1987;4:27–33.

95. Ojemann GA, Whitaker HA. The bilingual brain. *Arch Neurol.* 1978;35:409–412.

96. Ojemann GA. Individual variability in cortical localization of language. *J Neurosurg.* 1979; 50:164–169.

97. Haglund MM, Berger MS, Shamseldin M, *et al.* Cortical localization of temporal lobe language sites in patients with gliomas. *Neurosurgery.* 1994;34:567–576.

98. Hermann BP, Wyler AR. Effects of anterior temporal lobectomy on language function: A controlled study. *Ann Neurol.* 1988;6:585–588.

99. Davies KG, Weeks RD. Results of cortical resection for intractable epilepsy using intraoperative corticography without chronic intracranial recording. *Br J Neurosurg.* 1995;9:7–12.

100. Heilman K, Wilder BJ, Malzone WF. Anomic aphasia following anterior temporal lobectomy. *Trans Am Neurol Assoc.* 1972;97:S65–S76.

101. Ojemann GA, Dodrill CB. Verbal memory deficits after left temporal lobectomy for epilepsy. *J Neurosurg.* 1985;62:101–107.

102. Rausch R, Crandall PH. Psychological status related to surgical control of temporal lobe seizures. *Neuropsychologia.* 1982;24:191–202.

103. Chelune G. Hippocampal adequacy versus functional reserve: Predicting memory functions following temporal lobectomy. *Arch Clin Neuropsychol.* 1995;10:413–432.

104. Barr WB, Goldberg E, Wasserstein J, *et al.* Retrograde amnesia following unilateral temporal lobectomy. *Neuropsychologia.* 1990;28:243–255.

105. Rausch R. Psychological evaluation. In: Engel J, ed. *Surgical Treatment of the Epilepsies.* New York: Raven Press; 1987:181–195.

106. Fedio P, Martin A. Ideative–emotive behavioral characteristics of patients following left or right temporal lobectomy. *Epilepsia.* 1983;24:S117–S130.

107. Davidson RA, Fedio P, Smith BD, *et al.* Lateralized mediation of arousal and habituation: Differential bilateral electrodermal activity in unilateral temporal lobectomy patients. *Neuropsychologia.* 1992:30:1053–1063.

Psychiatric Considerations in Patients with Epilepsy

Jacob C. Holzer, M.D., and David M. Bear, M.D.

This chapter focuses on psychiatric and behavioral aspects of epilepsy. Rather than presenting an exhaustive review of the subject, the chapter provides a framework for the evaluation and management of frequently encountered psychiatric symptoms and behavioral problems. The chapter addresses major clinical topics related to behaviors during the ictal and interictal periods, seizure subtypes, psychiatric syndromes, diagnosis, and treatment interventions.

DOES EPILEPSY PREDISPOSE PATIENTS TO PARTICULAR PSYCHIATRIC ILLNESSES OR BEHAVIORAL PROBLEMS?

This question reflects a long-standing controversy about the relationship between behavioral conditions and epilepsy. Until the early 20th century, seizures were often considered a form of psychopathology and persons with epilepsy were routinely confined to asylums. Perhaps in response to this extreme and inaccurate belief, some advocates for the epilepsy community have argued that there is no increased risk of psychiatric or behavioral symptoms among epilepsy patients.

Data from a wealth of clinical and research studies now support a balanced position, concluding that patients with epilepsy are at higher risk for certain types of psychiatric and behavioral symptoms. It is important to note that, despite this increased risk, severe psychiatric illness or maladaptive behavior do not develop in the majority of patients with epilepsy. However, it is critical for the clinician who takes care of patients with epilepsy to consider the possibility of epilepsy-related psychiatric symptoms for which specialized evaluation and treatment may be helpful.

Conditions with increased prevalence among epilepsy patients include depression and other mood disorders, psychosis, dissociative disorders, anxiety and panic states, interictal behavior changes, and temper-related problems. In some patients with epilepsy, remarkable creative behaviors develop that should not be classified as psychopathologic.

The Comprehensive Evaluation and Treatment of Epilepsy
Copyright © 1997 by Academic Press. All rights of reproduction in any form reserved.

Although evidence supports a neurobiologic basis for many of the conditions mentioned, other predisposing factors deserve consideration in any patient with epilepsy. One important factor is the environment the patient experienced while growing up. For example, parental overprotectiveness or overrestrictiveness, the necessity for the child to adhere to specific medication regimens or to take regular blood tests, limitations on the child's participation in sports or other activities, and repeated seizures might have restricted the child's social development and intellectual functioning. Neurologic disorders may result in other symptoms in addition to seizures, causing added difficulty in negotiating everyday life. Social stigma, restrictions, and biases have an adverse effect on self-esteem and limit involvement in academics, employment, and social activities. These factors may play a major role in the development or severity of psychiatric complications in some patients.

ARE THERE DIFFERENCES BETWEEN ICTAL AND INTERICTAL BEHAVIORAL SYMPTOMS?

Distinguishing the ictal from the interictal period is critical to understanding the various psychiatric and behavioral symptoms that can develop in epilepsy. The peri-ictal period includes the preictal, ictal, and postictal stages, distinct from prolonged interictal periods when patients are not experiencing seizures. Peri-ictal psychiatric and behavioral phenomena tend to occur in the setting of partial seizures emanating from the temporal or frontal lobes. Simple partial seizures, by definition, do not produce a loss of or alteration in consciousness, and transient psychiatric or behavioral symptoms may be the simple partial seizure's most prominent manifestation. By contrast, sustained (interictal) changes in disposition, mood, or thought occur in some patients with long-standing temporal lobe epilepsy (TLE).

HOW DO PSYCHIATRIC OR BEHAVIORAL SYMPTOMS VARY IN PATIENTS WITH SIMPLE AS OPPOSED TO COMPLEX PARTIAL SEIZURES?

Focal seizures can produce a wide range of symptoms and experiences, including motor, sensory, autonomic, psychiatric, behavioral, and cognitive events. Maintenance of consciousness during the event separates a simple partial from a complex partial seizure. In a simple partial seizure, the seizure focus is localized, the patient maintains awareness of the environment and memory for events occurring during the seizure, and specific ictal symptoms can be experienced and recalled for the duration of the spell. In contrast, a complex partial seizure involves an alteration in consciousness, the patient being unable to interact with and respond

Table 7.1

Comparison of Simple and Complex Partial Seizures

Feature	Simple Partial	Complex Partial
Duration	Brief (30–120 s)	Similar to simple partial
Consciousness	Preserved	Impaired
Postictal phase	Absent	Present
Automatisms	Often absent	Present
Ictal EEG changes	Low yield[a] (approximately 25% of patients)	High yield (approximately 90% of patients)
Interictal abnormal EEGs	Unclear	Frequent
Increased prolactin	Often absent	Absent or present

[a] Especially for pure sensory symptoms.

Motor Symptoms
  Focal clonic motor activity
  Speech arrest
Somatosensory and Special Sensory Hallucinations
  Somatosensory
  Unformed visual
  Unformed auditory
  Olfactory
  Gustatory
  Vertiginous-vestibular
Autonomic Symptoms
  Abdominal sensation, nausea
  Chest sensation
  Unusual head sensation
  Hypersalivation
  Diaphoresis
  Cold or warm sensation
  Pallor or flushing
  Piloerection
  Palpitations

Psychic–Cognitive Symptoms
  Fear
  Anxiety
  Depression
  Anger
  Irritability
  Pleasure
  Dysphasia
  Déja vu
  Jamais vu
  Derealization
  Depersonalization
  Dissociation
  Speeding of thoughts
  Incoherence of thoughts
  Distortion of time
  Distortion of body image
  Distortion of odor intensity or quality
  Distortion of sound intensity or quality
  Distortion of color intensity or quality
  Distortion of size or shape
  Distortion of distance
  Formed visual hallucinations
  Formed auditory hallucinations
  Mystical experience

Figure 7.1   Partial-seizure phenomena. (Adapted with permission from Devinsky O, Vasquez B. Behavioral changes associated with epilepsy. *Neurol Clin.* 1993;11:127–149.[1])

to the environment or to recall ongoing events. Consciousness may be assessed during a patient's seizure by asking the patient to respond to a simple motor command or to remember a word. Some clinical differences between simple and complex partial seizures are summarized in Table 7.1.

Peri-ictal symptoms experienced during partial seizure activity may include motor symptoms, such as focal clonic activity; somatosensory phenomena, including unformed hallucinations and perceptual changes; autonomic changes, including diaphoresis and palpitations; abdominal sensations; and emotional–cognitive symptoms, including fear, anxiety, depression, anger, dissociation, déja vu, environmental distortions, and formed hallucinations. Figure 7.1 lists symptoms of partial seizures.

ARE THERE DIFFERENCES BETWEEN TEMPORAL AND FRONTAL LOBE EPILEPSIES?

Subtle clinical distinctions between seizures originating in temporal versus frontal brain regions have been identified. Complex partial seizures originating in temporal regions (TLE) have an average duration of 1–3 min, are followed by a distinct post-ictal period of confusion, and occur three to five times per month on average. Automatisms (stereotypic movements) tend to involve the face and upper extremities more than the lower extremities. Patients with frontal lobe epilepsy (FLE) also experience impaired consciousness and automatisms during seizures, although motor automatisms may involve the lower extremities more frequently. The average seizure frequency in patients with FLE is approximately 10 per day; the seizures often occur in clusters, each lasting an average of one-half minute with little or no postictal confusion. Peri-ictal behavioral presentations in FLE may suggest a loss of the ability to regulate behavior according to social norms; symptoms can include shouting, cursing, laughing, and sexually provocative behaviors. The presentation may initially be confused with psychogenic nonepileptic seizures (hereafter referred to as nonepileptic seizures). Table 7.2 summarizes some of the clinical differences between TLE and FLE.

Table 7.2

Differences between Temporal Lobe Epilepsy (TLE) and Frontal Lobe Epilepsy (FLE)

Feature	TLE	FLE
Duration	1–3 min	Approximately 1/2 min
Frequency	3–5 times/month	Approximately 10/day
Automatisms	Face, upper extremities > lower extremities	Lower extremities > face, upper extremities
Clusters of seizures	No	Yes
Postictal confusion	Yes	± Postictal confusion
Peri-ictal behavioral symptoms	Sometimes	Frequently

Despite statistical differences between the presentations of TLE and FLE, differentiation in an individual case is not always possible. Limbic association areas in the anterior temporal and orbitofrontal regions are the anatomic substrate for the expression of psychiatric and behavioral symptoms during seizure activity. Because of rich interconnections between these regions and the greater sensitivity to seizure activity in limbic structures, seizures beginning in either the temporal or frontal regions can spread to involve both regions, therefore blurring any clinical distinctions.

WHY IS DEPRESSION A SERIOUS COMPLICATION OF EPILEPSY?

Depression, a prevalent condition in epilepsy, should be considered a serious problem because of its association with increased morbidity and potential for self-injury or suicide. An important tool in understanding the variety of depressive syndromes in epilepsy is the timing of the mood symptoms in relation to the ictus.

Preictal depression can have its onset hours to days before a seizure and is often ameliorated by a generalized convulsion. This phenomenon has been well documented in studies utilizing rating scales for depression and associated symptoms before and after seizures.

Fear and depression are the two most common mood auras in simple partial seizures. During the ictal phase, the mood change occurs suddenly and is not related to an environmental event or precipitant. Depression may extend beyond the seizure as a result of continuing subclinical seizure activity, altered neurochemistry, or psychologic associations to the depressive aura. The type of mood experienced, such as shame or embarrassment versus fear, may reflect underlying neurobiologic changes activated by a seizure focus.

Ictal crying (dacrystic seizures) occurs rarely, despite the prevalence of unpleasant or dysphoric mood auras. Ictal laughing (gelastic seizures) occurs more commonly, yet the experience of euphoria during an ictus (a "Dostoyevskian seizure") is extremely rare. The divergence may represent an uncoupling of emotional experience from the expression of affect during the ictal phase.

During the postictal phase, depression is a common yet often overlooked event, possibly obscured by cognitive impairments such as confusion, disorientation, or anterograde amnesia. Depression during this period can last from days to weeks.

Depression during the interictal phase is perhaps the most common psychiatric association in epilepsy and presents a unique treatment challenge. Although there is significant support for a neurologic basis for this phenomenon, other etiologies need to be considered, including psychosocial and pharmacologic factors. Interictal behavior changes, described later, may contribute to social isolation and the development of a complex depressive syndrome.

Treatment of ictal-related depression depends to a great extent on seizure control. Two commonly used antiepileptic drugs are carbamazepine and valproic acid, both of which tend to cause fewer cognitive and psychiatric side effects than phenobarbital, primidone, or phenytoin. Patients with sustained episodes of interictal depression may benefit from antidepressant medications. Despite the concern that particular antidepressants will compromise seizure control, this is rarely the case in clinical practice. Specific antidepressant treatment interventions are described later in the chapter.

WHAT TYPES OF PSYCHOSIS MAY DEVELOP IN PATIENTS WITH EPILEPSY?

A number of factors can contribute to the development of psychotic symptoms in persons with epilepsy. During the peri-ictal phase, seizure activity can result in cognitive, affective, and psychosensory disturbances, which may be perceived as psychotic. Memory distortions can include the sense of having had a particular experience before (déja vu) or the absence of an appropriate sense of familiarity (jamais vu), either of which may be perceived by the patient as disordered thinking. Forced thinking (a sudden intrusive thought) and thought blocking (a sudden interruption in thought) may be experienced. Illusions and formed and unformed hallucinations in different modalities (visual, auditory, olfactory, etc.) are other peri-ictal symptoms that may occur. Anger, irritability, paranoia, and affective or anxiety symptoms may all contribute to a patient's sense that his or her thoughts are "crazy." The patient may experience acute confusion during the peri-ictal period, and some complex automatisms may be perceived by others as manifestations of psychosis.

Interictal psychosis can develop as a schizophrenia-like state or can be associated with an affective disorder. The schizophrenia-like psychosis of epilepsy, which is believed to affect 10–30% of patients with long-standing complex partial seizures, has been associated primarily with TLE. Although this type of psychiatric presentation may appear similar to idiopathic schizophrenia, important distinctions can be made between the two conditions. Schizophrenia-like states in epilepsy include a more reactive affect than the restricted affect found in schizophrenia, more obsessional traits, an absence of psychosis in the patient's family, an absence of schizoid traits premorbidly, and a psychosis marked by ideas of reference, paranoid delusions, and hallucinations.

Psychosis may be associated with toxic-metabolic effects of antiepileptic medications, the use of other medications, medication withdrawal, and antiepileptic medication-induced folate deficiency. Other causes of psychosis include substance use and withdrawal and primary psychiatric conditions such as brief reactive psychosis.

The treatment approach to psychosis in epilepsy depends on the etiology of the symptoms and whether the psychosis is the sustained interictal type. Symptoms limited to the peri-ictal period may respond to antiepileptic drug treatment without the addition of an antipsychotic medication, whereas a schizophrenia-like syndrome during the interictal period requires both antiepileptic and antipsychotic medications. Although controversial, some reports have indicated that overaggressive antiepileptic treatment aimed at maximizing blood levels of medications, minimizing seizure symptoms, and "normalizing" the electroencephalogram (EEG) have resulted in an exacerbation of psychosis and other psychiatric symptoms. Theories about mechanisms remain unproved but include an antagonism between seizures and psychosis, toxic effects of antiepileptic medications, folate deficiency, and effects on the reticular formation.

WHAT OTHER PSYCHIATRIC SYMPTOMS MAY DEVELOP IN EPILEPSY?

Anxiety is an important and common condition associated with epilepsy and can have various causes. In addition to the direct anxiety produced by a seizure during the ictal phase, anxiety symptoms can develop during the postictal and interictal periods. Seizures can produce autonomic effects resulting in symptoms that mimic anxiety or panic, including increased heart rate, increased blood pressure, and flushing. In patients with epilepsy, anxiety may also develop as a response to anticipating a seizure, which could result in the development of secondary phobia. Certain medications (such as stimulants), medication withdrawal from barbiturates or benzodiazepines, and alcohol and substance abuse may also result in anxiety states. Various medical conditions, including thyroid disease, asthma, hypoglycemia, and adrenal dysfunction, may also produce anxiety. In summary, the clinician should consider all these potential causes when evaluating a patient with epilepsy in whom an anxiety condition has developed.

Fear during the ictal phase is a common affective symptom during partial seizures. The intensity can vary from slight nervousness to extreme horror and panic. The ictal fear reaction is usually of abrupt onset and brief duration (approximately 1/2–2 min), whereas an idiopathic panic attack may build up more gradually and last longer. During the postictal phase, anxiety or fear, like prolonged postictal depression, may persist for hours or even days. Antiepileptic drug therapy is the primary treatment for these postictal symptoms.

Anxiety conditions, such as generalized anxiety and panic disorder, are more prevalent in the epilepsy population than in persons who do not have epilepsy. The management of interictal anxiety conditions is similar to that of idiopathic anxiety and may include pharmacologic trials of anxiolytic and antidepressant medications and behavioral therapy, in addition to the use of antiepileptic medications.

Dissociative experiences, in which the patient's sense of identity and memory are disturbed, are another important class of symptoms that may develop during a partial seizure. Dissociative symptoms that may occur during a seizure include depersonalization, derealization, autoscopy (looking at one's body from outside), and multiple personalities. These symptoms tend to be limited to the peri-ictal phase; prolonged symptoms during the postictal phase may be a result of postictal confusion or psychosis.

HAVE SPECIFIC BEHAVIORS BEEN DESCRIBED DURING THE INTERICTAL PERIOD IN PATIENTS WITH TLE?

In many patients with epilepsy, interictal changes in personality do not develop; however, in some patients, a syndromic pattern of behaviors has been observed. *Behavioral change* is a more appropriate description than behavioral disorder, because some of the behaviors are not maladaptive or pathologic. This section will review behavioral changes described in the interictal period. These changes are summarized in Figure 7.2.

Some of the difficulty in studying behavioral and cognitive changes during the interictal period results from multiple variables that may be associated with epilepsy. These include structural brain lesions that may produce both behavioral symptoms and seizures (e.g., vascular lesions, tumors, scars), the use of antiepileptic medications, and psychosocial effects (including isolation, stigmatization, dependence, inability to drive).

Obsessiveness
Viscosity
Emotionality
Hypergraphia
Circumstantiality
Paranoia
Depression
Aggression
Anger
Dependence
Increased Religious Concerns
Increased Philosophic and Moral Concerns
Altered Sexual Interest

Figure 7.2   Interictal behavioral changes in TLE. (Adapted with permission from Devinsky O, Vazquez B. Behavioral changes associated with epilepsy. *Neurol Clin.* 1993;11:127–149.[1])

A distinct interictal behavioral syndrome associated with TLE was first described in the English literature over 20 years ago. The clinical features include altered sexual interests, religiosity, viscosity, and hypergraphia. Altered sexuality usually takes the form of hyposexuality. This symptom occurs in approximately half of TLE patients. A confounding variable may be the effect of antiepileptic medication on sexual functioning. However, hyposexuality has been reported to improve after adequate antiepileptic medication treatment or temporal lobectomy. Rarely, hypersexuality or other altered sexual behaviors may develop.

Increased religious beliefs and a heightened concern for morality have been highlighted in the literature. Viscosity, another frequently described finding, refers to an interpersonal style marked by increased verbalization, circumstantiality, and difficulty shifting topics in conversation. It has been suggested that subtle interictal language impairment may play a role in the development of viscosity, although a tendency to develop intense personal relationships (social cohesiveness) may be more critical. Hypergraphia (extensive writing) refers to an increase in the volume of written material a patient produces and a preoccupation with details within the content. Religious and moral themes tend to predominate.

ARE TEMPER PROBLEMS OR AGGRESSION ASSOCIATED WITH TLE?

Overt aggressive behaviors occur in a minority of epileptic patients. It is useful to distinguish between peri-ictal and interictal temper problems. Aggressive behavior during the ictal phase tends to be a rare event, and when it does occur, the aggressive behaviors are often unintended and secondary to stereotyped movements. Other signs and symptoms of seizure activity may be present, and electrophysiologic abnormalities may be captured during EEG monitoring.

During the postictal period, aggression occurs most frequently as an aspect of a postictal confusional state. Patients may be more likely to exhibit aggressive behavior if attempts are made to approach or restrain them. In some cases, postictal irritability, pain, or depression may result in an outburst of hostile behavior. As is true of ictal aggression, the behavior tends to be brief and is not directed toward particular persons.

Interictal aggressive behavior in patients with TLE typically develops in the context of other interictal behavior changes, especially a deepening of emotional valence and heightened moral or religious concerns that may fuel indignant feelings. In general, such a pattern of behavior will follow the development of epilepsy rather than precede it. Aggressive behavior may be more common in patients who were subjected to an early disruptive family life or physical abuse, or in patients who have histories of fire setting, animal torture, conduct disorder, or substance abuse. Patients with interictal aggression tend to be distinguishable from those with

Ictal Phase
  Rare, usually unintended or nondirected, related to stereotyped movements
  Other signs or symptoms of seizures may be present, including EEG abnormalities
Postictal Phase
  Present as part of postictal confusion, irritability, depression, or pain
  Tends to be brief, nondirected
  May intensify if the patient is approached or restrained
Interictal Phase
  Tends to occur as a component of other interictal behavioral changes
  Follows rather than precedes the onset of epilepsy
  Patient tends to take responsibility for his or her actions, espouse moral or religious
    convictions; may express remorse about the consequences of his or her actions

Figure 7.3   Typical features of aggression in TLE.

antisocial personality disorders, because the former typically assume responsibility for their actions, espouse moral or religious convictions, and feel sincere remorse about the consequences of their aggressive behavior. The neurobiology of interictal aggression may involve pathologic activation of the amygdaloid complex. Figure 7.3 summarizes some of the clinical features of aggression in TLE.

CAN EPILEPSY CONTRIBUTE TO CREATIVE BEHAVIOR?

The interictal behavioral changes previously described may, in some persons, result in a heightened, more productive level of functioning. Traits such as hypergraphia with attention to detail, a heightened sense of morality and religiosity, a sense of personal destiny, and a deepening of emotions may set the foundation for artistic creativity, political achievements, or military or religious leadership. People thought to have had TLE include Alexander, Caesar, Mohammed, Napoleon, Dostoyevsky, and Van Gogh. Although these famous persons were obviously exceptional, it is not uncommon for patients with TLE to produce written material, art, poetry, and other works that are creative and valued. This is in itself remarkable, considering the risk factors found in some patients with epilepsy, such as cognitive impairment, frequent seizure activity, comorbid neurologic impairment, and social restrictions.

HOW DO PHYSICIANS DISTINGUISH PSYCHOGENIC NONEPILEPTIC SEIZURES FROM TRUE EPILEPTIC SEIZURES?

Differentiating pseudoepileptic seizures from true epileptic seizures can be a challenging process (see Chapter 9). For seizures to be identified as psychogenic, data must be drawn from a number of sources, including clinical evaluations, EEG readings, and other diagnostic data (e.g., endocrine measures, therapeutic responses). It is important to note that psychogenic nonepileptic seizures and epileptic seizures are not mutually exclusive—a significant percentage of epilepsy patients experience psychogenic nonepileptic seizures at some point, and patients with psychogenic nonepileptic seizures can have significant neurologic illness. Although the distinction between these two states may be blurred, certain clinical features of each can help differentiate them.

In comparison to epileptic seizures, the following pattern may be more typical of psychogenic nonepileptic seizures. The onset may be gradual and the duration of the seizure prolonged. If movements are present, they may be uncoordinated, flailing, or struggling. The absence of movements, however, may indicate either psychogenic nonepileptic seizures or partial epileptic seizures with sensory symptoms and altered consciousness. Biting, which is atypical, tends to involve the arms or other body areas more than the tongue. Bladder and bowel incontinence and self-injury tend to be rare. During the peri-ictal phase, consciousness may be preserved, and postictal confusion may be absent. Verbal intervention and suggestion, initiating and ending the seizure, also suggest a psychogenic nonepileptic seizure.

The EEG can be useful in situations in which, during the seizure, epileptiform activity is present. A normal or nonepileptiform EEG may suggest a psychogenic nonepileptic seizure, but can also occur with a simple partial seizure undetected by surface leads. However, a normal EEG during a seizure in which the patient is displaying generalized motor movements would not be expected in a true epileptic seizure; this normal EEG may indicate a psychogenic nonepileptic seizure. The interictal EEG is not useful in making the distinction because it may be normal or abnormal in either case. Maneuvers aimed at stimulating seizures (e.g., use of a strobe light, hyperventilation) may not result in a clinical or diagnostic change in psychogenic nonepileptic seizures, in contrast to epileptic seizures. In some cases of epileptic seizures (generalized, complex partial), the prolactin level may be higher during the immediate postictal phase than at baseline, whereas after a psychogenic nonepileptic seizure or a simple partial seizure, the prolactin level should be at baseline. The patient's response to medication interventions may not help in making a distinction between an epileptic and a psychogenic nonepileptic seizure. However, tapering antiepileptic medications should not change the frequency of psychogenic nonepileptic seizures but may exacerbate epileptic seizures.

WHAT CONSTITUTES AN APPROPRIATE EVALUATION FOR THE EPILEPSY PATIENT WITH PSYCHIATRIC SYMPTOMS?

A thorough diagnostic evaluation will include careful psychiatric, neurologic, and medical examinations of the patient. It is usually helpful to have others (family, friends, etc.) provide collateral information. A clinical history is a crucial part of the evaluation. Patient demographic information should include marital status, handedness, ethnicity, religion, occupation, and language. The family history includes a description of immediate family members and home environment; the extended family history should include information on neurologic and psychiatric conditions. The perinatal history (if available) and early developmental history include information on early medical and neurologic problems, behavioral problems, and the course of developmental milestones. The educational history provides information on the highest grade the patient achieved; academic, social, and athletic abilities; and any difficulties in these areas, such as the need for special classes. The sexual history elicits information on the age of first contact, significant relationships, any unwanted sexual contacts, and any high-risk behaviors. The legal history provides information on any criminal behaviors, arrests and convictions, aggressive or assaultive behavior, and other legal difficulties. The history of military service includes information on combat exposure, achievements, any difficulties or disciplinary actions, and type of discharge. The occupational history provides information on jobs held and frequency of job changes, achievements and difficulties at work, and relationships with co-workers.

A critical part of the history is a thorough review of past and current substance use, including frequency, amount, effects, and related complications or problems (such as legal or medical complications). Substances to inquire about include tobacco, caffeine, alcohol, marijuana, cocaine, stimulants, depressants, hallucinogens, prescription medications, over-the-counter medications, and intravenous drugs.

The psychiatric history includes outpatient evaluations and treatment, inpatient hospitalizations, past medications and other treatments, and any suicidal and homicidal ideation or suicide attempts. A thorough neurologic and medical history, including current use of medications, is another critical component of the evaluation.

Each patient should receive a complete physical and neurologic examination. The mental status exam should include an assessment of current mood state and associated symptoms, thought content, thought process, perceptual problems, and suicidal and homicidal ideation, along with an evaluation of cognitive functions, including simple and complex attention, memory, language, visuospatial perception, and insight–judgment and other aspects of executive cognitive functioning. Laboratory and other diagnostic evaluations will depend in part on the type of clinical presentation. Common laboratory tests may include chemistries (e.g., electrolytes, renal functions, liver functions, glucose), blood counts, thyroid function tests, nutritional status, and specific tests for systemic illness. Structural and functional imaging studies, EEG recordings, and neuropsychologic testing will usually be indicated as part of a comprehensive evaluation. Other specific diagnostic tests will depend on the clinical situation but may include toxic screens, evaluations

---

Demographic Information   Marital status, handedness, ethnicity, religion, occupation, language

Family History   Description of immediate family; neurologic and psychiatric history of extended family

Perinatal and Early Developmental History

Educational History   Academic achievement, social and athletic skills, difficulties, special classes

Sexual History   Age of first contact, significant relationships, history of unwanted contacts, high-risk behaviors

Legal History   Criminal or aggressive behavior, other legal difficulties

Military Service History   Combat exposure, achievements or difficulties, type of discharge

Occupational History   Jobs, achievements or difficulties, relationships with co-workers

Substance Abuse History   Past and current use of caffeine, tobacco, over-the-counter and prescription drugs, and other substances

Psychiatric History   Outpatient and inpatient treatments, medication trials, suicidal or homicidal behavior

Medical and Neurologic Histories
Physical, Elementary Neurologic Exams

Mental Status and Cognitive Exams   Includes assessment of: (1) Current mood state and associated symptoms, thought content and process, perceptual symptoms, suicidal or homicidal ideation; and (2) attention, memory, language, visuospatial functions, and executive cognitive functions

Laboratory and Neurodiagnostic Evaluation   As indicated

Figure 7.4   Components of a neuropsychiatric evaluation in epilepsy.

for heavy metals, other neuroendocrine studies, evaluations for sexually transmitted diseases (including the human immunodeficiency virus), and cerebrospinal fluid analysis. The spectrum of laboratory and diagnostic studies appropriate to evaluate psychiatric and behavioral symptoms in medically and neurologically ill patients is broad, and the reader is referred to the text by Stoudemire and Fogel[2] for more detailed information on appropriate diagnostic studies. Figure 7.4 lists the components of a neuropsychiatric evaluation in epilepsy.

WHICH PSYCHOTROPIC MEDICATIONS MAY BE HELPFUL FOR PATIENTS WITH EPILEPSY?

Different types of psychotropic medications are available for treating psychiatric and behavioral symptoms in epilepsy patients, although some agents may adversely affect seizure control. Therefore, psychotropic agents need to be used with caution in patients with epilepsy. This section will address clinical indications for and side effects of these agents. A detailed discussion of the pharmacology of these drugs is beyond the scope of this chapter but is available in many standard pharmacology textbooks.

Antipsychotic medications are indicated for psychotic symptoms that extend beyond the ictal phase. As previously reviewed, these symptoms may include hallucinations, delusions, ideas of reference, and disorganized thought processes that approach a schizophrenia-like psychotic state. Other indications for antipsychotics include psychotic symptoms in the context of affective symptoms (such as depression or mania) and disorganized thought processes (such as those that may occur in delirium). These presentations should be differentiated from peri-ictal psychotic symptoms, for which the primary treatment should not be antipsychotics but antiepileptic medication. Additionally, other etiologies of psychoses in epilepsy (antiepileptic drug toxicity or withdrawal, folate deficiency, etc.) require a specific treatment approach.

Available antipsychotic medications are all essentially equal in efficacy, but they differ significantly in their side effect profiles. They can potentially exacerbate seizures in epileptic patients, although the various agents differ in this respect. The medications that carry the highest risk of exacerbating seizures include chlorpromazine and clozapine—these medications should generally be avoided in epilepsy patients. Molindone and fluphenazine appear to carry a lower risk of exacerbating seizures and are relatively safer to use. The side effects of antipsychotics depend on their potency and chemical class but include sedation, anticholinergic effects, and extrapyramidal symptoms.

Antidepressant medications are indicated for a variety of sustained mood disorders, including depression and anxiety states (such as panic disorder). Like antipsychotics, antidepressant medications should not be used to treat psychiatric symptoms limited to the immediate peri-ictal period but rather to treat sustained symptoms (such as prolonged postictal depression and interictal psychiatric symptoms). A wide range of antidepressant medications are available. They are divided into several classes, including tricyclic antidepressants, serotonin-reuptake inhibitors, atypical antidepressants, and monoamine oxidase inhibitors (MAOIs). Medications with a higher potential for inducing seizure activity include maprotiline, amitriptyline, nortriptyline, and clomipramine. Relatively safer antidepressants for the epilepsy population include desipramine, doxepin, and MAOIs. Some newer antidepressants (such as fluoxetine, paroxetine, and sertraline) may also be relatively safe but can influence antiepileptic drug levels. In some cases, use of an antidepressant may improve seizure control, possibly by treating symptoms related to the depression such as disturbed sleep and appetite. MAOIs may have anticonvulsant properties and can be a useful antidepressant medication in this population, although the clinician must be aware of potential drug and food interactions before prescribing MAOIs.

Mood-stabilizing medications (such as lithium carbonate, carbamazepine, and valproic acid) are indicated for periods of elevated mood and associated symptoms that may be consistent with "mania" during the interictal phase. For bipolar disorder, defined as a history of at least one episode of mania with or without a history of episodes of depression, lithium is the best-established mood-stabilizing medication; lithium, however, is associated with cognitive symptoms in some patients and has desynchronizing effects on the EEG. Lithium carbonate has been associated with increased seizure activity or behavioral deterioration in some patients. Carbamazepine and valproic acid have been used extensively in nonepileptic bipolar patients with success, and either one may be a more appropriate first choice in epileptic patients with bipolar mood symptoms.

IN ADDITION TO MEDICATION, WHAT PSYCHIATRIC INTERVENTIONS CAN BE HELPFUL FOR EPILEPSY PATIENTS?

Appropriate psychiatric interventions depend on a thorough diagnostic evaluation of the patient. As stressed earlier, psychiatric and behavioral problems in epilepsy may result from a variety of factors, which need to be identified before appropriate treatment can be given. Symptoms may be the result of an underlying medical condition that is causing both seizures and psychiatric disturbance; toxic-metabolic effects of medications or other substances; personal, social, or familial factors related or unrelated to the epilepsy; or the location of the seizure focus and the effect of the seizure activity, which may be producing the peri-ictal and interictal disturbances already reviewed. Identifying which factors may be operational in a patient with epilepsy is critical.

Psychotherapy (in one of the many forms available) may be an appropriate treatment intervention for some patients with identified problems, such as conflicts, adjustment problems, losses, emotionally traumatic experiences in the past, and persistent functional difficulties (e.g., in social or work situations). This modality is not appropriate as primary treatment for ictal symptoms (e.g., prolonged postictal depression) or interictal behavioral changes.

Behavioral therapy entails developing a strategy aimed at reducing or changing an unwanted symptom or behavior. It works well for some psychiatric conditions (such as obsessive–compulsive disorder) but is not appropriate for others (such as psychotic symptoms in acute schizophrenia). Behavioral therapy requires a significant amount of motivation on the part of the patient. Its use in patients with epilepsy depends on identifying specific behaviors or problems that might be reduced behaviorally.

Electroconvulsive therapy (ECT) is a well-accepted treatment for major depression, usually when the symptoms are refractory to medications. One contraindication to ECT is increased intracranial pressure. In patients with epilepsy, ECT may be an appropriate treatment intervention for refractory depression or mania. One effect of ECT is a temporary increase in the seizure threshold, which commonly results in the need for a higher stimulus intensity during the course of ECT.

A complicating factor in the epileptic patient is the need to reduce antiepileptic medication blood levels during the course of ECT, with the risk of exacerbating the underlying seizure disorder. Despite this, ECT can be a useful treatment modality in some patients with severe psychiatric symptoms refractory to other treatments.

WHAT EFFECT DOES EPILEPSY SURGERY HAVE ON PSYCHIATRIC SYMPTOMS?

Patients may be considered for temporal lobectomy if their seizures are medication-refractory, if their symptoms significantly interfere with the ability to lead a productive life, and if a resectable seizure focus is identified. The primary effect of surgery is a reduction in the severity and frequency of seizure activity in the majority of patients who undergo the procedure. Positive outcomes for some patients include increased productivity and an improvement in social functioning and cognition. Associated peri-ictal psychiatric symptoms, such as depression, fear, anxiety, and psychotic symptoms, may also improve as seizure activity is reduced. A decrease in the number or dosage of antiepileptic medications may also result in improvement in psychiatric and cognitive symptoms.

Although surgery may reduce certain ictal and medication-related symptoms, it can cause other clinical problems, such as decreased mobility and pain in the immediate postoperative period and psychiatric effects from certain postoperative medications, such as steroids. Depression is a common postoperative complication that can persist for several months after surgery. Interictal behavioral symptoms, as described earlier, often do not change with surgery. Patients with a schizophrenia-like interictal psychosis may worsen after surgery; therefore, surgery is not recommended for these patients.

WHAT EFFECTS DO ANTIEPILEPTIC MEDICATIONS HAVE ON PSYCHIATRIC SYMPTOMS IN EPILEPSY?

A growing number of antiepileptic medications are now available, each with differing indications and side effect profiles. These medications are reviewed in detail elsewhere in this text; this chapter will focus on antiepileptic medication effects relevant to psychiatry.

As a rule, carbamazepine and valproic acid are two antiepileptic medications useful for treating epilepsy associated with psychiatric or behavioral symptoms. Both medications are effective against partial seizures and have less impact on cognition than barbiturates. In addition, both medications have been extensively used with success in patients who have affective disorders or impulse control problems but not epilepsy. Carbamazepine is indicated for the treatment of partial and generalized seizures. Side effects can include nausea, ataxia, sedation, dyskinesias, and dystonias. Rare but serious hematologic complications can develop. Valproic acid is indicated for generalized epilepsy but is also effective in the treatment of partial and secondarily generalized tonic-clonic seizures. Side effects include gastrointestinal symptoms, sedation, and tremor, along with rare but serious hematologic and hepatic complications. Both of these medications have interactions that affect the availability of other antiepileptic and psychotropic medications when used concurrently. Benzodiazepines have antiepileptic properties and may be useful in treating psychiatric and behavioral symptoms linked to fear, anxiety, and panic.

Among frequently prescribed antiepileptic drugs, phenobarbital has negative effects on cognitive functioning, producing sedation, diminished attention, poor short-term memory, and impaired impulse control. Especially in patients with preexisting cognitive disorders, these effects may result in an exacerbation of psychiatric symptoms.

REFERENCES

1. Devinsky O, Vazquez B. Behavioral changes associated with epilepsy. *Neurol Clin*. 1993;11:127–149.
2. Stoudemire A, Fogel BS. *Psychiatric Care of the Medical Patient*. New York: Oxford University Press; 1993.

SELECTED READINGS

Cummings JL. Epilepsy: Ictal and interictal behavioral alterations. In: *Clinical Neuropsychiatry*. Boston: Allyn & Bacon; 1985:95–116.

Devinsky O, Bear D. Varieties of aggressive behavior in temporal lobe epilepsy. *Am J Psychiatry*. 1984;141:651–656.

Holzer J, Bear D. Epilepsy and psychosis. *Harvard Mental Health Lett*. 1993;9:5–6.

Smith DB, Treiman DM, Trimble MR. Neurobehavioral problems in epilepsy. In: *Advances in Neurology, Vol. 55*. New York: Raven Press; 1991.

Tisher P, Holzer J, Greenberg M, *et al*. Psychiatric presentations of epilepsy. *Harvard Rev Psychiatry*. 1993;1:219–228.

Waxman SG, Geschwind N. The interictal behavior syndrome in temporal lobe epilepsy. *Arch Gen Psychiatry*. 1975;32:1580–1586.

CHAPTER 8

Status Epilepticus

Frank W. Drislane, M.D.

Fortunately, most epileptic seizures stop within minutes. A patient who has continuous seizures or does not recover between recurrent seizures that are "so frequently repeated or so prolonged as to create a fixed and lasting condition"[1] is considered to have status epilepticus (SE). Clinical and experimental data indicate that seizure activity for 30 min is a reasonable criterion for use of the term, at least for recurrent seizures. SE has been recognized for centuries, but until the last few decades the term has been applied primarily to generalized convulsive seizures. Just as there are many types of epileptic seizures, there are many forms of SE. The simplest classification is that of convulsive or nonconvulsive status epilepticus, but a description of syndromes based on partial (focal) or generalized onset of seizures provides more insight into pathophysiology and clinical management (Table 8.1).

WHAT IS GENERALIZED CONVULSIVE STATUS EPILEPTICUS AND WHAT CAUSES IT?

Generalized convulsive status epilepticus (GCSE) is the most dramatic, most dangerous, and best studied type of SE. It is potentially life-threatening but also treatable, so it is important for the clinician to have an appreciation for its etiology, electrophysiology and pathophysiology, course, and consequences. Having a plan for medical management and pharmacotherapy is crucial.

Convulsive SE is readily recognizable. It may start with focal or complex partial seizures but often begins with a generalized convulsion. Convulsions recur, most lasting only a minute or so, along with intervals of persistent unresponsiveness. Each convulsion may begin with several seconds of a tonic phase with tensing of extensor muscles and forced expiration, followed by a clonic phase with gradually slowing clonic movements. Both phases usually involve bilateral and symmetric movements, although there may be a focal onset with head or eye deviation, even without unilateral limb movement. Consciousness is impaired, at least from the time of tonic seizures. Less often, convulsions are continuous. In this case clonic movements eventually diminish, often being replaced by repetitive jerking movements of the eyes, eyelids, or facial muscles alone or sometimes with intermittent

The Comprehensive Evaluation and Treatment of Epilepsy
Copyright © 1997 by Academic Press. All rights of reproduction in any form reserved.

Table 8.1

Types of Status Epilepticus

Type	Comments
Generalized	
Generalized tonic-clonic	"Grand mal"; may be secondarily generalized from a focus
Absence	"Petit mal"; "spike-wave stupor"
Myoclonic	May be primary or secondary
Tonic	Pediatric; often with Lennox–Gastaut syndrome
Atonic, akinetic	Pediatric; often with Lennox–Gastaut syndrome
Clonic	Infants
Partial (focal) onset	
Simple partial	Motor: epilepsia partialis continua
	Sensory (rare or rarely diagnosed)
	Autonomic (rare or rarely diagnosed)
	Psychic (fear, emotional content)
	Aphasic
Complex partial	Includes impairment of consciousness
Special types	
Neonatal–pediatric	Includes electrographic SE of sleep, infantile spasms
"Subtle" status	

limb jerking. These signs constitute "subtle" SE and imply continuing epileptic brain activity with a "decoupling" of electrical and motor systems.

The incidence of convulsive SE is usually estimated to be about 60,000 cases each year in the United States (probably over half of them in children), but population-based surveys suggest that it may occur several times as often.[2,3] The incidence of other forms of SE is less well documented.

Convulsive SE is not a disease itself but is rather a serious manifestation of some underlying disorder. Table 8.2 lists several causes of SE and is an amalgamation of many studies. No morbidity or mortality figure is worth reporting without a precise description of the population studied. Causes of convulsive SE vary tremendously; for example, alcohol and drug-related SE are generally more frequent in studies from urban hospitals.[4] Causes or precipitants of convulsive SE are also different in patients with known epilepsy than in those with acute, new illness. Table 8.2 focuses on adult cases. Congenital abnormalities and infection increase in importance in children.

Often, there is an interaction between acute systemic illness and earlier neurologic disease, including epilepsy and other earlier neurologic insults.[5] A history of epilepsy is often assumed, but in actuality about two-thirds of SE cases occur in patients who have not had previous seizures. About 1% of patients with epilepsy will have an episode of SE in a given year. Anticonvulsant withdrawal is often

Table 8.2

Causes of Status Epilepticus

Factor	Patients (%)[a]
Anticonvulsant withdrawal	25
Alcohol withdrawal	25
Cerebrovascular: including stroke, anoxia, hemorrhage	22
Metabolic: acute encephalopathy (e.g., hypoglycemia, systemic infection)	22
Trauma	15
Drug toxicity	15
CNS infection	12
Tumor	8
Congenital lesion	8
Prior epilepsy	33
Idiopathic	30

[a] Total of percentages exceeds 100% because of multiple causes (e.g., a patient with a congenital lesion and chronic epilepsy with anticonvulsant withdrawal or infection).

assumed in patients with epilepsy, although this may be less frequent than presumed.[6] Physician-changed regimens may cause withdrawal seizures as often as patient noncompliance. Infections may have a role in epileptogenicity, but several antibiotics can also precipitate seizures and alter anticonvulsant metabolism. New anticonvulsants may alter metabolism and lead to subtherapeutic or toxic levels of prior medications.

The epidemiology of convulsive SE has several clinical implications. First, there is usually an identifiable cause, and this should be sought. Trauma, new or prior vascular disease, metabolic derangements, drug toxicity (due to prescribed or "recreational" drugs), and infection not only help to explain the SE but often determine the subsequent course; the cause must be found for the SE to be treated appropriately. Alcohol abuse and benzodiazepine withdrawal are common contributors.[7,8] Second, there is often more than one cause or precipitant; medication withdrawal, infection, or sleep deprivation may add to an earlier illness and precipitate convulsive SE. In some series, up to 50% of patients have either an infection or a recent medication change. Conversely, even in acute illness, convulsive SE occurs more often in people with prior neurologic deficits. Third, despite the many known causes of SE, it can be the first sign of neurologic disease, especially in children, in whom up to 10% of initial seizures, particularly febrile seizures, may be SE.

WHAT COMPLICATIONS CAN OCCUR WITH CONVULSIVE STATUS EPILEPTICUS?

Convulsive SE can cause numerous complications (Table 8.3).[9,10] Autonomic changes, which can be severe, include hypertension, tachycardia, arrhythmias, diaphoresis, hyperthermia, and vomiting. Many changes are caused by increased circulating catecholamines. Hyperthermia may result from excessive convulsive muscle contractions as well as from hypothalamic effects. The electrocardiogram (ECG) may show conduction abnormalities or ischemic patterns.[11] Autonomic dysfunction and cardiac arrhythmias may explain much of the mortality of SE and some other unexplained sudden death in epilepsy patients.

Blood flow and cerebral metabolism are elevated in early SE but decline eventually, and the excessive metabolism of discharging neurons may outstrip the oxygen and glucose supply.[12] As seizures continue, autoregulation may break down and contribute to cerebral edema, particularly in children. Many physiologic changes of early SE appear to reverse after about 30 min, with subsequent hypotension, hypoxemia, hypoglycemia, and increasing acidosis and hyperkalemia. There

Table 8.3

Complications of Status Epilepticus

Classification	Complications
Systemic sequelae:	
Cardiac	Hypertension, tachycardia (reversing after 30 min), arrhythmias, cardiac arrest
Pulmonary	Apnea, respiratory failure, hypoxia, neurogenic pulmonary edema, aspiration pneumonia
Autonomic	Fever, sweating, hypersecretion (including tracheobronchial), vomiting
Metabolic	Hyperkalemia, hyperglycemia then hypoglycemia, volume depletion, venous stasis, possible thrombosis
Endocrine	Increased prolactin and cortisol
Other	Leukocytosis, cerebrospinal fluid pleocytosis, vertebral and other fractures, physical injury, rhabdomyolysis, renal failure, disseminated intravascular coagulation
Cerebral	Neuronal damage similar to that of hypoxia, hyperthermia: cortical layers 3 and 5, cerebellum, and hippocampus Cerebral edema, raised intracranial pressure Cortical vein thrombosis
Neurologic sequelae:	Increased seizure frequency, recurrent status epilepticus Decreased cognitive funtion (controversial) Drug effects, increased exposure to anticonvulsants

is a progressive loss of inhibitory γ-aminobutyric acid (GABA) receptors during SE, which may help to determine this critical period at which SE becomes more refractory to treatment and more dangerous physiologically. Hypotension and bradycardia may be worsened further by anticonvulsants and other medications. Cardiac arrhythmias may be precipitated by lactic acidosis and elevated catecholamines. Hypotension or volume depletion may complicate medical and metabolic disorders or lead to venous stasis and even cerebral venous thrombosis.

Status epilepticus prompts cortisol and prolactin release, although prolactin may become exhausted and return to normal levels in prolonged SE. Leukocytosis and spinal fluid pleocytosis may occur,[9,13] but these problems should not be attributed to the SE itself until infection or some other cause of inflammation has been excluded. Aspiration pneumonia is common if airway protection is not assured. Respiratory failure is probably more often due to medications than to SE itself.

Status epilepticus may cause subsequent intellectual impairment,[14] but studies suggesting that this is the case have generally been retrospective and have usually included only subjects who have had prolonged SE, who have had prior substantial neurologic and intellectual impairment, and who were taking several anticonvulsants. SE may worsen chronic epilepsy.

Abundant experimental animal evidence indicates that convulsive SE (whether induced by electrical stimulation, kainic acid, or lithium and pilocarpine) leads to neuronal damage caused directly by the neuronal epileptic activity.[12,15–16] The cellular activity of SE releases excitatory amino acids, which are, in turn, neurotoxic in excessive amounts. Hippocampal damage[17] and a subsequent recurrent seizure disorder are among the consequences. Systemic factors, however, especially hypotension, respiratory failure, and hypoxia, worsen the prognosis and contribute to cerebral damage. Repetitive electrical stimulation produces SE after approximately 30 min—the same time at which human homeostasis appears to deteriorate during convulsive SE.[14,18] Thus, both clinical and experimental data implicate 30 min as a critical time before which convulsive status should be interrupted if damage is to be avoided. Experimental data using electrical stimulation-induced SE also suggest that phenobarbital is far more effective than phenytoin at breaking this SE. These effects are more difficult to substantiate in humans, but pyramidal cell loss in the hippocampus has been identified after SE in humans.[17]

Patients may also exhibit an orderly sequence of electroencephalogram (EEG) changes in SE: discrete seizures, then merging seizures, then seizures interrupted by flat periods, and finally, periodic discharges.[19] Clinical convulsions abate as the EEG progresses. Patients in later EEG stages have seizures that are particularly refractory to the usual anticonvulsants, and these patients have a worsened prognosis. This fact suggests that EEG evidence of SE warrants aggressive treatment as the sign of continuing and damaging SE, even without motor phenomena. The EEG can show whether comatose patients are in a postictal state or are still having seizures.

Despite the many complications, the underlying disease is the most important prognostic factor in GCSE. Mortality has declined in recent decades and should be below 2% from the SE *itself* with reasonable treatment. Mortality due to the condition causing GCSE may be substantially higher, often about 30%. Anoxia, stroke, drug toxicity, advanced age, central nervous system (CNS) infection, and severe metabolic derangements portend a worse outcome.[4] The presence of more than one medical complication, especially cardiac arrhythmias, hypotension, kidney or liver failure, and intracranial hypertension, also predicts a worsened outcome. The prognostic gravity of tumors and head injury varies with the series. SE due to alcohol abuse or drug withdrawal has a better outcome. SE lasting longer than 1 h is associated with 10 times the mortality of briefer episodes of SE.[20] Systemic complications, such as hypotension, and delayed effective treatment also worsen outcome. Patients whose SE does not respond to initial treatment with one or two anticonvulsants (patients with "refractory" SE) have a worse prognosis.

It has become increasingly clear that SE in patients with prior epilepsy and SE in those with a new diagnosis are almost different conditions. Patients who have had prior epilepsy or whose SE has been precipitated by withdrawal from an anticonvulsant or another medication fare far better. The reason may be earlier detection and diagnosis, partial treatment from earlier anticonvulsants, or the absence of acute severe insults that worsen the prognosis in other patients. Children also fare far better than adults; older patients are often prey to underlying illnesses with a higher associated morbidity and mortality.[21]

Clinical lessons also emerge from pathophysiologic and prognostic studies of convulsive SE. First, the longer the duration of SE, the more refractory it becomes and the more neuronal damage occurs. Second, although systemic factors, including hypotension, hypoxia, and acidosis, may add to the neurologic complications, some damage appears to accrue from the epileptic neural activity itself. Persistent EEG discharges generally indicate the need for treatment, so an EEG is necessary when a patient's convulsions have ended and the patient has not awakened. Third, clinical and experimental data suggest that 30 min of convulsive SE is a critical duration in neurologic function and probably in prognosis. This figure is far less certain in other, particularly nonconvulsive, forms of SE.

WHAT ARE THE OTHER TYPES OF STATUS EPILEPTICUS?

Convulsive SE is rarely difficult to diagnose. Other forms of SE may be less obvious, and they may be mistaken for other causes of altered mental status or movement disorders. The management of other forms of SE is often similar, though less urgent, than the management of convulsive SE. The other forms can be divided into generalized seizures and those with a partial or focal onset. This chapter covers generalized forms of SE and those without convulsions (some general and some of potential focal onset).

ABSENCE (PETIT MAL) STATUS EPILEPTICUS

The terminology related to absence SE is confusing, including such descriptions as "spike-wave stupor" and "epileptic twilight states." Absence SE implies generalized epileptiform EEG discharges (Fig. 8.1). Because of the difficulty of detection, it is hard to know how often absence status occurs. It may occur one-fourth as often as convulsive SE. It typically affects patients with prior primary generalized (inherited) epilepsy, but patients may be otherwise healthy and seizure-free and may have been off medication for years. When the disorder occurs in an older person with a remote history of epilepsy and no recent treatment, it may appear to the office physician to be merely confusion or limited responsiveness caused by an infection or other systemic illness. Older patients have a higher incidence of de novo absence SE than younger ones. Metabolic and pharmacologic precipitants exist, particularly benzodiazepine withdrawal in the elderly.[22] Persistent epileptic unresponsiveness with generalized EEG discharges also explains some persistent coma after generalized convulsions.[23]

Onset may be sudden or gradual. Patients may be awake, walking and talking, although they are often confused. Motor activity may be preserved but clumsy.[24,25] There is occasionally some blinking or myoclonus. Absence SE can persist for days or weeks without being recognized. A history of epilepsy is suggestive. It is entirely possible that most cases are missed, but the diagnosis can be readily confirmed by EEG. Some EEGs show generalized 3-Hz epileptiform discharges. Some may be secondarily generalized from a focus.

Especially in younger patients with primary generalized epilepsies, benzodiazepine therapy is often successful rapidly. Valproic acid may be more efficacious in preventing recurrences. Most patients return to normal, although recurrence of absence SE is relatively common. In older patients and those whose SE has a less certain cause, the response to anticonvulsant therapy can be delayed. The typical absence status of patients with prior epilepsy is not thought to be life-threatening, but occasionally episodes end with a generalized convulsion. Absence SE is probably the most benign type of SE in terms of potential neuropathophysiologic consequences and may warrant less aggressive treatment than other forms of SE.

MYOCLONIC STATUS EPILEPTICUS

Myoclonic status epilepticus (MSE) also occurs in several forms. The most severe form, which is virtually always fatal, occurs after anoxia. Persistent myoclonus

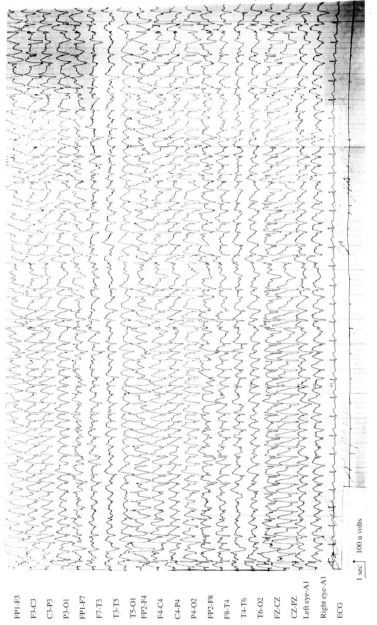

FP1-F3
F3-C3
C3-P3
P3-O1
FP1-F7
F7-T3
T3-T5
T5-O1
FP2-F4
F4-C4
C4-P4
P4-O2
FP2-F8
F8-T4
T4-T6
T6-O2
FZ-CZ
CZ-PZ
Left eye-A1
Right eye-A1
ECG

1 sec | 100 u volts

Figure 8.1 EEG of a 33-year-old woman with a history of epilepsy, now ambulatory and speaking, but confused at the time of office visit; approximately 3-Hz generalized spike-and-slow wave discharges with a frontal and central emphasis.

due to a severe encephalopathy without MSE is potentially reversible.[26] The EEG helps determine whether myoclonus is the sporadic sign of an encephalopathy or part of MSE. The former has a better prognosis. After anoxia, MSE is better considered a sign of a severely damaged brain than a treatable epileptic condition.[27] MSE may have motor manifestations limited to "subtle" status, also an ominous sign after anoxia.[28]

MSE also occurs as a manifestation of generalized epilepsies such as juvenile myoclonic epilepsy; it may include prolonged epileptic myoclonus without loss of consciousness.[29] The EEG shows a characteristic generalized polyspike and slow wave discharges with a normal background between episodes. Episodes may go on for hours (with preserved consciousness), but the prognosis is excellent given the prior normal neurologic function. Patients can also return to baseline in the MSE of progressive myoclonus epilepsies, although the epilepsy may be part of a progressive debilitating disease.[30] In all these conditions, the EEG can help distinguish MSE from encephalopathies with less rhythmic abnormalities.

TONIC STATUS EPILEPTICUS

Tonic SE, which is rare, is seen primarily in children, particularly those with Lennox–Gastaut syndrome. Treatment of the potentially injurious seizures is often frustrating, as is the associated mental retardation. Rarely, benzodiazepines have been cited as triggering tonic status. Tonic (and atonic) SE is distinctly uncommon in adults and certainly in those with normal neurologic function interictally. Similarly, generalized clonic SE is a pediatric condition. Clonus is often of low amplitude; both sides of the body are usually involved but may move asynchronously.

COMPLEX PARTIAL STATUS EPILEPTICUS

Complex partial status epilepticus (CPSE) implies impairment of consciousness caused by seizures with a focal cortical origin. The disorder is sometimes called fugue states or psychomotor status. Confusion is the most common symptom. A sudden alteration in behavior, particularly in a patient with prior epilepsy, should suggest the possible diagnosis of CPSE. A diagnosis of CPSE is frequently invoked to explain bizarre behavior, but this type of SE is actually uncommon. Some patients may have complex partial seizures with a prolonged postictal phase. CPSE may be continuous or include frequent discrete seizures without recovery between them; the latter series of spells account for some of the prolonged episodes. CPSE can go on for weeks or even months, and patients may have prolonged cognitive deficits after CPSE. CPSE can be difficult to distinguish from absence SE. Patients with CPSE may exhibit more bizarre behavior during seizures and, thus, their disorder may be confused with psychiatric disease or metabolic encephalopathies with delirium.

The usual site of origin is assumed to be mesial temporal structures with limbic connections, but recordings obtained from implanted electrodes have shown that frontal lobe onset is common.[31] The EEG may show the seizure clearly (but this is less likely in frontal areas without implanted electrodes) or may show just persistent focal slowing. Seizures may spread rapidly, and nonconvulsive SE with generalized discharges ("absence SE") may actually arise from a focus.[32]

Increasing reports of cognitive and other sequelae from prolonged CPSE have lent a greater urgency to its interruption, but treatment is usually not as aggressive as for GCSE. Most CPSE responds relatively rapidly to anticonvulsants but may recur frequently and even regularly in the same patient, even with adequate anticonvulsant therapy.[33,34]

NONCONVULSIVE STATUS EPILEPTICUS

Nonconvulsive status epilepticus (NCSE) includes many of the syndromes previously described. Most patients have absence SE; fewer have CPSE. SE with simple partial sensory or autonomic symptoms and all SE without convulsions are included. The EEG can vary tremendously in NCSE, often exhibiting slower discharges than expected, and usually showing generalized rather than focal abnormalities.

ELECTROGRAPHIC STATUS EPILEPTICUS

In patients with electrographic SE (ESE), the significance of the continuous epileptic discharges evident on the EEG is unknown or controversial. Children with ESE during sleep (ESES) may have no clear clinical concomitant, but most have mental retardation and epilepsy.[35] Many of these children have markedly impaired language function. In waking, they tend to be healthier than patients with Lennox–Gastaut syndrome. Medications may improve the EEG without affecting overall health or behavior. ESES can be associated with neuropsychologic regression after previously normal development.[36]

ESE can also be seen in adults, in some cases representing absence SE or occurring after GCSE. In other cases it may be an unexpected finding in patients with severe medical illness with encephalopathies and is of uncertain clinical significance. Some patients have subtle motor phenomena, but in others coma is the only manifestation. Diagnosis rests on the EEG.[37] Anticonvulsant therapy can be helpful but may be unrewarding, primarily because of the severe underlying illness.

HOW IS STATUS EPILEPTICUS DIAGNOSED?

As in all other areas of medicine, effective treatment is facilitated tremendously by the correct diagnosis! Convulsive SE is rarely a diagnostic difficulty, but NCSE, including after generalized seizures, may be difficult to recognize or may be missed altogether. Conversely, shaking and responding poorly do not always suggest epilepsy (Table 8.4). Movement disorders, including chorea, myoclonus, tremors, and tics, have all been treated as SE, the treatment potentially causing greater harm than the disease.

"Pseudo status" is particularly troublesome. Complicating diagnosis, these nonepileptic episodes often occur in patients with epileptic seizures as well.[38] Out-of-phase limb movements and more complicated vocalizations correlate with nonepileptic spells.[39] An EEG recording can be diagnostic if it can be arranged during the events; the absence of epileptiform features is suggestive, although it may be impossible to exclude seizures totally, because some (especially frontal seizures) can leave the surface EEG unaffected. Quick reversion to a normal background also suggests pseudoseizure. Iatrogenic morbidity is common in these patients, and spells may persist until treatment causes respiratory arrest.[40] Recurrence is common. Psychiatric management is appropriate but not always successful.

Table 8.4

Differential Diagnosis of Apparent Status Epilepticus

With prominent motor abnormalities:	
Movement disorders	Myoclonus, tremors, chorea, tics, dystonic reactions
Structural disease	Decerebrate, decorticate posturing
Psychiatric disorders	Pseudoseizure–conversion, acute psychosis
Usually "nonconvulsive":	
Epilepsy-related disorders	Postictal state, periodic lateralized epileptiform discharges with acute structural lesions
Acute encephalopathies	Toxic: metabolic (e.g., hypoglycemia, organ failure delirium related to drugs, alcohol, or infection)
Psychiatric disorders	Catatonia, acute psychosis
Sleep disorders	Narcolepsy, cataplexy, parasomnias
Syncope	Cardiac, vagal, hypovolemia, medication toxicity
Vascular disease	Strokes, transient ischemic attacks
Head injury	Stupor, coma, amnesia
Transient global amnesia	Usually clears quickly; rare recurrence

The patient's history often reveals the reason for SE (Table 8.2). Trauma, drug overdose, alcohol use, medical illness, stroke, or epilepsy may be uncovered through discussions with the patient's family members and companions or by the patient's medical bracelet and personal possessions. Physical examination focuses on the underlying cause of SE and localization of the neurologic abnormality. Vital signs are crucial, given the cardiovascular complications; respiratory failure is an occasional complication of SE but more often is a result of medications. The general examination can show signs of infection (by fever, nuchal rigidity, or skin lesions) or systemic illness, such as kidney or liver disease. Signs of head injury or coagulopathy are also important. The neurologic examination also assesses whether seizures are actually continuing in subtle ways.

Appropriate laboratory studies include a search for metabolic abnormalities, particularly of sodium, calcium, magnesium, and glucose; kidney, liver, and coagulation assays are also important. Toxicology screening and measuring anticonvulsant levels and arterial oxygen tension are often helpful, but treatment must begin before these levels are known. Blood gas and prolactin levels can be useful in considering the possibility of pseudoseizures. Women of childbearing age should have a pregnancy test, in part so that they can be counseled about the effects of SE and medications on the fetus, on the mother, and on implications for treatment and management. Pregnant women should be assessed for eclampsia. Urgent computed tomography scans are prompted by concerns about head injury, by an asymmetric neurologic exam, or by seizures with a focal origin. Any source of infection must be found. Lumbar puncture is mandatory if there is any suggestion of central nervous system (CNS) infection or when SE is of unknown cause or is difficult to control.

GCSE is diagnosed without an EEG, and treatment begins without it. An EEG is necessary for the diagnosis of NCSE, although treatment may begin based on clinical suspicion. EEGs are mandatory when a patient does not respond to initial treatment, because it may be impossible to ascertain clinically whether the patient is postictal or still seizing.

As in other emergencies, attention to airway, breathing, and circulation (the ABCs) is crucial. Patients with GCSE or coma from other forms of SE usually need intubation, at least for airway protection. Physical safety and prevention of further injury must be assured. Use of a soft oral airway tube is reasonable, but forced insertion or the use of hard objects is not. Intravenous access must be assured. Thiamine and a bolus of 50% glucose should be infused after a reliable normal saline intravenous line is established. ECG monitoring should be continued to watch for arrhythmias and ischemia. The goal of medical management is to normalize blood pressure, volume status, temperature, ventilation, and oxygenation. Hypomagnesemia may worsen seizures, and magnesium is appropriate for alcoholic or malnourished patients. Drug overdoses may prompt gastric emptying or even hemodialysis.

HOW ARE ANTICONVULSANTS USED TO TREAT STATUS EPILEPTICUS?

The choice of anticonvulsants for SE is still controversial. Few studies have compared different medications, and it is important to stress that most describe GCSE alone. Almost all published protocols and guidelines refer to GCSE; differences for other forms of SE will be pointed out. Generalized NCSE after convulsions should probably be considered as much an emergency as GCSE. Other forms of SE are of less certain morbidity and urgency. Medication use is generally similar, if less immediate. Nevertheless, the pathophysiologic underpinnings of many different types of SE (with the possible exception of absence SE) argue for urgent treatment in almost all cases. Other forms of SE can lead to convulsions, and a casual approach is inappropriate.

Rather than trying to decide on "the best anticonvulsant," it may be more useful for the physician to consider medications in two groups. One group consists of rapidly acting anticonvulsants, largely limited to benzodiazepines, which are often necessary for the interruption of SE, especially when the physiologic and pathologic consequences of GCSE are imminent. Benzodiazepines are invaluable in interrupting continuous seizures but may not be necessary when seizures are discrete, even with incomplete recovery. The other group of anticonvulsants (led by phenytoin and phenobarbital but including most other anticonvulsants) work less rapidly but provide continued protection against the reemergence of SE and are almost always necessary after the first few minutes. The goal must be to stop continuous convulsions or other seizures and to interrupt continuing EEG discharges.

PHENYTOIN

Phenytoin is probably the most frequently used anticonvulsant for SE but is often given in inadequate doses.[4] Its major disadvantage is the length of time required for a loading infusion (Table 8.5). However, the drug may be beneficial before reaching "therapeutic levels." The advantage of minimal sedation is generally overstated but may be pertinent for patients with head trauma, hemorrhage, or raised intracranial pressure, for whom it is important to monitor alertness; patients with GCSE are unconscious, and the most immediate concern is stopping the seizures. In the absence of acute structural lesions, phenytoin may be successful alone in up to 80% of patients with GCSE.[41] It can then become a long-term maintenance medication without the necessity of changing or adding drugs. Patients may need adjunctive benzodiazepines to interrupt convulsions if they occur during phenytoin infusion. Many authorities recommend phenytoin as the primary treat-

Table 8.5

Properties of Anticonvulsants Used in the Treatment of Status Epilepticus

Medication	Doses	Kinetics	Complications	Comment
Phenytoin	15–20 mg/kg <50 mg/min Maintenance level >20 μg/ml	Effect in 10–30 min Peak effect in 1 h Elimination $t_{1/2}$: 24–48 h	Cardiac arrhythmias Hypotension	Bolus lasts 6–24 h Best in following level of consciousness Worse for cardiac disease
Phenobarbital	10–20 mg/kg <100 mg/min Maintenance level >40 μg/ml	Effect in 5–20 min Peak in 1 h Elimination $t_{1/2}$: 120 h	Respiratory depression, hypotension (possible synergy with benzodiazepines)	Slower than benzodiazepines Depression of consciousness can be prolonged after loading
Diazepam	10 mg (0.25 mg/kg) Repeat q15 min; up to possibly 40 mg <5 mg/min	Effect in 1–2 min Peak in 20–30 min Metabolite $t_{1/2}$: 36 h	Sedation, respiratory depression, hypotension Recurrent symptoms as it wears off	Rapid interruption of convulsions Needs to be followed by maintenance anticonvulsants
Lorazepam	4–8 mg (0.1–0.2 mg/kg) <2 mg/min	Effect in 2–5 min Peak in 15–30 min Elimination $t_{1/2}$: 12–15 h	Same as diazepam; less sudden	More prolonged protection (up to 12 h) against seizure recurrence No active toxic metabolites
Pentobarbital	Load 3–5 mg/kg Maintenance 1–4 mg/kg/h	Effect in minutes Elimination $t_{1/2}$: 20–40 h	Respiratory depression Hypotension Hypothermia	Uniformly effective High mortality due to underlying disease Duration of treatment unknown (possibly 24–48 h)

ment of GCSE, sometimes after initial interruption of convulsions with a benzodiaz-epine.

A usual loading dose is 15 mg/kg, but 20 mg/kg is reasonable before conclud-ing that phenytoin is insufficient. It should be given by intravenous bolus or in saline solution at a maximum rate of 50 mg/min; it may precipitate in glucose solutions. Intramuscular phenytoin is poorly absorbed and should not be used.

Conduction defects are the primary cardiac toxicity, but hypotension is not rare. Cardiac monitoring is appropriate during phenytoin infusion. Elderly patients or those with cardiac disease may not tolerate phenytoin as well as phenobarbital. Acute toxicity is more closely related to the infusion rate than to total dose; patients with possible complications may tolerate greater doses in slower infusions. A new phenytoin prodrug without the propylene glycol carrier may allow rapid infusion without toxicity.

PHENOBARBITAL

Phenobarbital, which is often used if phenytoin is insufficient, is frequently avoided out of fear it will cause sedation, but its advantages include a relative lack of cardiac toxicity until very high doses are reached. Aside from phenytoin, it is the major anticonvulsant available intravenously for longer-term management. Up to 20 mg/kg is reasonable. Loading is faster than with phenytoin, but its lipid solubility is lower and brain penetration is slower.[42] Nevertheless, phenobarbital may act quickly, even before therapeutic levels are established. In addition, although some SE may be refractory to phenytoin, high enough doses of phenobarbital will control almost all seizures. Very high doses require artificial ventilation and may cause hypotension, but they may be tolerated better than expected.[43] Sedation must be expected with high doses, but levels below 40 μg/mL should not produce prolonged coma.

Phenobarbital has been compared favorably with a combination of diazepam and phenytoin in one prospective trial; clinical response was actually faster with phenobarbital.[44] Barbiturates and benzodiazepines may be particularly likely to cause respiratory depression and hypotension when used together.[45]

DIAZEPAM

Diazepam is a common first treatment for SE, but conservative management would restrict it to patients with continuing convulsions or those having another convulsion during infusion of a maintenance medication. Different reviews have shown widely varying efficacy rates in SE: from 38–83%. Diazepam can interrupt convulsive SE rapidly but should not be used alone. The usual practice is to administer 10 mg intravenously over a few minutes, repeating if necessary. Rectal administration has been effective, particularly in children. Intramuscular diazepam is absorbed slowly. Diazepam is lipid soluble, enters the brain rapidly, and may have an anticonvulsant effect within a minute. Nevertheless, it redistributes to many tissues, and its CNS effect declines in 20–30 min; recurrent seizures or SE is common when longer-acting anticonvulsants are not used concomitantly. Repeated doses may lose effectiveness but produce metabolites with prolonged elimination half-lives and potential toxicity, including prolonged coma. Continuous infusion of diazepam (generally 4–8 mg/h) is often discussed for the management of SE but is rarely practiced, probably because the optimal doses have not been clearly established, and rapid acute tolerance may develop.[46] Continuous infusion should be used in intensive care units only. Iatrogenic apnea can occur suddenly; it is often ascribed to seizures or to "tongue swallowing."

LORAZEPAM

Lorazepam has several advantages. It acts rapidly enough to interrupt seizures quickly and still has a more prolonged anticonvulsant effect; some physicians consider it to satisfy the requirements for both the acute interruption of SE and prolonged protection against recurrence. Doses are approximately half as large as those of diazepam. Its lipid solubility is half of diazepam's, and its brain penetration is slower but still rapid.[42] Its effect declines less rapidly than diazepam's, but it has no active, troublesome metabolites.

Many epileptologists prefer lorazepam because of its favorable pharmacokinetics, but direct comparative studies are few. A double-blind, randomized trial found lorazepam marginally more effective than diazepam in controlling SE, with an onset of action not significantly different.[47] Adverse effects are similar to those of diazepam, although perhaps less sudden. Lorazepam may provide 12 h of anticonvulsant effect, but acute tolerance may occur and reduce its maintenance value.

MIDAZOLAM AND CLONAZEPAM

Midazolam has proved effective in some particularly refractory cases of SE after failure of other benzodiazepines and phenytoin.[48] In such cases, the use of midazolam may prevent the adverse effects of barbiturate-induced coma. Its action is extremely rapid because of high lipid solubility, but its effect is short-lived, and relapses of seizures may be expected. It may be utilized in 0.2 mg/kg (5–20 mg) intravenous boluses. The short duration of action allows clinical assessment soon after its discontinuation. It may be the best intramuscular treatment of SE when this is the only available route. Clonazepam appears similar to other benzodiazepines and is popular in Europe, but it is not available in intravenous form in the United States for the treatment of SE.

PARALDEHYDE

Paraldehyde has fallen out of favor in clinical trials but remains a popular alternative, especially in patients who are allergic to other anticonvulsants and in whom intravenous access is limited. Five to ten mL may be given rectally mixed with mineral oil. Intramuscular use yields a faster effect but may produce sterile abscesses. The physical preparation is important because of its rapid decomposition and reaction with plastic and rubber tubing. The onset of action of paraldehyde is slower than that of medications described earlier. Its effective half-life is 6 h. It may be more effective for SE prompted by alcohol withdrawal,[49] but this has not been well studied. Oral administration of paraldehyde in the setting of possible aspiration can lead to serious pulmonary toxicity. Its smell causes some of its unpopularity.

VALPROIC ACID AND CARBAMAZEPINE

Valproic acid is generally available in rectal form only in the treatment of SE.[50] Rectal doses of 17 mg/kg are generally recommended. Peak concentrations may lag by hours, and the effect may be even more delayed.[51] Many patients never achieve therapeutic levels. It may be a useful adjunct in the long-term treatment of refractory or intermittent SE, and it is helpful in preventing the recurrence of absence SE.[52] Currently, valproic acid has a minimal role in the acute management of SE. Similarly, enteral carbamazepine may be useful in long courses of refractory seizures but is not available intravenously nor is it helpful in acute management of SE. Felbamate, gabapentin, and lamotrigine are not currently available intravenously and have not been well studied for SE.

PENTOBARBITAL

When GCSE has continued for 30–45 min or when other forms of SE must be stopped (although no one knows exactly when that is), pentobarbital (or thiopental) can provide definitive treatment.[53,54] Short-acting barbiturates act rapidly but require intensive care unit treatment. Loading doses of 3–5 mg/kg followed by infusion of 1–4 mg/kg/h are typical.[55] Effectiveness is assayed by effect on the EEG, with an attempt to eliminate seizures or aim for a "burst suppression" or flat record; most authors seek a burst suppression pattern. The half-life of pentobarbital is approximately 20 h (shorter than phenobarbital's, so it dissipates sooner) but may be extended at higher levels. Accordingly, prolonged coma after pentobarbital treatment should not be attributed to a "burnt-out" brain before the medication has had time to dissipate. Blood levels are more useful for indicating residual toxicity than for assessing therapeutic effect.

All SE should be suppressible with adequate pentobarbital doses, but hypotension is common. Usually, volume replacement and low doses of vasopressors are sufficient.[56] Myocardial function and temperature regulation can be impaired. Most reports of pentobarbital use show a high mortality,[57] usually attributed to severe underlying diseases causing SE to be refractory enough to require pentobarbital. An advantage of pentobarbital, besides its invariable effectiveness when used in large enough doses, is that it reduces cerebral metabolism and blood flow. The infusion is also easy to adjust. The optimal duration of barbiturate-induced coma has not been established; recommendations range from 4–72 h. Patients should probably have therapeutic blood levels of two other anticonvulsants before pentobarbital is withdrawn. Pentobarbital should be considered the definitive treatment of GCSE after 30–45 min of convulsions or when earlier medications have failed or are unavailable. A few investigators have found higher doses of benzodiazepines, including lorazepam and midazolam, a reasonable alternative to pentobarbital and one with less effect on blood pressure.

INHALED ANESTHETICS

Inhaled anesthetics are less well studied and far less convenient than the drugs already described, but may be useful for patients who are allergic to pentobarbital. Most inhaled anesthetics increase cerebral blood flow, which is a theoretical disadvantage. This problem probably applies least to isoflurane, which is possibly the most effective anesthetic with the least cardiovascular effect in the setting of SE.[58] Halothane is used relatively frequently,[59] but isoflurane may produce a burst suppression EEG tracing with less severe cardiovascular morbidity. Both agents may necessitate the use of vasopressors.[58] Nitrous oxide does not appear effective. Enflurane can precipitate convulsions.

LIDOCAINE AND PROPOFOL

Lidocaine can have a rapid effect without causing significant respiratory depression.[60] Several reports describe successful use of this agent in focal motor SE. At higher doses, however, it can also cause convulsions and must remain a last resort. Similarly, intravenous propofol, a nonbarbiturate anesthetic, is extremely lipid soluble and fast acting. It can cause severe respiratory depression and nonepileptic involuntary movements[61] and can also precipitate seizures.

NEUROMUSCULAR BLOCKING AGENTS; STEROIDS AND OSMOTIC AGENTS

Neuromuscular blocking agents eliminate motor activity, but they are not anticonvulsants. They may provide false reassurance when SE continues on an electrical and metabolic basis. They can help when excessive movement impairs oxygenation, acid-base balance, or temperature regulation, but adequate doses of anticonvulsants, particularly pentobarbital, will obviate these problems. Steroids and osmotic agents may be used to treat cerebral edema that results from prolonged SE, particularly in children, but their efficacy has not been established. Rarely, a persistent seizure focus causing refractory partial SE may be resected surgically.[62]

TREATMENT SUMMARY

Most medication trials have studied patients with GCSE. The same medications may treat other forms of SE. Intravenous benzodiazepines usually interrupt absence SE, and subsequent treatment may be unnecessary. For patients with continuous generalized discharges and coma, however, intravenous benzodiazepines are often insufficient. For partial or nonconvulsive SE, enteral valproate and carbamazepine are more valuable, although the response may take days; rarely will pentobarbital or anesthetics be necessary. In children, phenobarbital is often preferred to phenytoin because of better absorption, greater efficacy, and possibly fewer long-term side effects.

WHEN SHOULD ELECTROENCEPHALOGRAPHY BE USED?

The use of electroencephalography in SE depends on the seizure type and vigor of treatment. It is generally unnecessary with generalized convulsions but is mandatory when motor activity has ceased and the patient has not returned to normal; the physician needs to know if the seizures are actually continuing. An EEG is necessary to assess medication effect with high doses of anticonvulsants, particularly pentobarbital. Certainly, with neuromuscular blocking agents, an EEG is required to tell whether SE has been treated at all.

WHEN AND HOW SHOULD THE PATIENT'S CONDITION BE REEVALUATED DURING TREATMENT?

Protocols for the treatment of SE emphasize the ABCs of cardiorespiratory support in acutely ill patients, followed by one of several orders of standard anticonvulsants, often emphasizing diazepam, lorazepam, phenytoin, and phenobarbital. Rather than choose one protocol for all patients, the physician should keep in mind the principles detailed in Figure 8.2.

Continual reassessment of the patient's clinical condition and electroencephalography are necessary, as is continued reevaluation of the diagnosis and medication effectiveness. When SE does not respond to treatment as expected, the clinician's attention should refocus along several lines. First, the diagnosis of SE must be

---

1. Be sure of the diagnosis. Distinguish from myoclonus, other movement disorders, decerebrate posturing, and pseudoseizures. Blood gases and EEG may be helpful. After 30 min of recurrent seizures without recovery, the patient should be considered in SE. The same urgency is appropriate when convulsions are continuous for more than 2 min.
2. Determine the cause of SE through history, examination, and appropriate laboratory tests.
3. Note airway, respiration, blood pressure, and cardiac rhythm. Most patients with GCSE require intubation. Patients with other forms of SE often do not. Establish an intravenous line with saline, thiamine, and glucose. Administer antibiotics when infection is a possibility. Draw blood for metabolic studies, determination of anticonvulsant levels, and toxic screens.
4. Use a long-acting medication. Phenytoin, the most frequently used maintenance medication, should be given in saline at 50 mg/min, with attention to the cardiogram, to a dose of 18–20 mg/kg rather than the commonly used 1000 mg. Phenobarbital is more often used for children, elderly patients, or persons with cardiac rhythm disturbances, at 10–20 mg/kg, up to 100 mg/min, with attention to blood pressure.
5. Administer rapidly acting anticonvulsants (i.e., benzodiazepines) if GCSE has lasted 30 min, if convulsions are continuous, if convulsions occur during the infusion of phenytoin or phenobarbital, or if phenytoin or phenobarbital is not successful. Lorazepam, 5–10 mg in adults, can be administered at a rate of 2 mg/min and repeated if necessary.
6. In the intensive care unit after intubation, provide definitive treatment with pentobarbital after 30–45 min or if the previously mentioned agents are unsuccessful. Use 5 mg/kg for induction and attempt to eliminate epileptiform activity on the EEG; many physicians proceed to burst suppression EEG tracings. Maintenance dosage is 1–5 mg/kg/h as needed to control seizures and to attain the desired EEG recording. Some physicians have found higher doses of lorazepam or midazolam a reasonable alternative with less effect on blood pressure. When used, pentobarbital might be discontinued after 24–48 h, assuming clinical and electrographic seizures have ceased and that two longer-acting anticonvulsants are at high therapeutic levels.
7. Continue to reassess clinical and EEG activity and attend to the diagnosis and medical complications, until the patient returns to normal.
8. Choose maintenance medications and establish them at therapeutic levels. Attend to complications such as hypothermia, acidosis, hypotension, rhabdomyolysis, renal failure, infection, and cerebral edema.

Figure 8.2   Guidelines for the treatment of status epilepticus.

correct. Second, correct assessment of the underlying cause is crucial; SE is most likely to continue when trauma, hemorrhage, or infections such as encephalitis remain untreated. Third, medications must be given in adequate doses; for example, the 1000-mg standard phenytoin infusion may be insufficient. Fourth, medication absorption must be adequate; that may not be the case if there are problems with intravenous access or if the drug is given via another route. Finally, SE may be treated successfully and then recur, most often because of inadequate attention to maintenance levels of longer-acting anticonvulsants or to lack of treatment of the underlying disease.

REFERENCES

1. Gastaut H. Clinical and electroencephalographic classification of epileptic seizures. *Epilepsia.* 1970;11:102–113.
2. Hauser WA. Status epilepticus: Epidemiologic considerations. *Neurology.* 1990;40(suppl. 2):9–13.
3. DeLorenzo RJ, Pellock JM, Towne AR, *et al.* Epidemiology of status epilepticus. *J Clin Neurophysiol.* 1995;12:316–325.
4. Lowenstein DH, Alldredge BK. Status epilepticus at an urban public hospital in the 1980s. *Neurology.* 1993;43:483–488.
5. Barry E, Hauser WA. Status epilepticus: The interaction of epilepsy and acute brain disease. *Neurology.* 1993;43:1473–1478.
6. Barry E, Hauser WA. Status epilepticus and antiepileptic medication levels. *Neurology.* 1994;44:47–50.
7. Alldredge BK, Lowenstein DH. Status epilepticus related to alcohol abuse. *Epilepsia.* 1993;34:1033–1037.
8. Fialip J, Aumaitre O, Eschalier A, *et al.* Benzodiazepine withdrawal seizures: Analysis of 48 case reports. *Clin Neuropharm.* 1987;10:538–544.
9. Aminoff MJ, Simon RP. Status epilepticus: Causes, clinical features, and consequences in 98 patients. *Am J Med.* 1980;69:657–666.
10. Walton NY. Systemic effects of generalized convulsive status epilepticus. *Epilepsia.* 1993;34(suppl. 1):S54–S58.
11. Boggs JG, Painter JA, DeLorenzo RJ. Analysis of electrocardiographic changes in status epilepticus. *Epilepsy Res.* 1993;14:87–94.
12. Wasterlain, CG, Fujikawa DG, Penix L, *et al.* Pathophysiological mechanisms of brain damage from status epilepticus. *Epilepsia.* 1993;34(suppl. 1):S37–S53.
13. Barry E, Hauser WA. Pleocytosis after status epilepticus. *Arch Neurol.* 1994;51:190–193.
14. Dodrill CB, Wilensky AJ. Intellectual impairment as an outcome of status epilepticus. *Neurology.* 1990;40(suppl. 2):23–27.
15. Lothman EW, Bertram EH. Epileptogenic effects of status epilepticus. *Epilepsia.* 1993;34:S59–S70.
16. Meldrum BS, Brierley JB. Prolonged epileptic seizures in primates. Ischemic cell change and its relation to ictal physiological events. *Arch Neurol.* 1973;28:10–17.
17. DeGiorgio CM, Tomiyasu U, Gott PS, *et al.* Hippocampal pyramidal cell loss in human status epilepticus. *Epilepsia.* 1992;33:23–27.
18. VanLandingham KE, Lothman EW. Self-sustaining limbic status epilepticus. I. Acute and chronic cerebral metabolic studies: Limbic hypermetabolism and neocortical hypometabolism. *Neurology.* 1991;41:1942–1949.

19. Treiman DM, Walton NY, Kendrick C. A progressive sequence of electrographic changes during generalized convulsive status epilepticus. *Epilepsy Res.* 1990;5:49–60.

20. Towne AR, Pellock JM, Ko D, *et al.* Determinants of mortality in status epilepticus. *Epilepsia.* 1994;35:27–34.

21. DeLorenzo RJ, Towne AR, Pellock JM, *et al.* Status epilepticus in children, adults, and the elderly. *Epilepsia.* 1992;33(suppl. 4):S15–S25.

22. Thomas P, Beaumanoir A, Genton P, *et al.* "De novo" absence status of late onset: Report of 11 cases. *Neurology.* 1992;42:104–110.

23. Fagan KJ, Lee SI. Prolonged confusion following convulsions due to generalized nonconvulsive status epilepticus. *Neurology.* 1990;40:1689–1694.

24. Andermann F, Robb JP. Absence status: A reappraisal following review of thirty-eight patients. *Epilepsia.* 1972;13:177–187.

25. Niedermeyer E, Khalifeh R. Petit mal status ("spike-wave stupor"): An electroclinical appraisal. *Epilepsia.* 1965;6:250–262.

26. Celesia GG, Grigg MM, Ross E. Generalized status myoclonicus in acute anoxic and toxic-metabolic encephalopathies. *Arch Neurol.* 1988;45:781–784.

27. Young GB, Gilbert JJ, Zochodne DW. The significance of myoclonic status epilepticus in postanoxic coma. *Neurology.* 1990;40:1843–1848.

28. Simon RP, Aminoff MJ. Electrographic status epilepticus in fatal anoxic coma. *Ann Neurol.* 1986;20:351–355.

29. Jumao-as A, Brenner RP. Myoclonic status epilepticus: A clinical and electroencephalographic study. *Neurology.* 1990;40:1199–1202.

30. Berkovic SF, Andermann F, Carpenter S, *et al.* Progressive myoclonus epilepsies: Specific causes and diagnosis. *N Engl J Med.* 1986;315:296–305.

31. Williamson PD, Spencer DD, Spencer SS, *et al.* Complex partial status epilepticus: A depth-electrode study. *Ann Neurol.* 1985;18:647–654.

32. Thomson T, Svanborg E, Wedlund JE. Nonconvulsive status epilepticus: High incidence of complex partial status. *Epilepsia.* 1986;27:276–285.

33. Ballenger CE, King DW, Gallagher BB. Partial complex status epilepticus. *Neurology.* 1983;33:1545–1552.

34. Guberman A, Cantu-Reyna G, Stuss D, *et al.* Nonconvulsive generalized status epilepticus: Clinical features, neuropsychological testing, and long-term follow-up. *Neurology.* 1986;36:1284–1291.

35. Patry G, Lyagoubi S, Tassinari CA. "Subclinical status epilepticus" induced by sleep in children. A clinical and electroencephalographic study of six cases. *Arch Neurol.* 1971;24:242–252.

36. Jayakar PB, Seshia SS. Electrical status epilepticus during slow-wave sleep: A review. *J Clin Neurophysiol.* 1991;8:299–311.

37. Drislane FW, Schomer DL. Clinical implications of generalized electrographic status epilepticus. *Epilepsy Res.* 1994;19:111–121.

38. Lesser RP. Psychogenic seizures. *Neurology* 1996;46:1499–1507.

39. Gates JR, Ramani V, Whalen S, *et al.* Ictal characteristics of pseudoseizures. *Arch Neurol.* 1985;42:1183–1187.

40. Pakalnis A, Drake ME, Phillips B. Neuropsychiatric aspects of psychogenic status epilepticus. *Neurology.* 1991;41:1104–1106.

41. Wilder BJ, Ramsay RE, Willmore LJ, *et al.* Efficacy of intravenous phenytoin in the treatment of status epilepticus: Kinetics of central nervous system penetration. *Ann Neurol.* 1977;1:511–518.

42. Browne TR. The pharmacokinetics of agents used to treat status epilepticus. *Neurology.* 1990;40(suppl. 2):28–32.

43. Crawford TP, Mitchell WG, Fishman LS, *et al.* Very-high-dose phenobarbital for refractory status epilepticus. *Neurology.* 1988;38:1035–1040.

44. Shaner DM, McCurdy SA, Herring MO, *et al*. Treatment of status epilepticus: A prospective comparison of diazepam and phenytoin versus phenobarbital and optional phenytoin. *Neurology* 1988;38:202–207.

45. Browne TR, Penry JK. Benzodiazepines in the treatment of epilepsy. A review. *Epilepsia*. 1973;14:277–310.

46. Bell HE, Bertino JS Jr. Constant diazepam infusion in the treatment of continuous seizure activity. *Drug Intell Clin Pharm*. 1984;18:965–970.

47. Leppik IE, Derivan AT, Homan RW. Double blind study of lorazepam and diazepam in status epilepticus. *JAMA*. 1983;249:1452–1454.

48. Kumar A, Bleck TP. Intravenous midazolam for the treatment of refractory status epilepticus. *Crit Care Med*. 1992;20:483–488.

49. Browne TR. Paraldehyde, chlormethiazole, and lidocaine for treatment of status epilepticus. *Adv Neurol*. 1983;34:509–517.

50. Thorpy MJ. Rectal valproate syrup and status epilepticus. *Neurology*. 1980;30:1113–1114.

51. Vajda FJ, Mihaly GW, Miles JL, *et al*. Rectal administration of sodium valproate in status epilepticus. *Neurology*. 1978;28:897–899.

52. Berkovic SF, Andermann F, Guberman A, *et al*. Valproate prevents the recurrence of absence status. *Neurology*. 1989;39:1294–1297.

53. Krishnamurthy KB, Drislane FW. Relapse and survival after barbiturate anesthetic treatment of refractory status epilepticus. *Epilepsia*. 1996;37:863–867.

54. Van Ness PC. Pentobarbital and EEG burst suppression in treatment of status epilepticus refractory to benzodiazepines and phenytoin. *Epilepsia*. 1990;31:61–67.

55. Osorio I, Reed RC. Treatment of refractory generalized tonic clonic status epilepticus with pentobarbital anesthesia after high dose phenytoin. *Epilepsia*. 1989;30:464–471.

56. Yaffe K, Lowenstein DH. Prognostic factors of pentobarbital therapy for refractory generalized status epilepticus. *Neurology*. 1993;43:895–900.

57. Rashkin MC, Youngs C, Penovich P. Pentobarbital treatment of refractory status epilepticus. *Neurology*. 1987;37:500–503.

58. Kofke WA, Young RSK, Davis P, *et al*. Isoflurane for refractory status epilepticus: A clinical series. *Anesthesiology*. 1989;71:653–659.

59. Ropper AH, Kofke A, Bromfield EB, *et al*. Comparison of isoflurane, halothane, and nitrous oxide in status epilepticus. *Ann Neurol*. 1986;19:98–99.

60. Pascual J, Sedano MJ, Polo JM, *et al*. Intravenous lidocaine for status epilepticus. *Epilepsia*. 1988;29:584–589.

61. Shorvon S. Tonic clonic status epilepticus. *J Neurol Neurosurg Psychiatry*. 1993;56:125–134.

62. Gorman DG, Shields WD, Shewmon DA, *et al*. Neurosurgical treatment of refractory status epilepticus. *Epilepsia*. 1992;33:546–549.

GWENT HEALTHCARE NHS TRUST
LIBRARY
ROYAL GWENT HOSPITAL
NEWPORT

CHAPTER 9

Diagnosis and Management of Nonepileptic Seizures

A. James Rowan, M.D.

WHAT ARE NONEPILEPTIC SEIZURES?

Nonepileptic seizures (NESs) are episodic paroxysmal events that, in many respects, resemble epileptic seizures. Such events are often difficult if not impossible to differentiate from those due to epilepsy. Misdiagnosis is common; thus, in many cases, inappropriate treatment with antiepileptic drugs (AEDs) is inevitable. In arriving at an accurate diagnosis, the clinician's first task is to differentiate between the two major types of NESs: psychogenic and physiologic. Psychogenic NESs do not have a physiologic basis; rather, they are symptoms of an underlying psychiatric disorder. Physiologic NESs, on the other hand, are events that resemble epileptic seizures, but the cause is physiologic dysfunction—for example, cardiac arrhythmias, hypotensive episodes, or cerebrovascular disease. Such conditions may result in loss of consciousness, with or without associated motor manifestations. A detailed history and appropriate investigations (e.g., Holter monitoring, noninvasive carotid artery studies, or tilt-table testing) will usually reveal the true diagnosis.

The major portion of the following discussion will address the diagnostic and therapeutic problems posed by psychogenic NESs.

WHY IS AN UNDERSTANDING OF NONEPILEPTIC SEIZURES IMPORTANT?

NESs are relatively common. It is estimated that as many as 20% of the population seen in specialized seizure clinics suffer from NESs. Put another way, it is estimated that as many as 50,000 persons in the United States have NES. NESs may remain undiagnosed for long periods of time, sometimes years. In addition, if the patient has a past history of epilepsy and experiences a recurrence of seizures or currently has epilepsy and a new seizure type develops, the true diagnosis may be obscured. The clinician usually does not have an opportunity to observe the seizure in question and must rely on the information provided by the patient, an outside observer, or both. If NESs are misdiagnosed as epilepsy, treat-

The Comprehensive Evaluation and Treatment of Epilepsy
Copyright © 1997 by Academic Press. All rights of reproduction in any form reserved.

ment with AEDs will follow. NESs do not respond to AEDs. Indeed, continuing seizures in spite of increasing AED dosage or multiple AEDs is frustrating for the patient and physician alike. Moreover, AED therapy may lead to toxic side effects, resulting in additional disability and frustration. Thus, a correct diagnosis of NES is the critical factor that will lead to appropriate psychiatric intervention, discontinuation of AED therapy, and improvement in the patient's quality of life.

WHAT CAUSES NONEPILEPTIC SEIZURES?

Psychogenic NESs are manifestations of underlying psychiatric conditions and have diverse causes. Although a popular belief is that patients with NESs "fake" their seizures, this is not so in the vast majority of cases. The patient does not know why he or she has seizures and has little, if any, awareness of the influence of underlying emotional problems on their occurrence. The events are therefore regarded by the patient as real seizures. Some authors have viewed NESs as a cry for help—evidence of an underlying painful psychiatric condition that has not been addressed by family or physician. Others have viewed NESs as a coping mechanism for insoluble or intolerable life problems. The patient may have had a recent life crisis leading to NESs that suggests a direct relationship between the two. On the other hand, chronic psychiatric conditions or personality factors may lead to long-term, recurrent NESs. In such cases there may be no obvious triggering event.

WHAT CLUES TO THE DIAGNOSIS OF NONEPILEPTIC SEIZURES MAY BE PROVIDED BY THE PATIENT'S HISTORY?

Generally, there are many differences between the histories of patients with NESs and those of patients with epilepsy. NESs may occur only in the presence of others or, conversely, may never have been observed. In the latter case the clinician is dependent on the patient's description, which may be fragmentary and incomplete. Indeed, only loss of consciousness may be reported. If such a patient has a history of epilepsy, the probability of misdiagnosis is high. It is often said by clinicians that tongue biting and urinary incontinence do not occur with NESs. Unfortunately, many patients with documented NESs have reported these symptoms.

A clear emotional trigger for NESs may be discovered in the interview. Although this information may be suggestive, it should be noted that seizures are often ascribed to "stress" by patients with epilepsy. Thus, this criterion is not at all definitive.

The patient's reaction to his or her seizures may offer clues to the diagnosis. The classic description of the demeanor of the patient with NESs is *la belle indifference*. In the author's experience, however, such indifference is atypical. More commonly, the patient is concerned, sometimes excessively so, about the seizures. In fact, an *exaggerated* emotional response may provide a clue to NESs but should be considered in context with other information.

As noted earlier, NES treatment with AEDs, regardless of types or combinations, is unsuccessful. In fact, increasing doses of AEDs may lead to a paradoxical increase in seizure frequency. Sometimes, intolerance to AEDs poses a vexing problem for the clinician. Patients with NESs may complain of intolerable side effects at low doses or slow dose escalation of AEDs.

A history of abuse, either sexual or physical, is not uncommon in patients with NESs. At an appropriate time the clinician should inquire into this sensitive subject. Drawing firm conclusions from a history of abuse is perilous, however, because the incidence of abuse of persons with epilepsy, or indeed of persons in the general population, is not inconsequential. The author has also seen patients with epilepsy who have poignant histories of childhood or marital abuse.

Finally, suspicion is sometimes kindled by the patient's previous experience with other people who have epilepsy. The person may have encountered seizures in a professional capacity—for example, in a hospital setting. A family member or friend may have seizures, or the patient's own previous or current epileptic seizures may serve as templates for NESs. In addition, cultural influences may play a role in some cases.

DO NONEPILEPTIC SEIZURES HAVE CHARACTERISTICS THAT SUGGEST THE DIAGNOSIS?

If the clinician has an opportunity to observe one or more NESs, the phenomenology of the event may raise suspicion that the patient does not have epilepsy. Bear in mind that epileptic seizures typically start and end suddenly. For example, a simple absence seizure (formerly known as *petit mal*) begins with sudden loss of awareness, which continues for several seconds. The attack ends abruptly, at which time the person is fully aware and functional. Similarly, a tonic-clonic convulsion begins suddenly with a fall, loss of consciousness, and frequently an epileptic cry. Motor activity continues for a minute or so, progressing predictably and ending abruptly. At that point the patient is deeply comatose and flaccid. By contrast, NESs often have a gradual onset. For example, a nonepileptic seizure characterized by vigorous motor activity frequently builds in intensity as the event progresses. The event itself is often of longer duration than its epileptic counterpart, sometimes lasting many minutes or even hours. Moreover, the motor movements may have a waxing and waning quality through the course of the seizure—indeed, some NESs with motor manifestations are characterized by vigorous motor activity and intervening periods of quiet unresponsiveness. The event tends to subside gradually, and the postictal state, whether one of unresponsiveness or apparent confusion, is less profound than in the case of a tonic-clonic convulsion.

NESs that resemble true absence attacks are more difficult to differentiate from epilepsy than motor events. The staring, unresponsive state provides no obvious clues concerning the nature of the attack. However, if such attacks are of long duration, one might suspect that the diagnosis is other than epilepsy. The only way to confirm the true diagnosis is to record the event in question by EEG monitoring, preferably with simultaneous video monitoring.

Patients with NESs resembling complex partial seizures also present diagnostic difficulties because of the protean manifestations of the epileptic events. Such patients may exhibit confusional states with or without apparent automatic activities. Again, recording of the event is essential to confirm the diagnosis.

Additional features suggestive of NES include an emotional response during or after an event. Crying is not uncommon, nor is vocalization. Although crying may be observed in patients with epilepsy, it is more frequent in those with NES.

Typical NESs, especially motor events, do not seem to follow a "physiologic" progression. The motor activity tends to be chaotic, sometimes with flinging movements. Alternation of the movements, opisthotonus, pelvic thrusting, and dystonic posturing may be present. One important distinguishing feature of NES is that, in contrast to epileptic seizures, the face is often not involved.

Some patients with NESs exhibit avoidance behavior during events, especially during quiescent phases. For example, the patient may avoid striking himself or herself in the face if the patient's arm is held aloft and released. Such behavior suggests that the attack is nonepileptic.

ARE ANY OF THESE CLINICAL CHARACTERISTICS DIAGNOSTIC FOR NONEPILEPTIC SEIZURES?

Unfortunately, no pathognomic clinical features allow a definitive diagnosis of NES. Seizures originating in the frontal lobe, including the supplementary motor area, present a major diagnostic dilemma in differentiating NES from epilepsy. It is well documented that frontal lobe seizures may be characterized by prominent, chaotic, apparently "nonphysiologic" motor activity, such as flailing, alternating repetitive movements of the extremities, "bicycling" movements of the lower extremities, and tonic posturing. To most observers, such a picture appears to be clearly psychogenic or "hysterical." Moreover, the patient retains a degree of awareness during this stage. After the event subsides, there is little or no postevent confusion. These factors "confirm" to the unwary that the event indeed was not epileptic. An important aspect of the frontal seizure is a brief phase of tonic posturing that precedes the chaotic motor phase. This phase may take the form of abduction of the upper extremities or unilateral posturing with deviation of head and eyes. Forced downward deviation of the eyes has been observed. There may be accompanying vocalization. During this phase the patient is unresponsive, and the transition to the chaotic motor phase is rapid and abrupt. Inasmuch as the initial phase is frequently unobserved, whereas the prominent motor activity commands attention, the suspicion that the event may be epileptic is correspondingly diminished.

Pelvic thrusting movements have long been regarded as a sign of NES. It is therefore of interest that such movements can be seen in epileptic seizures, either as an accompaniment of tonic-clonic convulsions or as a manifestation of complex partial seizures. It has been observed that pelvic movements in tonic-clonic convulsions are more likely to be retropulsive, whereas those associated with NES are usually propulsive.

The features of gradual onset and gradual cessation, suggestive of NES, may be present in varying degrees in epilepsy. This is true both of generalized convulsions and complex partial seizures, although the "gradual" aspects of epileptic seizures may be more apparent than real. Certainly the electrographic seizure begins abruptly, but the clinical expression may seem to be otherwise. Although the duration of generalized tonic-clonic convulsions and complex partial seizures is usually relatively brief, on the order of 1–2 min, either seizure type may be prolonged. In addition, the seizures may appear to be intermittent—for example, in complex partial status epilepticus or in serial motor seizures.

In summary, the clinical expression of NES may raise one's index of suspicion but cannot be considered definitive. Only by recording the behavioral and electrographic characteristics of the event is it possible to be confident of the diagnosis.

DO NONEPILEPTIC SEIZURES SOMETIMES COEXIST WITH EPILEPSY?

The answer to this question is yes—frequently. The best available data suggest that in 20% of NES cases there is either a past history of epilepsy or coexisting epileptic seizures.[1] Unfortunately, the presence of both conditions complicates both diagnosis and management. Inasmuch as the physician usually does not have an opportunity to observe the event in question, reliance must be placed on observers in making diagnostic and therapeutic decisions. Because of the difficulty most people have in describing sudden or rapidly evolving events, it is likely that a presumptive diagnosis of epilepsy will be made. Moreover, if a patient suffers from both epilepsy and NES, it is probable that the seizure record in such patients, upon which changes in therapy will be based, will contain both epileptic seizures and NESs. Increases in the dosage of antiepileptic treatment is bound to follow reports of continuing seizures, even though the true problem may be superimposed NES. In such cases, if AED dosage increases are not accompanied by an alteration in seizure frequency or if seizures appear to increase in concert with an increased dose, the possibility of NES, or coexisting epilepsy and NES, should be considered.

HOW CAN ONE MAKE A DEFINITIVE DIAGNOSIS OF NONEPILEPTIC SEIZURES?

The so-called "gold standard" in the diagnosis of NES is the recording of a typical event during EEG–video monitoring (also see Chapter 10). This procedure is available at all centers specializing in epilepsy and is increasingly available at general hospitals and even in some neurologic group practices. Essentially, the EEG is recorded for a prolonged period, accompanied by continuous closed-circuit video observation. The EEG is digitized and conducted to a video monitor where recorded behavior and EEG are displayed simultaneously. It therefore is possible to make point-to-point correlations of recorded events and any accompanying electrographic changes.

Two types of monitoring are in general use: an outpatient procedure with a duration of 6–8 h (Daytime Monitoring, or DAYMON), and inpatient monitoring, which continues for 24 h or more. Each has its advantages. Outpatient studies are less expensive and more convenient than inpatient monitoring. Properly executed, there is evidence that DAYMON produces diagnostic yields comparable to those of longer studies. As a rule, DAYMON is appropriate for patients with relatively high seizure frequencies—at least three events per week. To increase yield, DAYMON should be carried out after the patient has been sleep deprived. During the procedure, which can be carried out in a living room, the patient wears an EEG transmitter connected to a wall outlet by coaxial cable. Wall-mounted video cameras provide continuous behavioral observation. Both EEG and video signals are transmitted to a control room where the EEG is reformatted and conducted to a video monitor. The EEG signal and video are displayed simultaneously for on-line observation, and both are recorded on videotape. The EEG may be recorded on paper or stored on optical disc. The patient is free to move about and carry out normal activities, such as talking, reading, and watching television. Participation by a family member or friend is encouraged, especially someone who has observed the patient's events in the past. The patient is invited to nap for at least an hour. Hyperventilation and photic stimulation are carried out. Although NES may occur spontaneously, the application of these procedures appears to increase diagnostic yield.

An important diagnostic aid is the use of suggestion techniques in an attempt to precipitate one of the patient's usual events. These techniques may take the form of placing alcohol pads over the carotid arteries or administering intravenous saline. The patient is informed that the procedure will be carried out for the purpose of inducing a seizure and that only by recording an event will a diagnosis be possible. If an event is precipitated and the event is typical of the patient's usual seizure, a diagnosis of NES is highly likely. False positives are rare. When DAYMON is performed in this manner, an overall success rate of approximately 60% can be expected.[2]

During NES there is no electrographic epileptiform activity, no initial EEG change such as premonitory spikes, and no postseizure slowing. Although the EEG tracing is frequently obscured by movement artifact, small interpretable segments containing alpha activity may be apparent, indicating that consciousness is preserved.

It should be emphasized that the interictal EEG in patients with NES may contain epileptiform discharges, even though the ictal record does not reveal electrographic seizure activity. Thus, the interictal EEG is of limited diagnostic value.

The most important task is to ensure that the recorded event(s) are typical of the patient's spontaneous attacks. This task can be accomplished only by reviewing the recorded attack with a person who has witnessed such events. If it is determined that the recorded and spontaneous attacks are similar, a presumptive diagnosis of NES can be made. Some workers require that more than one attack be recorded, although this is not always possible, especially with DAYMON. Nonetheless, in the author's experience, a single recorded event similar to previous attacks is sufficient to consider NES the most likely diagnosis. This diagnosis, of course, does not exclude the possibility of coexisting epilepsy, especially if the patient has attacks of apparently differing clinical characteristics.

If the patient's seizure frequency is relatively low, inpatient EEG-video monitoring for 24 h or more is indicated. This procedure requires hospital admission and a dedicated staff. Although more costly than DAYMON, inpatient monitoring is effective. More than one event may be recorded, increasing diagnostic certainty if the events are stereotyped. Inpatient monitoring also allows recording of a full night's sleep, increasing the possibility of recording sleep-provoked epileptiform activity as well as nocturnal clinical events. Several days of monitoring may be required before the diagnosis is made.

When the diagnosis of NES is confirmed, it is critical that it be presented to the patient in a positive, supportive, and nonthreatening manner. An empathetic, compassionate attitude on the part of the physician is an essential element in ensuring the patient's fealty and offering hope for the future.

NESs are presented as a paroxysmal disorder that cannot be treated with anticonvulsant medication. It is pointed out that NESs do not require chronic treatment with drugs that produce side effects. The disability associated with NES is emphasized, and the effect of the attacks on the patient's life are discussed. Also emphasized is that NESs have psychosocial consequences as profound as those of epilepsy.

The availability and indeed the success of treatment for NES is outlined. It is pointed out that many others suffer from NESs and that each person is unique, requiring tailor-made treatment. Finally, the patient is reassured that the outlook for improvement or complete recovery is excellent—even better than in the case of epilepsy. Such a conference is time-consuming but rewarding. In the author's experience, most patients are willing to accept a diagnosis of NES if it is presented in this manner, and they are eager to pursue an appropriate course of therapy.

WHAT IS THE DIAGNOSTIC ROLE OF PROLACTIN DETERMINATIONS?

Elevations in serum prolactin occur in the postictal phase (20–25 min after the seizure subsides) after most types of epileptic seizures. The most consistent increase is found after generalized tonic-clonic convulsions. At least a onefold to twofold increase in serum prolactin over baseline, and often a much greater increase, is found in 90–100% of patients after generalized tonic-clonic convulsions. After complex partial seizures, elevations of 43–100% have been found. The prolactin increase declines markedly to a 10% increase in simple partial seizures.[3] No prolactin elevation occurs after absence seizures. NESs do not usually raise prolactin levels, although this observation has been disputed. Thus, prolactin levels can be useful in some cases of NES, but they cannot be considered diagnostic unless elevated in the postictal period compared to baseline.

IF INTENSIVE EEG–VIDEO MONITORING IS NOT AVAILABLE, WHAT ALTERNATIVES CAN BE USED?

In fact, a diagnosis of NES can be made with reasonable assurance using commonly available tools. Probably the best method would be to obtain an EEG after the patient is sleep deprived. In addition, a video camera can be set up in the EEG room. During the recording, and after explaining the procedure, techniques of suggestion can be applied. Again, the importance to the patient of recording the event in question is emphasized. Although the probability of success with a relatively brief recording period is less than with DAYMON, some events will be captured.

The use of 24-hour ambulatory cassette EEG recording to diagnose NES is not recommended unless a home video unit is available. Without recording the behavioral aspects of the attack, there simply is too little diagnostic information. Moreover, excessive EEG artifacts during an attack renders the cassette EEG difficult, if not impossible, to interpret. If, on the other hand, the patient has attacks characterized by staring with little motor activity, cassette EEG can be useful. Certainly, differentiation of absence seizures from NES characterized by loss of awareness is relatively easy. Again, simultaneous video recording greatly enhances diagnostic power.

DO PATIENTS WITH NONEPILEPTIC SEIZURES HAVE A TYPICAL PSYCHOLOGIC PROFILE?

Attempts to characterize psychologic profiles of patients with NES have met with limited success. Perhaps the most consistent results have been derived from the application of the Minnesota Multiphasic Personality Inventory (MMPI). In particular, Dodrill[4] has reported that MMPI profiles differ between patients with epilepsy and those with NES. The typical findings in many NES patients are relatively high scores on the hysteria and hypochondriasis scales with a lower score on the depression scale. These characteristics differentiated NES from epilepsy in about 80% of cases.[4] Thus, the MMPI offers useful information but cannot be said to have sufficient power for diagnostic certainty. The results of psychologic testing, therefore, must be taken in concert with the results of other testing and must be considered supportive or nonsupportive of the diagnosis of NES.

WHAT ARE THE MOST COMMON PSYCHIATRIC DIAGNOSES ASSOCIATED WITH NONEPILEPTIC SEIZURES?

NES is classified as a conversion disorder in the *Diagnostic and Statistical Manual of Mental Disorders, 4th Edition* (DSM–IV)[5]. Conversion disorder is included in the broader category of somatoform disorders. Essentially, the patient exhibits symptoms suggestive of a neurologic or other general medical condition, preceded by conflicts or other stressors. The symptom is not feigned, and appropriate investigations fail to reveal evidence of a causative organic condition. The symptoms cause significant distress and interfere with the patient's general functioning. In some patients, NESs are part of a symptom complex subsumed under the rubric *somatization disorder*. In this condition the patient has a pattern of recurring multiple and significant somatic complaints beginning before the age of 30, extending for a prolonged period, sometimes many years.

Patients with NES also suffer from associated psychiatric disorders; in fact, more than one condition is often present. Anxiety disorders are commonly encountered, often unrecognized by patient or physician. In particular, many patients fulfill DSM–IV diagnostic criteria for panic disorder, with or without agoraphobia. The symptom complex of NES may be due solely to panic attacks, or the attacks may coexist with NES. Careful inquiry is essential in order to establish the diagnosis.

Depression is often seen in patients with NES. In some, it has been proposed that the pain of depression has been unrecognized or unaddressed by family or others. As a result, the development of NES may constitute a mechanism for bringing the patient's problems to the attention of the medical profession.

Psychosis such as schizophrenia is considered an uncommon accompaniment of NES, although it may be seen. Other conditions, even more infrequent, include malingering and factitious disorder.

A detailed psychiatric interview will usually bring out any associated psychiatric disorders. In some cases, however, application of the Structured Clinical Interview for DSM–IV (SCID) may be required to determine the number and extent of the patient's problems.

WHAT IS THE BEST APPROACH TO TREATMENT?

Unfortunately, neurologists usually have little interest in continuing to care for patients in whom NESs are diagnosed, considering these patients not to have neurologic disease. The problem is compounded by the fact that many psychiatrists are reluctant to take on patients with somatoform disorders. This reluctance represents a problem for these patients, who suffer from significant disability. When a psychiatrist is found who is willing to work with patients with NES, he or she should cooperate closely with the referring neurologist. The patient thus gains by receiving continuing support on the medical side while exploring the root causes of the psychiatric disability.

Probably the best approach to treatment for most patients is offered by a multidisciplinary team composed of specialists in the fields of neurology, psychiatry, psychology, and social work. Such a group addresses the multidimensional nature of NES including, in addition to diagnosis and management of the underlying psychiatric condition, problems of psychosocial functioning, occupational issues, and family interactions. Key to the team approach is a coordination of efforts in these several spheres, with the goal of restoring the patient to normal functioning in the shortest possible time.

The team approach can be carried out either on an inpatient or outpatient basis. In both cases the goals are the same. Inpatient programs are usually associated with epilepsy centers, two of the better known being located in Minneapolis and St. Paul, Minnesota. The major advantage to the inpatient approach is the intensity and focus that is possible at the onset of treatment. A major disadvantage, however, is the cost associated with hospitalization. The outpatient approach, as practiced at Mount Sinai in New York, is less intense but cost-effective. In the long run the two approaches probably produce similar outcomes. In the case of inpatient treatment, the patient is referred, on discharge, to a local psychiatrist, who carries out longer-term intervention. The outpatient approach combines regular team meetings with ongoing therapy. The principal therapist may be the psychiatrist, psychologist, or social worker, depending on the nature and extent of the patient's particular problem.

Clearly, each patient with NES requires an individualized treatment program. Those with significant depression may be treated with antidepressants along with ongoing psychotherapy. Patients with panic disorder may receive appropriate pharmacotherapy with an agent such as desipramine. Some will require only short-term psychotherapy. In those patients with somatoform disorder, supportive treatment and encouragement can aid overall functioning and bring to a halt "doctor shopping" for multiple somatic complaints. In the latter group, however, NESs are likely to continue.

WHAT IS THE OUTLOOK FOR PATIENTS WITH NONEPILEPTIC SEIZURES?

In general, the prognosis for patients with NES is favorable. Even without specific treatment, NESs tend to decline over time. A 1-year follow-up study of 80 patients in whom NESs were diagnosed during EEG–video monitoring revealed that 59% had become seizure-free in the interval, whereas an additional 20% reported a decline in event frequency. The literature is sparse with respect to the effectiveness of psychotherapy; but improvement in 60–90% of patients has been reported. Success rates appear to depend on the severity and duration of the psychiatric illness. Those with NES of relatively short duration, perhaps related to an intercurrent situation such as an acute loss, have a favorable prognosis. Indeed, short-term psychotherapy may be highly effective in these cases. On the other hand, prolonged duration of NES associated with severe psychopathology may be refractory to treatment. In these cases, supportive treatment may be all that can be offered. In any case, an optimistic attitude on the part of the caregivers is important and indeed justified; this should be conveyed to the patient at the outset and continually reinforced.

REFERENCES

1. Ramsay RD, Cohen A, Brown MC. Coexisting epilepsy and non-epileptic seizures. In: Rowan AJ, Gates JR, eds. *Non-Epileptic Seizures*. Boston: Butterworth–Heinemann; 1993:47–54.
2. French JA. The use of suggestion as a provocative test in the diagnosis of psychogenic non-epileptic seizures. In: Rowan AJ, Gates JR, eds. *Non-Epileptic Seizures*. Boston: Butterworth–Heinemann; 1993:101–109.
3. Pritchard PB. The role of prolactin in the diagnosis of non-epileptic seizures. In: Rowan AJ, Gates JR, eds. *Non-Epileptic Seizures*. Boston: Butterworth–Heinemann; 1993:93–100.
4. Dodrill CB, Wilkus RJ, Batzel LW. The MMPI as a diagnostic tool in non-epileptic seizures. In: Rowan AJ, Gates JR, eds. *Non-Epileptic Seizures*. Boston: Butterworth–Heinemann; 1993:211–219.
5. *Diagnostic and Statistical Manual of Mental Disorders,* 4th edition. Washington, DC: American Psychiatric Association; 1994:452.

CHAPTER 10

Ambulatory Electroencephalographic Monitoring
Technology and Uses

John R. Ives, B.Sc.

WHAT IS THE HISTORY OF AMBULATORY ELECTROENCEPHALOGRAPHIC MONITORING?

The first ambulatory electroencephalographic (EEG) recording on a patient with epilepsy was accomplished in the fall of 1973 by adding small neck-mounted EEG preamplifiers to a 4-channel, 24-hour continuous electrocardiogram (ECG) cassette recording device developed in the United Kingdom by Oxford Medilog Systems Inc.[1,2] This continuous EEG recording approach was pursued by Oxford Medilog, which developed an 8-channel system coupled with a scanning replay unit in the early 1980s. Before ambulatory monitoring, technical and methodologic advances were made in inpatient invasive (phase II) long-term monitoring (LTM) with the development of a 16-channel computer-based event recording system in the early 1970s for use with inpatients who were being evaluated with depth electrodes.[3] The innovative use of a buffer–delay memory system based on event monitoring with push-button capture of the clinical episode has now become the standard method for evaluating patients who are having surface (phase I) monitoring.[4] This efficient and successful design, along with the principle of event monitoring, was also used eventually for ambulatory and home monitoring upon the introduction of an event-based 16-channel ambulatory cassette recorder in the late 1980s.[5] As the power of computers increased, the events that could be monitored and automatically detected and recorded also expanded from interictal spikes and sharp waves to electrographic seizures. The continuous ambulatory recording technique has not evolved beyond 8 channels, unless two 8-channel systems are awkwardly worn together, whereas ambulatory event monitoring has continued to evolve from 16 to 18 and then 27 channels.[6-8] This evolution has been made possible by incorporating small, low-powered digital computer systems into the devices.

HOW DID THE EVENT RECORDING SYSTEM EVOLVE?

The first 16-channel ambulatory event system, referred to as "A1–A2," used a standard commercial "walkman" stereo cassette recorder as a permanent analog

The Comprehensive Evaluation and Treatment of Epilepsy
Copyright © 1997 by Academic Press. All rights of reproduction in any form reserved.

storage of the patient's EEG events.[5] Initially the memory capacity of the available low-powered static ram memory (SRAM) delay buffer was only 20 s. As this computer industry-driven SRAM technology expanded in capacity, eventually a clinically acceptable 2-min delay was possible. Finally, the SRAM capacity on board the waist-worn recorder allowed not only delay storage but also permanent storage of the events as well. This advance permitted replacement of the analog, mechanical cassette storage mechanism with a solid-state device in the form of a waist-worn recorder. As much as 16 megabytes of SRAM can be installed in the battery-operated waist-worn recorder, which can be used either to extend the amount of data captured to over 80 min (when the 18-channel system is being used) or to extend the channel coverage to 27 channels.

The waist-worn ambulatory recording system is supplemented by a toaster-sized dedicated computer that the patient takes home and connects to when convenient, particularly at night before going to sleep.[9] This "home computer" is a stand-alone, turnkey device that runs a version of the original spike-and-seizure-detection software that evolved from a relationship between Gotman and Telefactor. The current device is responsible for capturing four types of events: redundant push-button events, background samples, spikes, and electrographic seizures. These events are recorded on an internal hard drive, allowing for their recovery back at the laboratory into a host computer system, where further analysis, laser printing, and archiving are performed. This automatic detection device,[10,11] first developed in the mid-1980s, evolved from the original Digital PDP-12 room-sized computer,[3] first to a more transportable Digital PDP-45, and then to an IBM clone portable. Finally, a dedicated single-board 80186 microcomputer system, without any of the usual computer accessories such as display, keyboard, and diskette, was designed and built. Newer models have more than 0.5 to 2 gigabytes of hard disc storage and can be equipped with the fastest 80486 boards, if necessary, so that the ambulatory systems can emulate any in-hospital–based system.

HOW DOES AN AMBULATORY EEG MONITORING SYSTEM DIFFER FROM AN INPATIENT SYSTEM?

Designing and developing a system that is battery-operated, ambulatory, and unattended presents a number of engineering challenges. Essentially, an outpatient system has a subset of the features and functions of a line-voltage-supplied, attended, hospital-based EEG monitoring system. Examples of this are fewer channels (i.e., 8 to 27 as compared with 16 to 128) and no video coverage in the outpatient–home environment (but see discussion later in this chapter on future developments).

On the other hand, the more demanding home environment has promoted innovations that are beneficial to high-quality EEG recordings in general. An example is the development of bipolar-based, low-current, small, low-weight, battery-operated amplifiers that can be placed directly and comfortably on the patient's head. Placement on the head significantly reduces the amount of movement artifact, particularly during seizures. A bipolar amplifier has advantages of size and weight over an equivalent referential-based amplifier. Traditionally, the referential-based system had the advantage of being remontageable, but was always considered inappropriate for ambulatory unattended recordings, where the loss of the reference electrode during an ambulatory recording would adversely affect the quality of the total EEG recording. More recently, a method of remontaging from a specific bipolar montage has been developed.[12] This simple technique permits any other montage to be generated while indicating whether the process of remontaging is valid. If the process is not valid, one can still easily read the original "raw" bipolar EEG. Thus, ambulatory bipolar recordings can continue using a method that is superior in the harsher home environment but at the same time capable of being remontaged, similar to referential-based systems.

In the EEG shown in Figure 10.1A, a seizure has been recorded with the 27-channel system. In this case, some obscurity by muscle artifact was reduced by digital filtering, as shown in Figure 10.1B.[13,14] Because this is a 27-channel bipolar montage, it can be remontaged to any other montage. As seen in Figure 10.1C, the last channel has been used to represent the "error function," which is related to residual nonlinearities errors generated by mathematical subtraction of channels from each other. Because this channel is relatively flat, one is fairly confident that remontaging can be accomplished accurately. Unlike referential-based recordings, there is no "error function"; therefore, one does not know if remontaging from a referential-based raw EEG is valid or not. In the bipolar situation, if the "error signal" indicated problems, one could simply read the raw EEG as in Figures 10.1A and B. As it is, reading a bipolar montage is less a problem than reading a raw referential-based EEG, particularly during a seizure. Figure 10.1C illustrates this same seizure remontaged into a referential-based EEG, and as users of referential-based systems can appreciate, once a common reference-based EEG is obtained, any other montage can be realized.

WHAT ARE THE CLINICAL APPLICATIONS OF AMBULATORY MONITORING?

In our adult EEG laboratory, over one-third of all the EEGs performed are telemetries of one form or another. Of these 1200 telemetries, over 400 of them are done in the outpatient environment. We use the ambulatory telemetry equipment ubiquitously in many situations where the advantages of telemetry techniques are beneficial either to the efficient capture of relevant EEG information or to save on internal logistics. The majority of outpatient monitoring is done on patients for differential diagnostic purposes where the patient is having several events per week that may be more subjective than clinical. We have found that outpatient monitoring does not change the spontaneous frequency pattern of the patient's events as does hospitalization; therefore, in many cases the event yield in the outpatient environment is higher than that in the inpatient one.[15]

Because there is no difference in the equipment used in inpatient and outpatient monitoring, the methodology can be shifted without loss of quality from one environment to the other based on the clinical situation. This approach also makes it easy on the EEG technologist, because he or she needs only to learn one procedure, as well as on the electroencephalographer, who has only to get used to reading one medium.

HOW EFFECTIVE IS AMBULATORY OUTPATIENT EEG MONITORING?

The effectiveness of ambulatory outpatient monitoring is best illustrated by the following clinical example. A patient with intractable epilepsy was monitored as an inpatient for 14 days without recording any seizures despite the withdrawal of anticonvulsant medication. He was finally discharged back on medication, but told to call as soon as he had his first seizure, because he had a history of clustering. When he called, we hooked him up to the ambulatory system again with sphenoidal electrodes[16] and sent him home. The next day when he returned, he reported having two clinical seizures for which he pushed the event button (Fig. 10.2A). After evaluating the data, we also found one automatically detected seizure that was the same as the two clinical seizures. The system also captured many epileptic spikes (Fig. 10.2B) that were similar to those obtained during his hospital stay.

As stated earlier, ambulatory outpatient monitoring of surgical candidates has a role to play because it can efficiently record their 18 to 27 channel EEG (including sphenoidals) with the same qualities as any inpatient monitoring system.[17]

Figure 10.1   (A, p. 189) A 27-channel bipolar recording during the patient's seizure. The replay bandwidth is 100 Hz and thus the predominant marker of the seizure is initially some eye blinking followed by an obscuring buildup of muscle activity. The montage is a coronal sphenoidal (1–7), an EOG channel (8), then an A–P temporal left–right chain (9–12, 13–16). The last channels chain in the parasaggital, central, and T1–T2 electrodes into the original coronal chain (17–20, 21–22, 23–24). Finally a single channel of EKG is recorded, whereas the last two channels are unused. (B, p. 190) The same seizure shown in (A) has now been digitally filtered at 15 Hz. This now reveals the underlying slower rhythmic EEG activity. (C, p. 191) The same seizure of (A) and (B) has been remontaged; the last channel now provides an analog representation of the "error function" whose flatness indicates valid reconstruction, whereas large excursions indicate "error" or nonlinearities in the result. In this case the "error function" is relatively flat, indicating that the reading of the remontaged EEG is valid.

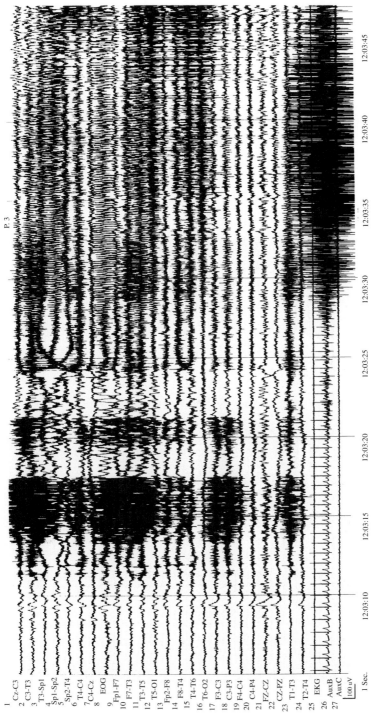

A

P. 3

1 Cz-C3
2 C3-T3
3 T3-Sp1
4 Sp1-Sp2
5 Sp2-T4
6 T4-C4
7 C4-Cz
8 EOG
9 Fp1-F7
10 F7-T3
11 T3-T5
12 T5-O1
13 Fp2-F8
14 F8-T4
15 T4-T6
16 T6-O2
17 F3-C3
18 C3-P3
19 F4-C4
20 C4-P4
21 FZ-CZ
22 CZ-PZ
23 T1-T3
24 T2-T4
25 EKG
26 AuxB
27 AuxC

1 Sec.

100 uV

12:03:10   12:03:15   12:03:20   12:03:25   12:03:30   12:03:35   12:03:40   12:03:45

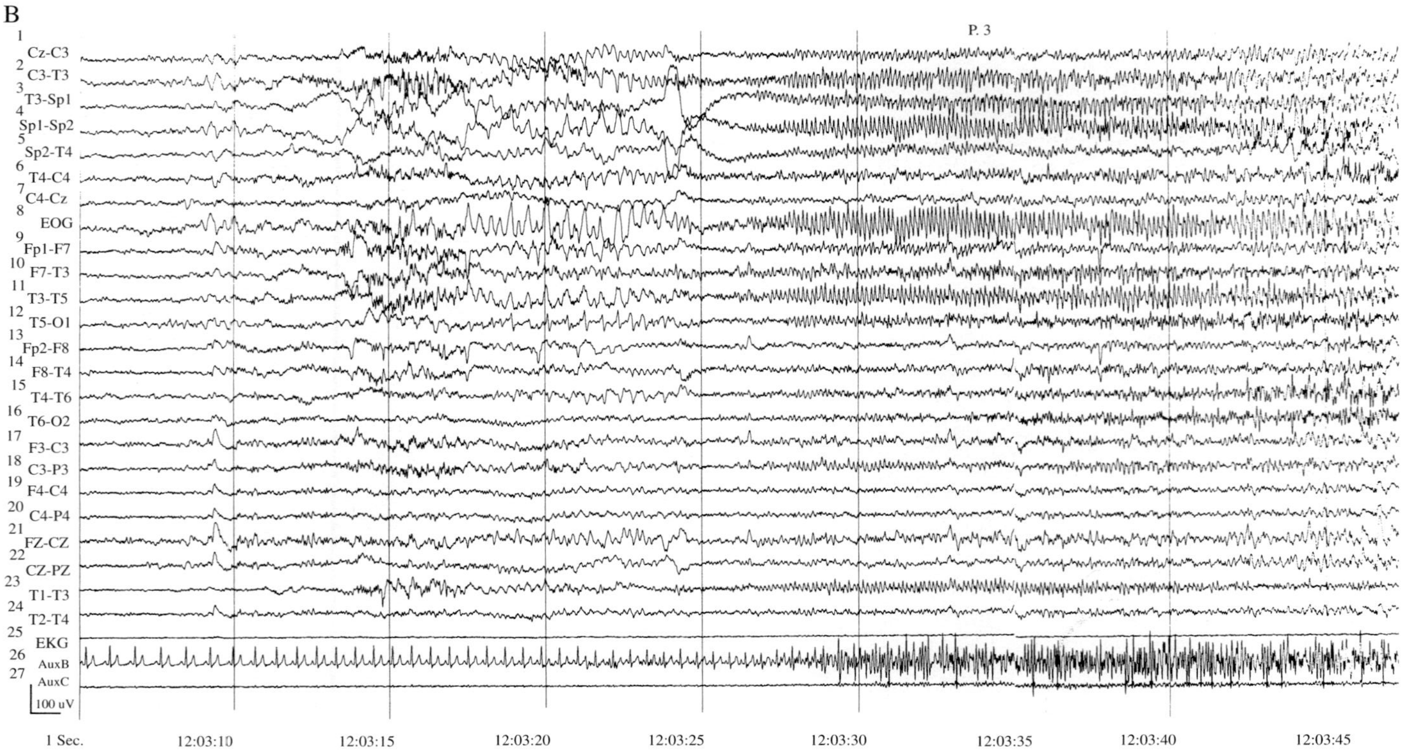

Figure 10.1 (*Continued*)

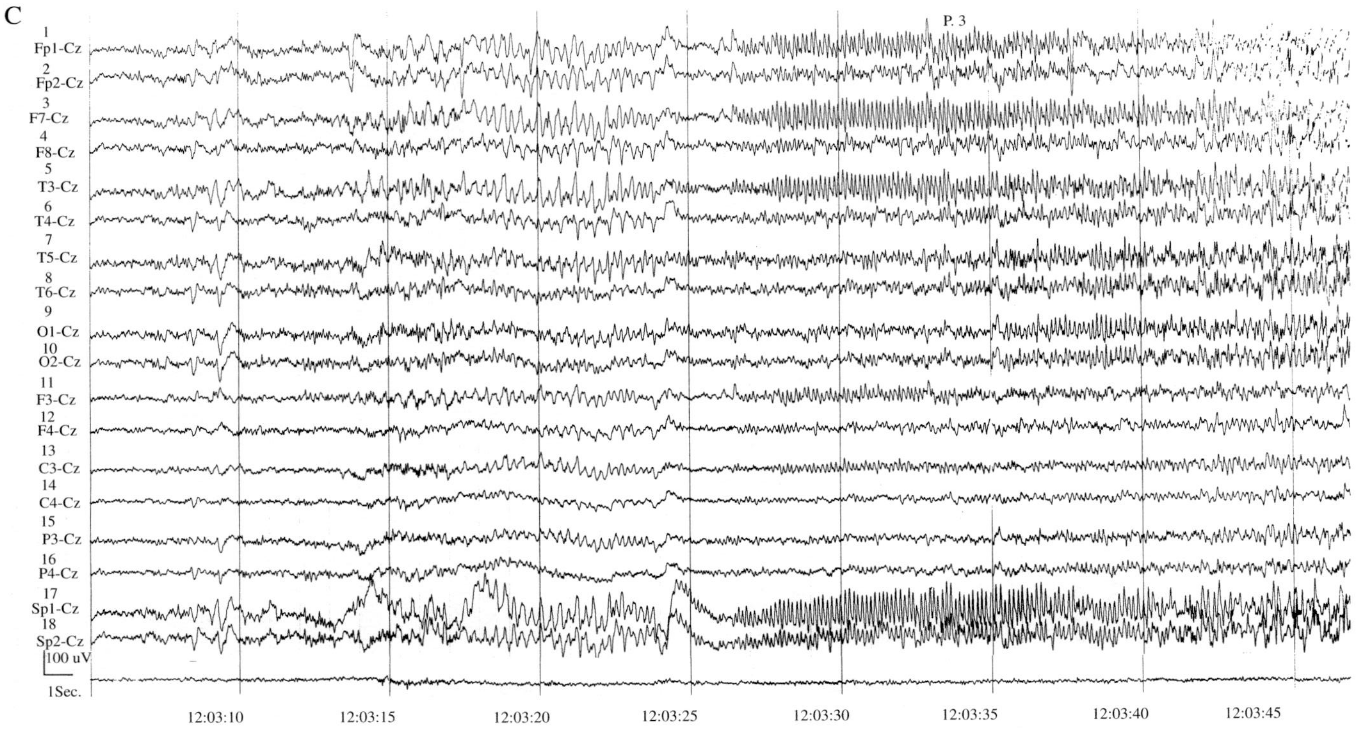

C

1 Fp1-Cz
2 Fp2-Cz
3 F7-Cz
4 F8-Cz
5 T3-Cz
6 T4-Cz
7 T5-Cz
8 T6-Cz
9 O1-Cz
10 O2-Cz
11 F3-Cz
12 F4-Cz
13 C3-Cz
14 C4-Cz
15 P3-Cz
16 P4-Cz
17 Sp1-Cz
18 Sp2-Cz

$\boxed{100 \text{ uV}}$

1 Sec.

P. 3

12:03:10   12:03:15   12:03:20   12:03:25   12:03:30   12:03:35   12:03:40   12:03:45

Figure 10.1 (*Continued*)

191

Patients need to be more carefully selected in this situation, and ambulatory outpatient monitoring is not appropriate for some patients and clinical circumstances. If video is not essential and the patient is aware of his events, or if there is a responsible person capable and willing to be with the patient all the time to push the button, then ambulatory outpatient monitoring will be appropriate and successful. In a situation in which the patient is not aware of his or her events, has no companion, and there is confusion about the description of the events, the inpatient environment with video is the best place to monitor the patient.

As more centers use digital, computer-based ambulatory monitoring, the scope and uses of this relatively new technique will be better delineated.[18] Some centers are already optimistic about its performance, particularly its potential use with pediatric patients.[19,20] To date, experience using this technique with children has been limited.

WHAT ADVANCES IN AMBULATORY OUTPATIENT EEG MONITORING CAN BE EXPECTED IN THE FUTURE?

VIDEO

In the past, video or clinical coverage has relied on continuous recording of the video image. This has been either accomplished by one 8-h tape being changed every 8 h, or by using three VCRs that automatically switch from one to the other. As the cable and TV industries evolve into digital video, this technique can be used by the EEG monitoring field. Already some investigators[21] as well as some long-term monitoring companies have either talked about or demonstrated early units (DigiTrace, NCS, Nicole/BMS, Telefactor). The significant data rate generated by digital video (up to 230 Mbytes/min) is overwhelming, but by again using an event-type approach with a significant delay or buffer, coupled with data compression techniques, the data flow can be contained in manageable sections. The analog and mechanical VCR are the last components of LTM that are unreliable because of their moving parts, so the future will see the elimination and improved reliability of this aspect. As in the past, once established in the hospital

---

Figure 10.2   (A, p. 193) One of two clinical seizures captured when the patient activated his "event" push button. A similar electrographic seizure was also automatically captured as well. This example also demonstrates the localization importance of the sphenoidal electrodes as well as their relative stability even in the ambulatory outpatient environment. (B, p. 194) The interictal spikes automatically captured on this patient during the same ambulatory outpatient recording session.

A

1 Cz-C3
2 C3-T3
3 T3-Sp1
4 Sp1-Sp2
5 Sp2-T4
6 T4-C4
7 C4-Cz
8 EOG
9 Fp1-F7
10 F7-T3
11 T3-T5
12 T5-O1
13 Fp2-F8
14 F8-T4
15 T4-T6
16 T6-O2
17 AuxA
18 AuxB

1 Sec.

100 UV

22:28:38   22:28:43   22:28:48   22:28:53   22:28:58   22:29:03

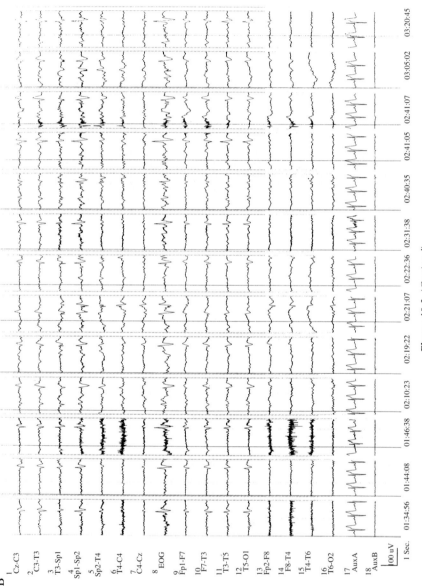

Figure 10.2 (*Continued*)

environment, miniaturization will enable a digital video system to go home with patients. In the interim, a continuous time-lapse system (10 frames/s) has been developed that integrates the EEG data acquisition and video by time locking the systems with a common clock. This unit is entering clinical trials and because of its integration and "turn-key" approach, it is demonstrating that it is an efficient and reliable approach to outpatient video–EEG monitoring.[22]

AMBULATORY OUTPATIENT MONITORING—THE FUTURE

With the digitization and establishment of a reliable, high quality ambulatory-based system with capabilities of 18 to 27 channels, coupled with the cost containment theme in the health care field, the use of ambulatory outpatient monitoring will continue to expand significantly in the future. As microcomputers become smaller and more integrated, with lower power consumption but with increased capabilities, the detection functionality and storage capacity of the toaster-sized take-home or bedside computer will migrate to the battery-operated waist-worn device.

Since the capital cost of a state-of-the-art EEG–video monitoring unit can be on the order of U.S. $100,000–$150,000 per patient-bed, these facilities will be reserved for selected patients who meet specific criteria to warrant hospitalization. A significant number of patients or a significant number of the person's monitoring days will be performed on an outpatient basis.

REFERENCES

1. Ives JR, Woods JF. 4-channel 24-hour cassette recorder for long term EEG monitoring of ambulatory patients. *Electroencephalogr Clin Neurophysiol*. 1975;39:88–92.
2. Marson GB, McKinnon JB. A miniature tape recorder for many applications. *Control Instrumentation*. 1972;4:46–47.
3. Ives JR, Thompson CJ, Gloor P. Seizure monitoring: A new tool in electroencephalography. *Electroencephalogr Clin Neurophysiol*. 1976;41:422–427.
4. Engel J Jr, Ebersole JS, Burchfiel JL, et al. Guidelines for long-term neurodiagnostic monitoring in epilepsy. *J Clin Neurophysiol*. 1985;2:419–452.
5. Ives JR. A completely ambulatory 16-channel cassette recording system. In: Stefano H, Burr W, eds. *EEG Monitoring*. Stuttgart: Gustav Fischer; 1982:205–217.
6. Stores G, Hennion T, Quy RJ. EEG ambulatory monitoring system with visual playback display. In: Woods JA, Penry JK, eds. *Advances in Epileptology, the Xth Epilepsy International Symposium*. New York: Raven Press; 1980:89–94.
7. Ives JR, Mainwaring NR, Schomer DL. An 18-channel solid-state ambulatory event recorder for use in the home and hospital environment. *Epilepsia*. 1992;33:63A.
8. Ives JR, Mainwaring NR, Gruber LJ, et al. A 27-channel bipolar based ambulatory EEG event recording system with remontaging capabilities. *Epilepsia*. 1993;34:81A.

9. Ives JR, Mainwaring NR, Gruber LJ, *et al.* Home computing: A remote intelligent EEG data acquisition unit for monitoring epileptic patients in the home environment. *Electroencephalogr Clin Neurophysiol.* 1988;69:49A.

10. Gotman J, Gloor P. Automatic recognition and quantification of interictal epileptic activity in the human scalp EEG. *Electroencephalogr Clin Neurophysiol.* 1976;41:513–529.

11. Gotman J. Automatic recognition of epileptic seizures in the EEG. *Electroencephalogr Clin Neurophysiol.* 1982;54:531–540.

12. Ives JR, Mainwaring NR, Gruber LJ, *et al.* Remontaging from bipolar recordings: A better way? *Muscle & Nerve.* 1993;16:1125–1126.

13. Gotman J, Ives JR, Gloor P. Frequency content of EEG and EMG at seizure onset: Possibility of removal of EMG artifact by digital filtering. *Electroencephalogr Clin Neurophysiol.* 1981;52:626–639.

14. Ives JR, Schomer DL. A 6-pole filter for improving the readability of muscle contaminated EEG. *Electroencephalogr Clin Neurophysiol.* 1988;69:486–490.

15. Riley TL, Porter RJ, White BG, *et al.* The hospital experience and seizure control. *Neurology.* 1981;31:921–915.

16. Ives JR, Gloor P. New sphenoidal electrode assembly to permit long-term monitoring of the patient's ictal and interictal EEG. *Electroencephalogr Clin Neurophysiol.* 1977;42:575–580.

17. Ives JR, Schomer DL, Blume HW. Pre-surgical evaluation using cassette EEG. In: Ebersole J, ed. *Ambulatory EEG Monitoring.* New York: Raven Press; 1989:195–216.

18. Morris GL, Galezowska J, Leroy R, *et al.* The results of computer-assisted ambulatory 16-channel EEG. *Electroencephalogr Clin Neurophysiol.* 1994;91:229–231.

19. Miles DK, Foley CM, Legido WD, *et al.* A comparative study of the efficacy of in-patient video-EEG and computerized out-patient longterm monitoring in a pediatric population. *Epilepsia.* 1994;35:48A.

20. Foley CM, Miles DK, Chandler D, *et al.* Role of computerized out-patient long-term EEG monitoring (CO-LTM) in the diagnosis and treatment of pediatric epilepsy. *Epilepsia.* 1994;35:147A.

21. Rector D, Burk P, Harper RM. A data acquisition system for long-term monitoring of physiological and video signals. *Electroencephalogr Clin Neurophysiol.* 1993;87:380–384.

22. Ives JR, Ives JD, Schomer DL. Home audio/video/EEG monitoring. *Epilepsia* (in press).

23. Ives JR, Mainwaring NR, Gruber LJ, *et al.* 128-channel cable-telemetry EEG recording system for long-term invasive monitoring. *Electroencephalogr Clin Neurophysiol.* 1991;9:69–72.

CHAPTER 11

The Surgical Treatment of Epilepsy

Howard Blume, M.D., Ph.D.

WHO IS A CANDIDATE FOR EPILEPSY SURGERY?

Appropriate candidates for epilepsy surgery have seizures that are not adequately controlled by medications and that are of such frequency, severity, or both, that they significantly interfere with the patients' lifestyles. The patient's perception of the severity of his or her epilepsy is a key determinant in the decision to operate. The process of evaluation and the experience of undergoing surgery are not easy for patients or their families, but the risks are low and the surgical outcome statistics are sufficiently favorable to weigh seriously the surgical option for patients who have repeated seizures. These patients can complete medication trials within 2–3 years and, if antiepileptic drug (AED) therapy proves unsuccessful, they can be evaluated for possible surgery (see also Chapter 5 for psychosocial considerations).

HOW DO SURGEONS KNOW THAT LOBECTOMY WILL HELP TO CONTROL OR ELIMINATE SEIZURES?

Electroencephalographic (EEG) data are the basis for determining the site of origin within the brain of a patient's seizures. Ideally, scalp electrode recordings, possibly including sphenoidal electrodes, obtained through telemetry will reveal a consistent origin of the seizures (see Chapter 10). If the seizures clearly arise from different sides of the brain on separate occasions, lobectomy is not likely to be of help. In these cases, successful removal of the "most active" or "worst" brain lobe often leads to increased seizure activity from the remaining site of seizure origin and no overall improvement in seizure incidence. Also, if the EEG data depict a generalized form of epilepsy onset, lobectomy will not be helpful.

Patients with generalized forms of epilepsy may be helped by sectioning of the corpus callosum, particularly if they have atonic seizures ("drop attacks"). If the scalp EEG data are ambiguous regarding the side or precise lobe of seizure onset, implanted electrodes may be necessary (see text that follows). Stereotaxic depth electrodes or grid electrodes with subdural strip electrodes may be placed

The Comprehensive Evaluation and Treatment of Epilepsy
Copyright © 1997 by Academic Press. All rights of reproduction in any form reserved.

to more precisely record seizure onset; these special electrodes are physically closer to the cortex than scalp and sphenoidal electrodes.

Regardless of whether scalp or invasive recording electrodes are used to record seizure onset and the pattern of seizure spread, after the accumulated data have shown that the area of seizure onset is consistently and repeatedly from the same portion of one of the frontal or temporal lobes, and it is further determined that the implicated lobe can be safely removed without affecting speech or fine sensory or motor cortical function, surgical intervention may be performed with a high probability of improvement. Intraoperative EEG recording before and after the cortical excision may further indicate the likelihood of success; a recording of active epileptiform activity in areas of the brain not operated on suggests a slightly less favorable situation than a postexcision recording that is free from epileptic discharges.

Magnetic resonance imaging (MRI) scans, positron emission tomography (PET) scans, and single photon emission tomography (SPECT) scans are all valuable in supporting the EEG data, particularly when they provide localizing information that correlates with the EEG findings (see Chapter 2). However, the static and dynamic information derived from these tests is perhaps most valuable in pointing to a possible conflict with the localization of seizure onset suggested by the scalp EEG data. For example, a lesion or an area of agenesis or atrophy visible on MRI may signal a possible false EEG localization if the ictal EEG shows seizure onset arising from the opposite side. Further EEG evaluation, perhaps with implanted electrodes, would then be advisable.

HOW IS A CORTICAL EXCISION PERFORMED?

The basic approach to excision of epileptogenic tissue is to coagulate the surface or pial vessels, sharply incise the pial membrane covering the cortex, and utilize fine suction or the Cavitron to cut through the tissue and define a resection line. The surgeon accomplishes these procedures by suctioning the cortex and white matter along the inner surface of the pial lining of the gyrus after making a sharp incision in the surface pia over a gyrus. In the frontal and temporal regions, it is important to keep the "pial barrier" as a protection over the main middle cerebral artery branches that course over the surface of the insula. Injury to or spasm of these vessels could lead to infarction of the frontoparietal cortex. The cranial nerves, brainstem itself, and major arteries of the circle of Willis are likewise protected from injury by leaving the medial pia as a protective structure and boundary. Various techniques may be used to tailor resection. When performing temporal lobectomies, some surgeons may choose to remove mainly medial temporal structures of the lower amygdala and hippocampus while leaving the lateral temporal lobe, a procedure that can be accomplished by making transcortical incisions down into the temporal horn of the lateral ventricle or by splitting the sylvian fissure. Most data suggest that leaving medial temporal structures while removing the lateral temporal lobe does not have as good an outcome as resections including the bulk of the hippocampus, even when specific lesions appear to involve only lateral temporal areas. Some neurosurgeons carry out the procedures with the patient under sedation but able to be easily awakened, using information gained from cortical mapping and intraoperative EEG recordings to decide precisely which areas to remove. Further recordings are sometimes made after initial removal of cortical tissue. Other neurosurgeons carry out a standard lobectomy, excising a defined amount of tissue without using intraoperative recordings and with the patient under general anesthesia.

HOW MUCH BRAIN TISSUE SHOULD BE REMOVED?

The main goal in performing cortical excisions is to remove as much of the epileptogenic tissue as possible without disturbing normal brain function. To achieve this goal, the surgeon must restrict the total amount of tissue removed. In both frontal and temporal brain tissue removals, the preservation of speech function often restricts the extent of removal, especially from the speech-dominant hemisphere. The area of speech function nearly always lies behind the rolandic fissure. In general, a safe margin of resection in temporal tissue removal is half a gyrus behind the rolandic fissure. The exact dimensions vary with each patient, many epilepsy patients having fairly small anterior temporal lobes on the affected side. The rolandic fissure usually lies about 5 cm from the anterior temporal tip, so that approximately 2 in., or 5 cm, of tissue is removed in a standard resection. Speech areas may be mapped out more fully with cortical stimulation and functional MRI. The frontal speech area, or Broca's area, is somewhat variable in size and shape but generally is a triangular-shaped gyrus along the base of the skull several gyri anterior to the rolandic fissure. This area, too, can often be mapped out by functional MRI or stimulation of the cortex during surgery. The supplementary motor speech area just anterior to the motor strip in the most medial portion of the frontal lobe along the midline can be removed, but this procedure often causes temporary speech impairment. This supplementary motor speech area is also variable in its location. Frontal resections, then, must skirt around Broca's area and the supplementary motor speech area if at all possible, sparing connecting white matter pathways to these regions as well as the surface cortex of these areas.

It is important to spare the uppermost part of the amygdala in the medial portion of a temporal removal so as to avoid injury to the optic tract on that side. In that way, a contralateral complete homonymous field cut may be avoided. Generally, only the lower two-thirds of the amygdala is removed, although some surgeons have reported removing as much as four-fifths of the amygdala with careful attention to microdissection. Another type of visual dysfunction may arise if removal of superficial white matter of the temporal lobe extends back as far as 7 cm. This extent of excision causes an interruption in the optic radiations of the temporal lobe that sweep around the temporal horn en route to the lower occiput below the calcarine fissure, resulting in an upper quadrant visual field cut on the side opposite the surgical site. The farther back the extent of the removal, the greater the degree of quadrant field cut into the more central portion of the visual field. Causing a slight visual field quadrant defect is often acceptable in removing a lesion or epileptogenic region that is posteriorly located in the lateral temporal region. However, when only a more medial excision is required, microsurgical techniques allow utilization of a small anterior temporal lobectomy in which up to 3 cm of the hippocampus is removed medially, along with the lower portion of the amygdala, but extensive lateral white matter is not removed. This procedure, then, prevents visual field defects and can be accomplished by an angled anterior-to-posterior approach.

WHAT IS THE LIKELIHOOD OF SUCCESS IN ARRESTING OR REDUCING SEIZURE ACTIVITY WITH CORTICAL EXCISIONS OR LOBECTOMIES?

The statistics on the success of epilepsy surgery vary, largely because of the patient selection process and not because of differences in surgical techniques. If patients referred for surgery include only those with well-localized, discrete epileptogenic areas of the anterior temporal lobe, seizure activity can be totally arrested in a high percentage of cases. If surgery is performed on patients who have more widespread epileptogenic brain areas, the percentage will be lower. Most centers are now reporting that 70–80% of patients undergoing temporal lobectomies have a marked reduction in seizures. Because frontal lobe epilepsy tends to involve more widespread brain regions than other types of epilepsy, successful lobectomy is more difficult to achieve in patients with frontal lobe onset seizures. The results of frontal lobectomy are less significant statistically because relatively few such procedures are performed in epilepsy surgery centers. However, frontal lobe removals produce total arrest of seizures in 30–40% of cases in most series.

WHAT ARE THE POSSIBLE COMPLICATIONS OF SURGERY?

Infection is the most frequent complication of epilepsy surgery, as it is for all operative procedures. The rate of infection is in the 1–2% range. Intraoperative or postoperative hemorrhage leading to severe deficits in speech or motor function or even to severe brain injury, coma, or death is extremely rare but not outside the realm of possibility when an intracranial procedure is carried out. Transient speech deficits can occur if the removal comes near speech areas or speech pathways. The risk of a permanent speech deficit, even with fine testing, is low as long as the guidelines for removal are followed. Loss of recent memory function, particularly for verbal material in dominant-side procedures and nonverbal material for nondominant-side procedures, for a few months to a year or more after surgical intervention is not infrequent. The results of long-term follow-up studies by precise cognitive testing indicate that the changes in function are fairly minimal in most patients. In contrast, the memory and speech functions of many patients are impaired by ongoing seizure discharges, so that many series demonstrate improvement in cognitive functioning after successful arrest of seizures by surgery. The loss of vision in a quadrant or a complete homonymous hemianopsia is a risk of surgery but an extremely low one if regular guidelines are followed.

WILL A PERSON WHO UNDERGOES LOBECTOMY FOR SEIZURES BE "DIFFERENT" AFTER SURGERY?

The uniqueness of the patient's personality and brain function characteristics are not changed by lobectomy. However, any problems the patient may have had in the past with depression or other emotional disturbances may recur and, in fact, be magnified in the early postoperative phase. In addition, it has been well documented that some patients whose seizures are successfully arrested have difficulty in adjusting to their new state and their new relationships to their family and to society as a whole. In some patients, this period of adjustment is so difficult that they require considerable support from their families and from a psychiatrist or psychologist for up to a year or more after surgery. For about 6 weeks to 6 months after surgery, most patients become easily fatigued and are often disturbed by crowds, noise, or activity around them. As is true of any patient who has had a brain injury or brain surgery, these patients may have difficulty performing sophisticated cognitive tasks, such as those required in a school environment, in the first 6–12 months after surgery; therefore, attempting challenging cognitive tasks is not usually advisable. Nevertheless, many patients who are employed can return to their previous work within 6–12 weeks after surgery as long as allowances are made for their limitations during the recovery process.

WHAT IS A HEMISPHERECTOMY?

Patients who have congenital hemiplegia and who lack development of one cerebral hemisphere may have broad areas of seizure discharges occurring almost continuously over one hemisphere, together with frequent intractable seizures. Some of these patients have seizure discharges that cross the corpus callosum to the opposite side, causing interferences in the function of the opposite hemisphere as well. Often, cognitive function in these patients, as well as normal fine movement in the foot and hand on the side opposite the affected hemisphere, is severely handicapped. However, as patients in whom this condition is congenital grow up, they become remarkably mobile despite their affected extremities. These patients will often experience dramatic improvement with removal of the atrophic or poorly developed cortex that is causing seizure discharges but is not critical for significant useful function. Formerly, the entire cortical mantle was removed. However, this technique tended to cause hemorrhaging into the large, empty removal cavity that became filled with spinal fluid after the cortical excision. This hemorrhaging could lead to sensorineural hearing loss as rising iron levels in the spinal fluid from the breakdown of blood gradually proved toxic to the eighth cranial nerve. Another complication was the occurrence of hydrocephaly in these patients. Current techniques entail sectioning through the white matter connections from the cortex to the opposite hemisphere and to the deeper brain structures while removing only the central frontal-parietal cortex and white matter. This method leaves minimal empty areas in the affected half of the cranium and eliminates the complications caused by excisions of all affected areas, but provides an equal degree of improvement. About 85–90% of these patients experience arrest of their seizures, accompanied in most cases by dramatic improvement in function, including further cognitive development. The risks are similar to those associated with any temporal lobe or frontal lobe resection.

WHAT IS A CALLOSOTOMY?

Callosal sectioning is interruption of the main white matter connections between hemispheres. Consisting of thick white matter, the corpus callosum is the most superior of the interhemispheric brain structures. Severing a part or all of this structure greatly reduces the spread of epileptic discharges from one hemisphere to the other and has the added benefit of halting or decreasing the frequency of "drop attacks" from certain types of generalized seizures. However, this procedure does not reduce partial seizures arising from either hemisphere.

In some centers, congenital hemiplegia and intractable epilepsy are treated with callosal sectioning. Although this procedure stops the spread of epileptic activity from the affected hemisphere into the other one, it does not tend to reduce the incidence of partial seizures nearly as well as the central excision and white matter sectioning of hemispherectomy. Callosal sectioning, then, is generally reserved for those patients who have generalized epilepsy with drop attacks; this procedure is effective in reducing seizure frequency in this selected population.

HOW IS CALLOSAL SECTIONING CARRIED OUT?

Callosal sectioning is often done in stages, the anterior one-third of the corpus callosum being sectioned initially and then, if necessary, the mid one-third sectioned in a second procedure. Generally, a craniotomy is performed adjacent to the midline and one hemisphere (generally the nondominant hemisphere) is gently retracted microsurgically to expose the corpus callosum lying between the two hemispheres. Suctioning and microsurgical instrumentation are used to section all the way through the corpus callosum. The surgeon must be sure to protect the underlying blood vessels and those on either side of the line of sectioning. After this procedure, the patient tends to neglect the nondominant extremities initially, but recovery usually occurs within a few weeks. If a second stage of surgery is carried out at the same time, neglect of the nondominant extremities is likely to be more profound, because the dominant hemisphere tends to send messages to the opposite hemisphere through the corpus callosum to give commands to the extremities on the dominant side. Other pathways of crossover do become more facile with time, allowing these commands to get across so as to permit normal function in a few weeks, as mentioned previously. Complete callosal sectioning can cause some permanent deficits such that, when the patient's eyes are closed, one side of the brain does not cooperate with the other even in simple tasks, with the result that the extremities of the right and left sides of the body may carry out conflicting movements. With eyes open, the patient can compensate for this problem.

The main complications associated with callosal sectioning are brain swelling from retraction of one hemisphere during the procedure, which causes local deficits or hemiparesis on the opposite side. In addition, hemorrhages into the spinal fluid or infarcts to underlying deep brain areas can occur, leading to coma or a vegetative state. These problems sometimes occurred in the early days of callosal sectioning, before the development of more modern techniques and advances in microsurgery. However, these complications are exceedingly rare.

WHAT ARE IMPLANTED EEG ELECTRODES?

As mentioned earlier, implanted EEG electrodes may be necessary to pinpoint the origin of epileptic seizures if scalp EEG recordings are inconsistent with other evaluations (such as MRI and neuropsychologic tests). These invasive electrodes are conductors placed inside the skull or brain that allow EEG recording from the surface of the brain or deep within the cortex. There are two main categories of implanted electrodes—subdural electrodes and stereotaxic depth electrodes. The first type of implanted electrode consists of a series of discs mounted in thin plastic and designed to lie on the surface of the cortex. These discs are often configured as linear strips consisting of a selected number of electrode contact points and are placed under the temporal or frontal lobes or along the medial surfaces of the hemispheres. Another arrangement is a grid composed of squares or rectangles, intended to cover large surface areas and to be placed over the cortical convexity surfaces after a craniotomy. Generally, strips are placed through small burr hole openings into the intracranial cavity. Some centers use only this latter configuration. Grid electrodes are used when there is a question about the site or lobe of origin of the seizures. Although grid electrodes were once placed on both sides in some instances, this practice required bilateral craniotomies, resulting in considerable morbidity. Today, there is probably no valid indication for this extreme practice.

Stereotaxic depth electrodes are the other main category of implanted electrodes. In the past, both rigid and flexible depth electrodes were used. Today, only flexible electrodes are employed. These fine plastic flexible electrodes are attached to wires that carry currents from deep and superficial brain structures. These currents are recorded through contact points mounted in the walls of the electrodes. Fine wires extending through the bores of the plastic electrodes are inserted with stylets placed in the bores. Stereotaxic depth electrodes are particularly helpful in determining the side of origin in temporal lobe epilepsy or, more commonly, in frontal lobe epilepsy in which the spread of abnormal discharges from one frontal lobe to the other is so rapid that the site or side of origin is difficult to ascertain. Various targets for the deepest contact points can be used but commonly include the cingulate gyrus, the subfrontal region, the amygdala, and several sites within the hippocampus. These electrodes are placed through stereotaxic techniques (see next section).

HOW ARE DEPTH ELECTRODES IMPLANTED?

A variety of techniques may be used to place depth electrodes. They may be placed from the convexity in angled trajectories from the surface of the skull, or they may be placed along the side of the head in trajectories that are all parallel if they are truly horizontal or perpendicular to the side of the skull. Generally, the patient is placed in a frame that is affixed to the skull with pins and then undergoes CT or MRI scanning of the head. Target sites for placing the electrodes are then selected using the scans of the head with reference to the frame. This technique allows calculations to be made that aid in placing the holes in the skull more precisely and in directing the implanted electrodes into the target area. Some centers use arteriography to visualize the blood vessels of the brain in conjunction with this frame, to try to ensure that the trajectories do not pass through areas where major blood vessels lie. At some centers, a local anesthetic plus a sedative is administered before these procedures are performed; at other centers, a general anesthetic is used. Computer-guided "frameless stereotaxy" can now be used with MRI of the brain and vasculature to place electrodes without fixing the head in a frame. After the electrodes are in place, they may be left there for a week or two, the wires projecting from under a dressing placed over the head. During that time, continuous telemetry is performed in an attempt to record the onset of a series of seizures. If necessary, medications may be tapered to try to increase the likelihood of seizures. In addition, both depth electrodes and grid electrodes can be use to stimulate the brain and to map out cortical and subcortical functions. In some cases, the stimulation of electrodes may trigger auras or seizures.

WHAT ARE THE RISKS OF IMPLANTING ELECTRODES?

The main risks associated with implanting electrodes are infection and hemorrhage. Passing electrode wires through the scalp creates a passageway through which spinal fluid may escape from the interior of the cranial cavity. That same passageway through the scalp can also allow bacteria to enter the head and cause an infection. The infection may take the form of meningitis or, more serious, a brain abscess. Brain abscesses may occur late, but their incidence is less than 1%.

Electrode placement can cause hemorrhaging on the surface or deep within the brain. Angiography may be used to circumvent this complication by guiding placement of the targets and pathways in areas where there are no major blood vessels. In reality, small implanted electrodes may push aside any major blood vessels in their path rather than perforate them, but significant intracerebral hemorrhages have been reported, although the incidence is 1% or less. Direct brain injury due to the passing of electrodes has not been demonstrated because the electrodes are so fine and normally push aside the neural tissue and do not penetrate or injure the neurons themselves.

CONCLUSION

Epilepsy surgery is an appropriate option for patients whose seizures are inadequately controlled by AEDs and are so frequent, severe, or both, thay they interfere significantly with their lifestyles. The surgical options are cortical excision or lobectomy, callosal sectioning, and hemispherectomy. In general, the success rate of epilepsy surgery is high, especially when the epileptogenic region is a discrete area within the anterior temporal lobe. With most surgical procedures used to treat epilepsy, the incidence of complications is low, usually between 1–2%.

REFERENCES

1. Engel J, ed. *Surgical Treatment of the Epilepsies, 2nd Ed.* New York: Raven Press; 1993.
2. Cascino GD. Surgical treatment of the epilepsies. In: Hopkins A, Shorvon S, Cascino G, eds. *Epilepsy, 2nd Ed.* London: Chapman & Hall Medical; 1995:221–242.
3. Wyllie E, ed. *The Treatment of Epilepsy: Principles and Practice.* Philadelphia: Lea and Fibiger; 1993.

CHAPTER 12

Endocrine Aspects of Partial Seizures

Pavel Klein, M.B., B.Chir., and Andrew G. Herzog, M.D., M.Sc.

HOW DO HORMONES AND EPILEPSY INTERACT?

Hormones affect seizures, and seizures affect hormonal regulation and secretion. Thyrotoxicosis, hyponatremia associated with the syndrome of inappropriate antidiuretic hormone secretion (SIADH), and hypoglycemia all lower seizure thresholds in epileptic patients and may trigger de novo situational seizures. These facts are noted in the standard medical textbooks and do not need to be discussed here. However, more subtle manifestations of hormonal influences on seizures and vice versa may easily be overlooked because they are not usually emphasized in the training of neurologists. Awareness of how different hormones relieve or exacerbate seizures may lead to improvement in the treatment of seizures with the use of adjunctive hormonal therapy. Seizure effects on hormonal physiology, for instance reproductive and sexual functioning, may result in significant impairment of the patient's life in addition to the effect of the seizures themselves—for instance infertility or impotence. Treatment of these complications may significantly improve the patient's life.

In women with epilepsy, the most commonly encountered endocrine problems relate to the effects of their gonadal steroids on seizures, as in the case of catamenial epilepsy; to the change in seizure expression during changes in endocrine status such as menarche, pregnancy, and menopause; and to the effect of seizures on endocrine reproductive function, such as ovulation and sexuality. In men with epilepsy, the most commonly encountered endocrine problem is altered sexuality, usually hyposexuality. In both men and women, seizures cause acute as well as chronic alterations in hormonal secretions. These alterations can be used as diagnostic aids in seizure evaluation, for instance in the case of a postictal increase in prolactin secretion. In both men and women with epilepsy, antiepileptic drugs (AEDs) may affect endocrine function, producing clinically important consequences. Finally, in both men and women, hormonal treatment may in certain settings be successfully used as adjunctive anticonvulsant therapy. This chapter will address these issues.

The Comprehensive Evaluation and Treatment of Epilepsy
Copyright © 1997 by Academic Press. All rights of reproduction in any form reserved.

CATAMENIAL EPILEPSY: WHAT IS IT AND HOW SHOULD IT BE EVALUATED AND TREATED?

Catamenial (from the Greek word *katamenia: kata,* by; *men,* month) epilepsy refers to seizure exacerbation in relation to the menstrual cycle. Traditionally, the term has been used to refer to seizure exacerbation at the time of menstruation. In its purest form, catamenial epilepsy may cause seizures only at the time of menstruation. This form is uncommon. More commonly, a woman may tend to have seizures at particular times during her menstrual cycle, usually just before or during the onset of menstruation or at the time of ovulation.[1-3] In this case, the best way of establishing whether or not the patient's seizures tend to worsen at certain points of the menstrual cycle is to have her keep a careful seizure diary in relation to her menstrual cycle (using the first day of menstrual bleeding as the first day of the cycle). The menstrual cycle is then divided into four phases: (1) menstrual, counting days -3 to $+3$; (2) follicular, days $+4$ to $+9$; (3) ovulatory, days $+10$ to $+16$; (4) luteal, days $+17$ to -4; the number of seizures in each phase is counted. The average daily number of seizures for each menstrual phase is then compared with the average daily number of seizures for the whole month to see whether a pattern of exacerbation or remission at certain phases of the menstrual cycle is present. We define seizure exacerbation as a twofold or greater increase in average daily seizure frequency during the affected part of the menstrual cycle over the remainder of the cycle.

Three patterns of catamenial seizure exacerbation may be observed[2] (Fig. 12.1): perimenstrually, at the time of ovulation, or throughout the whole second half of the menstrual cycle. The former two patterns occur in women with normal menstrual cycles. The latter pattern, which is the most difficult one to distinguish because the time of seizure exacerbation is prolonged rather than focused, occurs in women with abnormal menstrual cycles. Such women have anovulatory cycles and inadequate luteal phase syndrome.[4] Because they do not ovulate, no corpus luteum is formed during the second (luteal) half of the menstrual cycle and no progesterone is secreted.

Menstrually related hormonal fluctuations in estrogen and progesterone underlie these different patterns of catamenial seizure exacerbation. Estrogens, in particular estradiol, the most important of the different estrogen forms, have potent proconvulsant properties. They exert an excitatory effect on neurons by stimulating the N-methyl-D-aspartate type glutamate receptor.[5] When administered intraperitoneally, intravenously, or topically to the brain surface, estrogens cause seizures, including fatal status epilepticus, in various animal seizure models.[6-9] In female rats, temporolimbic seizures are most easily elicited at the time of ovulation, when serum estrogen levels are at their highest.[10] In women with epilepsy, intravenous administration of conjugated estrogens activates epileptiform discharges and may result in seizures.[11]

Progesterone has the opposite effect. It hyperpolarizes neurons, acting via one of its natural endogenous metabolites, allopregnanolone, as an agonist at the

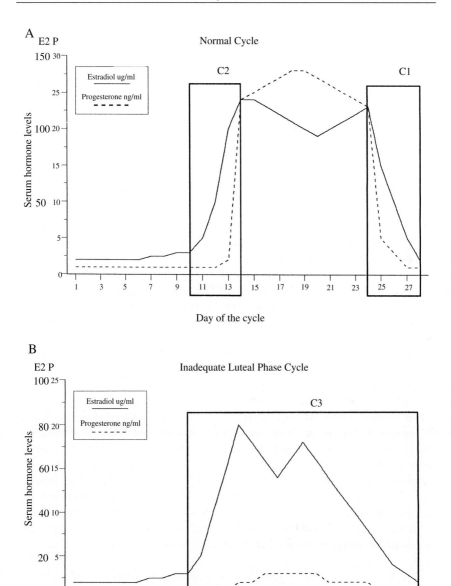

Figure 12.1   The three patterns of catamenial exacerbation of epilepsy—(A) C1, C2, and (B) C3—in relation to serum estradiol (E2) and progesterone (P) levels.

γ-aminobutyric acid (GABA)-α receptor with a potency almost a thousandfold greater than that of pentobarbital and greater than the most potent benzodiazepine, nitroflurazepam.[12,13] In animal seizure models, progesterone lessens epileptiform discharges, inhibits preexisting seizures,[9,14] and protects against the development of seizures.[8] In women with partial seizures, intravenous infusion of progesterone, resulting in luteal phase plasma levels, suppresses interictal epileptiform discharges.[15]

Thus, estrogens facilitate seizures, whereas progesterone protects against seizures. During the menstrual cycle, serum levels of estradiol and progesterone fluctuate (Fig. 12.1). In a normally menstruating woman, the surge of serum estrogen levels at the time of ovulation may be associated with increased seizure tendency; as may the fall in serum progesterone levels premenstrually–perimenstrually. In a woman with an anovulatory cycle, estrogen levels rise at the end of the follicular phase and stay elevated throughout the luteal phase until premenstrually, as in normally menstruating women; but there is little or no progesterone secretion (hence the term *inadequate luteal phase syndrome*). Thus, there is estrogen–progesterone (E–P) imbalance with a relative excess of estrogen (or deficiency of progesterone) throughout the whole second (luteal) half of the menstrual cycle, with associated seizure exacerbation.[16] A number of studies have suggested that it is both progesterone deficiency and estrogen excess relative to progesterone that contribute to the catamenial pattern of seizure exacerbation in both normal women and in women with menstrual irregularities[1,2,16] and that the E–P ratio is the determining factor of overall reproductive hormonal effect upon seizure frequency.[16]

In addition, premenstrual exacerbation of seizures may also be related to a decline in anticonvulsant medication levels.[17,18] In women with catamenial epilepsy, phenytoin (DPH) levels decline premenstrually, by up to one-third.[17,18] This decline may be due to an increased rate of clearance, with an associated reduction in the half-life of DPH from 19–13 h.[17] Hepatic microsomal enzymes metabolize both gonadal steroids and anticonvulsants such as DPH, with competition between the two. The premenstrual decline in gonadal steroid secretion may therefore permit increased metabolism of AEDs, resulting in lower serum levels.[17] However, it is not certain whether all AEDs are thus affected; phenobarbital is not, and catamenial fluctuation in serum levels of other AEDs has not been studied.

HOW SHOULD CATAMENIAL EPILEPSY BE EVALUATED?

We suggest the following steps in evaluating catamenial epilepsy[2]:

1. Establish the presence of a catamenial pattern of seizure exacerbation using a careful seizure and menstrual diary, as previously outlined.

2. Establish the clinical menstrual pattern: normal or abnormal menstrual cycles.
3. Check midluteal serum progesterone levels (e.g., on day 22 of a 28-day menstrual cycle) to see whether an inadequate luteal phase is present.
4. If type I (perimenstrual) catamenial seizure exacerbation is present, check trough AED levels on day 22 (when estradiol and progesterone levels are high and AED level should be "normal") and day 1 (menstrual, when estradiol and progesterone levels are low) to see whether the level is low at this time and could be the cause of perimenstrual seizure exacerbation.

For a discussion of the treatment of catamenial seizures, see the section on hormonal treatment in epilepsy at the end of this chapter.

MENARCHE, PREGNANCY, MENOPAUSE: DO THEY AFFECT SEIZURES?

Changes in reproductive hormonal status associated with menarche,[19] pregnancy,[20,21] and menopause[22] may all affect clinical manifestation of seizures.

MENARCHE

Menarche may be associated with the resolution of some forms of partial seizures and the exacerbation of others. The former group includes the "primary" partial seizures, such as benign rolandic epilepsy of childhood and benign occipital epilepsy of childhood,[23,24] which resolve spontaneously in both sexes in the mid-teens, almost invariably by 16 years of age. The explanation for this phenomenon is not clear and has not been investigated. Changes in both the reproductive hormones and adrenal steroid hormones associated with puberty and adrenarche could be involved.

Secondary partial seizures (idiopathic or lesional) may show exacerbation in relation to menarche. A number of investigators have observed that late childhood and adolescence are peak periods for the first manifestation of epilepsy.[19,25] This tendency is particularly strong among women with catamenial epilepsy, up to two-thirds of whom may experience the onset of seizures within 3 years of menarche.[11,25] Preexisting complex partial seizures in women may increase in frequency at the time of menarche.[26] The finding that oophorectomy in rats before sexual maturation decreases their susceptibility to seizures in adulthood suggests that increased neuronal excitability, associated with the elevation of estrogens at the time of menarche, may provide an explanation for this observation.[9]

In one study, no effect of menarche on seizures was found.[27] An explanation for this finding may be that the menarche effect is difficult to distinguish from the adrenarche effect.

PREGNANCY

Pregnancy may have variable effects on epilepsy. A small number of women experience seizures for the first time during pregnancy and have seizures only during pregnancy.[20] In about one-third of women, seizures worsen during pregnancy, probably because of decreased levels of AEDs, related to a greater volume of distribution and a higher rate of clearance.[20,21] In about one-sixth of women, seizure frequency decreases, possibly because of increased medication compliance.[20,21]

MENOPAUSE

The generally accepted belief is that menopause has little effect on epilepsy. Earlier this century, for instance, castration was used unsuccessfully to treat epilepsy in women.[28] In some patients seizures may cease at the time of menopause, whereas in other patients seizures may worsen.[22] The term *menopause* refers to a complex process and a variable end point that may differ significantly from person to person. Although estrogen levels decline as ovarian function diminishes, progesterone declines before estrogen, with resulting elevation of E–P serum ratios.[29] Early during menopause, for example, anovulatory cycles may develop and lead to increased E–P ratios that would be expected to promote the occurrence of seizures. At the end of the process, estrogen production by the ovaries may become essentially undetectable and may potentially lead to a beneficial effect.

Another menopausal effect upon seizures may be due to associated hormone replacement therapy. In particular, the triggering of seizure exacerbation in women with epilepsy by the initiation of estrogen replacement therapy is relatively common. This effect occurs usually even if progesterone replacement therapy is used concomitantly, because the progesterone commonly used is a synthetic progestin with little or no anticonvulsant activity. *Synthetic* progestins are much less effective anticonvulsants than *natural* progesterone. If a menopausal woman with epilepsy needs to be given estrogen replacement therapy (e.g., for osteoporosis or to prevent ischemic heart disease), we suggest simultaneous use of natural progesterone to mimic normal luteal phase serum levels; for example, 100–200 mg t.i.d. cyclically 2 weeks/month[30] (see section on hormonal treatment).

IN WHAT OTHER WAYS MAY HORMONES AFFECT SEIZURES?

HORMONE-CONTAINING MEDICATION

Isolated reports exist of estrogenic oral contraceptives exacerbating and progestin-containing oral contraceptives ameliorating seizures, particularly in women with catamenial epilepsy.[11,25] For the most part, however, oral contraceptives have not been shown to have a significant direct effect upon seizures, other than affecting the levels of certain AEDs.

PATHOLOGIC HORMONAL STATES

Reproductive endocrine disorders may favor the development of temporal lobe epilepsy (TLE) in women. Conditions in which serum estrogen levels and E–P ratios are chronically elevated may be associated with an increased incidence of seizures by causing constant exposure of temporal lobe structures to estrogen without the normal luteal elevation of progesterone, thus heightening interictal epileptiform activity and the possibility of "kindling." In this regard, more than 50% of women with anovulatory cycles or amenorrhea may have EEG abnormalities that may normalize after treatment with the antiestrogen clomiphene citrate and restoration of ovulation.[31] It is possible that partial seizures of temporal lobe focus (TLE) may themselves promote the development of polycystic ovarian syndrome (PCOS) and hypothalamic hypogonadism (HH), two of the conditions associated with inadequate luteal phase syndrome.[32] Thus, epilepsy may alter the hormonal environment in such a way as to further facilitate seizures, as discussed in the text that follows.

HOW DOES PARTIAL EPILEPSY AFFECT ENDOCRINE REPRODUCTIVE FUNCTION IN WOMEN?

Reproductive dysfunction and endocrine disorders are unusually common among women with epilepsy.[32] Fertility is reduced by 20–30% of the expected number of offspring among married epileptic women, although the reduction may affect only women whose seizures began before the age of 10.[33] Thirty-five percent of women with partial seizures of temporal lobe focus have anovulatory cycles.[34] About 60% of women with TLE have menstrual cycle abnormalities, such as amenorrhea, oligomenorrhea, or abnormally long (>32 days) or short (<26 days) menstrual cycle intervals.[32] These abnormalities are often associated with distinct reproductive endocrine disorders. PCOS and HH are present in 20% and 12%, respectively, of women with TLE, as compared with 5% and 1.5% of women in the general population. Premature menopause and functional hyperprolactinemia are present in 4% and 2%, respectively, of women with TLE, as compared with fewer than 1% (for either condition) of women in the general population.[32]

The pathogenic mechanism of these disorders has not been established. It may relate to the effect of temporal lobe seizures or interictal epileptiform discharges upon the functioning of the hypothalamo-pituitary-gonadal hormonal axis. No structural lesions in the hypothalamus or in the pituitary have been found in epileptic patients with reproductive endocrine disorders.[32]

Ovulation is controlled by luteinizing hormone (LH) and follicle-stimulating hormone (FSH), which are regulated by luteinizing hormone–releasing hormone (LHRH) secreted by hypothalamic LHRH-containing neurons.[35] The LHRH neurons release LHRH into the portal hypophyseal circulation, which carries it to the anterior pituitary. There, LHRH stimulates LH and FSH release into the systemic circulation. FSH acts on the ovary to stimulate the maturation of the follicle. This process is associated with production by the ovary of estrogen during the follicular phase of the menstrual cycle. When the follicle is mature, a surge of estrogen production stimulates a surge in LH secretion from the pituitary by a positive feedback. This is followed by ovulation, the release of the ovum from the follicle. The remaining follicle now becomes transformed into corpus luteum, which secretes progesterone and estrogen during the luteal half of the menstrual cycle. At the end of this phase, production of both estrogen and progesterone fall, leading to menstruation.[29]

LHRH, LH, and FSH are secreted in a pulsatile manner (see Ref. 29 for a review). LH pulses in the peripheral blood are controlled by LHRH pulses.[29] Alteration in the normal pulsatile pattern of LHRH and LH secretion may be important in the pathophysiology of reproductive disorders with abnormal ovulation, including PCOS and HH. Both diminished and excessive LH pulsatile secretion can lead to loss of ovulation. Ovulation starts only after the LH pulsatile pattern becomes established during puberty[29] and is lost when LH pulsatility is lost (e.g., in secondary amenorrhea caused by anorexia nervosa) or becomes excessive.[29] Women with PCOS may have increased LH pulse frequency.[29] Women with hypothalamic hypogonadism have decreased LH pulse frequency.[36]

The control of the pulsatile release of LHRH by LHRH cells is subject to modulatory influences from different parts of the brain,[37] including the amygdala. There are direct anatomic and physiologic connections between the amygdala and the preoptic area and the mediobasal hypothalamus, the sites of the LHRH-containing neurons.[38,39] The amygdala can be divided, anatomically and functionally, into two distinct parts: the corticomedial and the basolateral divisions. The basolateral amygdala exerts an inhibitory influence on gonadotropin function and on ovulation, whereas the corticomedial amygdala stimulates hypothalamic gonado-tropin function and ovulation (see Ref. 40 for a review).

LH pulsatile secretion is altered in women with epilepsy. Women with untreated epilepsy have higher LH pulse frequency than normal controls.[41] Women with TLE and PCOS tend to have left-sided epileptiform discharges and increased LH pulse frequency, whereas women with TLE and HH usually have right-sided epileptiform discharges and diminished LH pulse frequency.[36,42] Thus, involvement of temporal lobe structures, namely the amygdala, by ictal or interictal epileptiform discharges may disrupt normal limbic modulation of the hypothalamic endocrine regulation, thereby altering the frequency of LH pulse secretion and promoting the development of reproductive endocrine disorders. More particularly, discharges involving the left amygdala may lead to increased secretory activity of the hypotha-lamic LHRH neurons and their terminals, resulting in increased LH pulse frequency and PCOS. In contrast, discharges involving the right amygdala may lead to reduced activity of the LHRH neurons, reduced LH pulse frequency, and hypothalamic hypogonadism.[36]

Reproductive endocrine disorders may, in turn, affect TLE. They may promote its development de novo in women with anovulatory cycles and lead to its exacerbation in women with TLE in whom reproductive endocrine disorders develop as a consequence of the TLE. Estrogen receptors are present in the amygdala as well as in the hippocampus.[43] As noted earlier, estrogen enhances excitatory neuronal activity[5] and facilitates seizure development in animal models[6,8] and EEG spikes in epileptic patients.[11] Progesterone acts in the opposite manner to potentiate inhibitory synaptic transmission,[12] exert an anticonvulsant effect in animal models,[8] and attenuate the appearance of interictal spikes in epileptic pa-tients.[15] PCOS and HH are characterized by anovulatory cycles, with failure of progesterone secretion during the luteal phase. Such cycles may, therefore, expose the amygdala and the hippocampus to continuous estrogen without the normal cyclical progesterone effects, and thereby may promote interictal epileptiform activity and seizures. In fact, anovulatory cycles are associated with more frequent seizures.[16] Thus, the hormonal changes associated with anovulatory cycles may exacerbate seizures. A positive feedback cycle may be envisaged whereby TLE leads to endocrine reproductive disorders with failure of ovulation, which in turn further exacerbates the seizure disorder (Fig. 12.2).

HOW SHOULD WOMEN WITH EPILEPSY AND REPRODUCTIVE DYSFUNCTION BE EVALUATED?

The most common reproductive complaint of women with partial epilepsy that may be related to epilepsy is an irregular menstrual cycle—usually prolonged

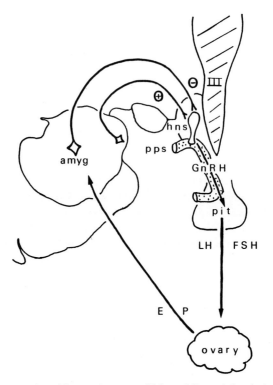

Figure 12.2 A cross-section of the anterior temporal lobe and diencephalon depicting direct projections from the two anatomically distinct functional divisions of the amygdala (amyg) to the same ventromedial hypothalamic neurons. The different influences of these projections on hypothalamic neurosecretory cells (hns) modulate pulsatile gonadotropin-releasing hormone (GnRH) secretion. Releasing hormones enter the pituitary portal system (pps) and regulate the pattern of luteinizing hormone (LH) and follicle-stimulating hormone (FSH) secretion by the pituitary (pit). These gonadotropins induce ovulation and stimulate estradiol (E) and progesterone (P) production. Gonadal steroids, in turn, bind to specific amygdaloid hormone receptors and influence neural activity, including epileptiform discharges.

but sometimes shortened (or both). The two most common epilepsy-related causes of this irregularity are PCOS and HH. Other possible causes are functional hyperprolactinemia and premature menopause. Of course, if a woman complains of secondary amenorrhea, pregnancy or menopause should not be forgotten as a possible cause. We suggest the following approach:

1. History and examination to:
   a. Rule out pregnancy and menopause.

b. Evaluate for PCOS, HH, and hyperprolactinemia; hirsutism; acne (for PCOS-associated hyperandrogenism); and galactorrhoea (for hyperprolactinemia).

2. Endocrine evaluation:

a. During follicular phase—for example, menstrual cycle day 4: LH, FSH, estradiol, total testosterone, free testosterone (FT), androstenedione (A), dehydroepiandrostenedione sulfate (DHEAS), prolactin, and thyroid function tests:

   i. In PCOS, one or more of the androgens (FT, A, or DHEAS) are elevated; the usual LH/FSH ratio of 1 is increased to >2.5, and prolactin may be increased (in about 25% of cases). FT as well as total testosterone need to be checked, because the latter may be affected by several AEDs and FT is the functionally relevant parameter (see later section on AEDs and hormonal functioning).

   ii. In HH, LH, FSH, and estradiol are all low.

   iii. In hyperprolactinemia, remember that psychotropic medications—including benzodiazepines when used as AEDs (e.g., clonazepam)—as well as TLE are a possible cause.

   iv. Hypothyroidism is a common cause of menstrual irregularities.

b. During the midluteal phase (e.g., menstrual cycle day 22), progesterone and estradiol:

   i. In inadequate luteal phase syndrome of all causes, progesterone level is low, less than the normal 5 ng/ml. In PCOS, estradiol is normal.

   ii. In HH, both estradiol and progesterone are low.

3. Radiologic evaluation:

a. Pelvic ultrasound:

   i. For PCOS if indicated by the preceding laboratory values.

b. Magnetic resonance imaging (MRI) of the brain (coronal views of the hypothalamus and pituitary):

   i. For HH and hyperprolactinemia; to be done only if the history and examination point to a structural (i.e., TLE-unrelated) cause of HH and hyperprolactinemia.

HOW DOES EPILEPSY AFFECT WOMEN'S SEXUALITY?

Hyposexuality is seen more often in epileptic women than in the general population; 25–65% of women with TLE are estimated to be affected.[44] As with epileptic men, hyposexuality in epileptic women is seen much more often in those with TLE than with primarily generalized epilepsy. Hyposexuality is characterized by lack of libido and difficulty in achieving orgasm. The disorder may be a result of a number of factors, including psychosocial disability, medications (see text that follows), and epilepsy-related dysfunction of limbic structures, in particular of the amygdala. In this respect, hyposexuality occurs more commonly with right-sided TLE. In that setting, it is associated with hypothalamic hypogonadism and low serum LH level.[32] By contrast, it has been our experience that women with left-sided TLE are rarely hyposexual.

HOW DO SEIZURES AFFECT REPRODUCTIVE ENDOCRINE FUNCTION IN MEN?

Reproductive endocrine dysfunction is common in men with epilepsy.[45–48] Hyposexuality, the most common clinical finding, is often a cause of great concern and, not infrequently, of marital difficulties. Its recognition is thus important, particularly because it is often treatable.

Hyposexuality is present in one-third to two-thirds of all men with TLE.[47] Causes include hypogonadotropic hypogonadism (about 25%), hypergonadotropic hypogonadism (about 10%), and hyperprolactinemia (about 10%).[47] Reproductive dysfunction may be confined to the patient's sexuality with reproductive potential remaining normal. Unlike women with epilepsy, men with epilepsy have mostly normal fertility,[33,45] although isolated cases of infertility have been observed.[47] In most epileptic men with sexual dysfunction, the dysfunction is hyposexuality; rarely is hypersexuality observed.[47,48] Both impotence with normal libido and global hyposexuality with decline in both libido and potency are seen.[46,47]

The pathogenesis of sexual dysfunction in epileptic men, as in epileptic women, is likely to be multifactorial. Alteration of temporal lobe function by an underlying pathologic lesion, alteration of temporal limbic structures by ictal or interictal discharges, associated neuroendocrine changes, and medication effects may all play a part.

In lesional TLE, the underlying pathologic process may be important. In cases of TLE secondary to neoplasm, for instance, hyposexuality has been noted to precede the onset of seizures by several months.[46]

Although several AEDs can cause hyposexuality (a detailed discussion follows), epilepsy-related alteration of limbic structures may be directly involved. Thus, hyposexuality is commonly seen in TLE but not in other types of epilepsies,[48] may occur in patients with untreated TLE,[47] and may improve with AED treatment even if it involves higher AED dosing.[46,48]

Sexual behavior is controlled by the sexually dimorphic regions of the hypothalamus and the amygdala[43]—the same regions that regulate reproductive endocrine physiology. Alteration in the function of these structures by ictal or interictal epileptiform discharges may affect both the behavioral and the endocrine aspects of sexual behavior.

Hormonally, sexual behavior is promoted by LH and androgens in men and women and by estradiol in women; it is inhibited by prolactin. Men with TLE who have reproductive and sexual dysfunction tend to have right-sided lateralization of seizures,[49] reduced LH pulse frequency compared with men with left-sided TLE (unpublished personal observation), and increased risk of hypogonadotropic hypogonadism and hyposexuality. Thus, epilepsy may alter temporolimbic modulation of the frequency of LHRH and LH pulses in relation to the lateralization of the paroxysmal discharges and thus affect gonadal androgen secretion and androgen-dependent sexual behavior. Moreover, this behavior may depend not only on the serum levels of androgens but also on the responsiveness to androgens by brain structures such as the androgen receptor-containing amygdala and hippocampus.[43] It is possible that alterations in these structures by ictal or interictal epileptiform discharges could alter the responsiveness to androgens, resulting in hyposexuality or hypersexuality.

In addition, elevated prolactin levels may also be a contributing factor to hyposexuality in epileptic men. Chronic hyperprolactinemia in nonepileptic men is associated with decreased libido and impotence.[50] Men with both complex partial and primary generalized seizures have increased prolactin levels interictally.[51] Prolactin antagonizes LHRH release from the hypothalamus, with a resulting reduction in LH and FSH secretion. Epilepsy-associated hyperprolactinemia could thus result in hypogonadotropic hypogonadism with associated hyposexuality.

The effects of AEDs on sexuality and the evaluation of hyposexuality are discussed later, in the section on AED effects on hormonal function.

WHAT EFFECTS DO SEIZURES HAVE ON HORMONE PRODUCTION ACUTELY, AND WHAT CLINICAL RELEVANCE DO THESE EFFECTS HAVE?

Transient postictal elevation of serum prolactin occurs after primarily or secondarily generalized tonic-clonic seizures and after partial complex seizures, but rarely after partial simple seizures.[52–54] Prolactin rises within 10–30 min after the seizure, the level gradually returning to normal over the subsequent hour. The elevation occurs in 80% of tonic-clonic, 45% of complex partial, and 10% of simple partial seizures.[55] Depth electrode recordings in patients with partial seizures show that a rise in serum prolactin is always associated with partial complex seizures involving the temporal lobes and often with partial simple seizures with high-frequency discharges and widespread involvement of the mesial temporal limbic structures.[56] The prolactin elevation after simple partial seizures is about 45% lower than that seen after partial complex seizures.[56]

The prolactin rise presumably reflects modulation of hypothalamic function by the temporal lobe ictal discharge. Prolactin secretion by the anterior pituitary gland is controlled by neurons in the arcuate nucleus of the hypothalamus; the fibers of these neurons travel through the median eminence to reach the hypophyseal portal circulation.[57] Dopaminergic neurons in the arcuate nucleus tonically inhibit the release of prolactin from the pituitary; as yet unidentified prolactin-releasing factor-secreting cells activate prolactin release. These neurons are subject to a modifying influence from the amygdala.[39] The amygdala stimulates prolactin secretion via beta-adrenergic receptors and inhibits it via dopaminergic receptors.[58] Seizures are accompanied by dopamine release and depletion. Thus, ictal dopamine depletion in the hypothalamus may perhaps lead to the transient postictal rise in prolactin secretion.

OF WHAT CLINICAL UTILITY IS POSTICTAL PROLACTIN TESTING, AND HOW SHOULD IT BE DONE?

Transient postictal serum prolactin elevation has been used clinically to distinguish primarily or secondarily generalized tonic-clonic seizures and partial complex seizures of temporal lobe origin from pseudoseizures (nonepileptic seizures). Prolactin levels, unlike cortisol levels,[59] are infrequently elevated in nonepileptic seizures. When they do rise, they do not rise above the twofold level that can accompany stress or occur postprandially. By contrast, in tonic-clonic or partial seizures involving the temporal lobe there is at least a threefold, and often higher (e.g., fivefold to twentyfold), postictal rise in serum prolactin level.[55]

Several factors limit the usefulness of postictal serum prolactin elevation as a test in distinguishing bona fide seizures from "pseudoseizures." First, postictal serum prolactin elevation cannot be used to differentiate simple partial seizures from pseudoseizures. Second, in partial complex seizures, only those arising from the temporal lobe lead to prolactin elevation. Third, even 10–20% of patients with tonic-clonic seizures may not show a postictal prolactin rise. Fourth, ambiguous test results, such as a twofold elevation, are not helpful. Finally, prolactin level rises predictably only after a single seizure. Repeated seizures (i.e., more than two seizures in 12 h) may be associated with progressively smaller elevations (presumably because of exhaustion of stored prolactin from the pituitary lactotrophs).

With these caveats, however, the test is a useful one. A positive test result—that is, greater than threefold postictal prolactin elevation—suggests the presence of an epileptic seizure, and a negative result makes it unlikely that an ictal event was epileptic if the event was a tonic-clonic seizure. We follow a simple protocol of checking serum prolactin level 20 min and 12 h postictally (24 h in outpatient settings) in patients whose seizure frequency is less than 1 in 12 h. The 12-h (or 24-h) postictal value serves as the patient's own post-hoc baseline.

IS THE CHECKING OF OTHER HORMONE LEVELS POSTICTALLY WORTHWHILE?

Other hormones show less consistent postictal changes. Serum cortisol is elevated after both bona fide and simulated generalized seizures.[59] The cortisol rise follows that of corticotropin, beta-endorphin, and beta-lipotropin, all products of a common precursor molecule, proopiomelanocortin.[60] Elevated vasopressin after seizures has also been reported.[60] Because all these hormones are secreted in response to stress, their postictal elevation may not be specific to epileptic seizures. Inconsistent findings of postictal changes in LH and FSH have been revealed by different authors.[53,54,60] No consistent significant postictal change has been seen in serum levels of growth hormone or TSH.[54,60] Thus, postictal testing of hormones other than prolactin is at present not clinically useful.

ARE ANY OTHER HORMONAL SYSTEMS CLINICALLY AFFECTED BY PARTIAL SEIZURES?

The function of the hypothalamo-pituitary-adrenal axis may be altered chronically as well as acutely in seizure patients.[59,60] Cortisol has been shown to be elevated interictally in some studies[61] but not in others.[51] Corticotropin is also elevated interictally in patients with temporal lobe seizures,[61] a finding that appears to be related specifically to abnormal functioning of the anterior temporal lobe,[61] where the amygdala is located, and to be limited to TLE that involves the amygdala. For instance, stimulation of the amygdala in TLE patients[62] as well as in animals[63] leads to a rise in serum corticosteroids and corticotropin, but stimulation of the hippocampus inhibits their secretion.[62]

Corticotropin is secreted by the anterior pituitary in response to corticotropin-releasing hormone (CRH) produced by neurons in the paraventricular nucleus of the hypothalamus. These neurons receive a direct input from CRH-containing neurons in the amygdala.[64] Postictal and interictal elevation of corticotropin and cortisol after seizures is thus most likely due to activation of the hypothalamic-adrenal axis by the amygdala as a result of ictal and interictal epileptiform discharges.

What are the clinical consequences of this activation? Few have been appreciated to date, but that may be because they have not been specifically sought. We have reported three cases of reversible Cushing's syndrome and myopathy in patients with refractory complex partial seizures. The Cushing's syndrome and myopathy fluctuated in parallel with seizure exacerbations and remitted with normalization of glucocorticoid levels upon treatment with ketoconazole, an inhibitor of adrenal steroidogenesis.[65] Ketoconazole also successfully treated the seizures.

Experimental data suggest that interictal activation of the CRH-corticotropin-corticosteroid axis may lead to exacerbation of seizures[66,67] and may also contribute to some of the chronic sequelae of poorly controlled chronic TLE associated with hippocampal damage, such as memory impairment.[68] However, no clinical data exist to support this hypothesis.

Anticonvulsant medications may affect endocrine function in a number of different, clinically significant ways. The most prominent effects are those on the reproductive function, chiefly on sexuality.

WHAT IS THE EFFECT OF AEDs ON SEXUALITY IN MEN AND WOMEN AND ON REPRODUCTION IN MEN?

The hepatic enzyme-inducing AEDs, namely, phenobarbital, primidone, carbamazepine (CBZ), and DPH, may all contribute to or cause reproductive and sexual dysfunction in men with epilepsy.[69,70]

Androgens are important in regulating potency and libido.[71] Testosterone is the most important androgen. Its serum concentration is affected by the barbiturates, DPT, and CBZ. Serum testosterone exists in three forms: free testosterone (FT, 2–3% of total), albumin-bound (55%), and sex hormone-binding globulin (SHBG)-bound (43–45%) (see Ref. 72 for a review). The SHBG-bound fraction is not biologically active, but the albumin-bound and free fractions are. Reduction in free but not total testosterone is associated with diminished libido[69,70] and potency. Testosterone increases potency (see Ref. 72) and libido, whereas estradiol *lowers* it (see Ref. 72). Although estradiol constitutes only 1% of male gonadal steroids, it exerts almost 50% of the negative feedback on male LH secretion (see Ref. 72). Hepatic enzyme-inducing AEDs lower the amount of free or biologically active testosterone available to stimulate sexual function; at the same time they increase the serum level of estradiol, which actively inhibits it.

Barbiturates, DPH, and CBZ affect serum testosterone and estradiol levels by at least four distinct mechanisms:[72]

1. CBZ and DPH act directly on the testis to inhibit testosterone synthesis by the Leydig cells of the testis.[73]

2. Barbiturates, CBZ, and DPH induce the hepatic p-450 enzymes that catabolize both AEDs and testosterone. Induction of those enzymes leads to increased clearance of testosterone from the body and lowering of its level.

3. These drugs induce the liver production of SHBG.[69,70] Thus, serum SHBG is elevated, more of the total testosterone gets bound to SHBG, and less of it remains available as free or biologically active testosterone. The increase in SHBG-bound testosterone may result in normal or even elevated levels of total testosterone, even while the concentration of free or bioactive testosterone is reduced.[69,70] Clinically manifest hyposexuality corresponds to the duration of AED therapy,

being more likely to occur after 5 or more years of treatment with CBZ or DPH.[74] The reason may be that SHBG levels increase progressively over time during chronic treatment with these medications.[74]

4. These drugs induce the liver production of the enzyme aromatase, which converts estradiol to testosterone (the final common path of all natural estradiol production). Its induction by the AEDs leads to an elevated serum level of estradiol[75] and, by shunting of FT to estradiol, to further reduction of serum-free testosterone. Thus, the ratio of FT to estradiol (FT–E2) is lower in epileptic men with hyposexuality than in sexually normal epileptic patients or in normal controls.[76] Because estradiol exerts a potent negative feedback upon male LH secretion, suppression of LH secretion leads to hypogonadotropic hypogonadism. Estradiol may also produce premature aging of the hypothalamic arcuate nucleus (see Ref. 72) and, with it, hypothalamic hypogonadism. Both these effects may result in impaired testosterone secretion. Moreover, estradiol stimulates SHBG synthesis, whereas testosterone inhibits it. Thus, AED-induced elevation of estradiol could have a downward-spiraling effect of decreased testosterone and testosterone–E2 ratio, stimulating SHBG synthesis, with resultant further depression of bioactive testosterone over time.

WHAT ARE THE LABORATORY FINDINGS IN HYPOSEXUAL PATIENTS WHO ARE GIVEN AEDs?

Total serum testosterone levels may be normal or occasionally even elevated.[69] However, levels of FT—or biologically active testosterone (BAT)[77]—are reduced. Serum estradiol is frequently elevated. In summary, the laboratory findings show: (1) Usually normal serum total testosterone; (2) reduced serum-free or biologically active testosterone; (3) elevated SHBG; (4) often elevated serum estradiol.

In practical terms, the following endocrine tests should be administered to hyposexual men who are receiving AEDs: total testosterone, FT, and estradiol levels in all patients; and bioactive testosterone level in those patients in whom results of the former two tests are normal.[77] In addition, serum LH and FSH should be checked to evaluate the possibility of hypothalamic hypogonadism.

HOW CAN AED-RELATED HYPOSEXUALITY BE TREATED?

Treatment of AED-related hyposexuality consists of several options and is usually successful. Obviously, changing anticonvulsant medications from the hepatic enzyme-inducing category to hepatic enzyme-inhibiting ones such as sodium valproate can be considered. In patients with previously hard-to-control seizures that are well controlled with the hyposexuality-causing AEDs, however, changing AEDs may not be desirable. In those patients, treatment with testosterone to restore normal FT levels (aiming for the high end of the normal range) would be the first step. Intramuscular depotestosterone, usually at 400–600 mg every 2–3 weeks, or the much more expensive cutaneous androderm patch, applied daily, can be used. Rarely, aggressive tendencies may develop with testosterone. This treatment may be sufficient. In some patients, however, there may be no response or, more commonly, initial improvement may be followed by a relapse. Relapse may be caused by rising levels of serum estradiol after testosterone treatment, because more testosterone is available for conversion to estradiol via the enzyme aromatase. If a relapse occurs, addition of the aromatase inhibitor testolactone to the testosterone will lower the serum estradiol level and will restore normal libido and potency.[77] In some patients, lowering estradiol levels with testolactone may even lead to improved seizure control.[77] Finally, treatment with the antiestrogen clomiphene may restore sexuality[78] as well as improve seizure control[78,79] (see also the text that follows).

WHAT ADDITIONAL EFFECTS MAY AEDs HAVE ON REPRODUCTIVE FUNCTION IN WOMEN?

Sodium valproate may be associated with increased occurrence of PCOS.[80] In PCOS, the patient has anovulatory cycles and hyperandrogenism. Characterized by hirsutism and menstrual disorders, the condition is more frequent in obese women (see Refs. 29 and 81 for reviews). Isojarvi et al.[80] have noted PCOS to be more common in epileptic women treated with sodium valproate (approximately 45%) than in those who are treated with CBZ (20%). They suggest that valproate causes weight gain, insulin resistance, and hyperinsulinemia, which then cause hyperandrogenism,[82] which leads to PCOS. Hyperinsulinemia may indeed cause hyperandrogenism by directly stimulating ovarian steroidogenesis[29] and by inhibiting the synthesis of SHBG with a consequent increase in the availability of bioactive androgens. Interestingly, for poorly understood reasons, weight gain is much more likely to occur if valproate treatment is started before the age of 20 than after that age, irrespective of the duration of treatment or of seizure severity.[80]

On the other hand, we have argued that PCOS is related to the underlying epilepsy (see previous section) and that the difference in the incidence of PCOS between valproate-treated women and women treated with other AEDs may be due to a beneficiary effect upon PCOS by hepatic enzyme-inducing AEDs such as barbiturates, DPH, and CBZ.[81] Thus, PCOS is less common in treated women (13%) than in untreated women (30%) with TLE when treatment does not include sodium valproate.[32] Hepatic enzyme-inducing AEDs lower biologically active androgen levels, whereas valproate does not. AEDs other than valproate, therefore, may treat epilepsy-related hyperandrogenism and thus PCOS, whereas valproate therapy may not. This mechanism could contribute to the higher occurrence of PCOS in valproate-treated women with epilepsy.[81]

It is possible, however, that both mechanisms have an effect; that is: (1) That valproate may, by virtue of causing hyperinsulinemia, cause or exacerbate PCOS in some epileptic women; and (2) that AEDs such as barbiturates, DPH, and CBZ may treat PCOS by treating hyperandrogenism. Other effects of valproate on reproduction may include amenorrhea and pubertal arrest seen transiently after initiation of valproate therapy.[83,84]

WHICH OTHER HORMONAL SYSTEMS ARE AFFECTED BY AEDs?

THYROID HORMONES

Thyroid function test results are frequently abnormal in patients who are given CBZ or DPH. Thyroxine (T_4) and free thyroxine (FT_4) are often lowered, down to 70% of their normal values (see Refs. 85 and 86 for reviews). TSH- and TRH-stimulating test results usually remain normal, however, and the patients remain clinically euthyroid. Only two patients given CBZ and CBZ plus DPH have been reported to have overt hypothyroidism.[85] The observed changes may be due to increased conversion of T_4 to T_3, induction by the hepatic enzyme-inducing AEDs of peripheral metabolism of the thyroid hormones,[85] and competition by CBZ and thyroid hormones for thyroid-binding globulin.[85] In clinically asymptomatic patients, the changes are of little clinical importance and require no treatment. In thyroxine-substituted hypothyroid patients, the increased peripheral metabolism of thyroid hormones with CBZ may necessitate adjusting upward the dose of thyroxine used.[85]

ANTIDIURETIC HORMONE

CBZ causes water retention and hyponatremia because of an SIADH-like effect. This effect is more likely to occur with CBZ serum levels above 6 μg/ml and in the elderly. It may be a result of a combination of action: a direct ADH-like effect on the renal tubule (which is reversed by demeclocycline), and a promoting effect at the hypothalamus (see Ref. 85 for a review). By contrast, DPH inhibits ADH release,[85] and concomitant treatment of DPH in CBZ-treated patients with inappropriate ADH may reverse the latter.[85]

CORTISOL

CBZ causes a clinically asymptomatic increase in free cortisol levels.[85] DPH in large doses may increase corticotropin and cortisol levels initially.

CAN HORMONES BE USED TO TREAT EPILEPSY?

Endocrine treatment of seizures may rationally be aimed at those endocrinologic aspects of seizures that act either to exacerbate or to ameliorate them. As already discussed, progesterone may have an anticonvulsant effect, whereas estrogen, CRH, and cortisol may have proconvulsant effects. Thus, treatment with progesterone, estrogen antagonists, and medications that suppress the activity of the hypothalamo-pituitary-adrenal axis may prove to be useful adjunctive treatments in appropriate patients.

GONADAL HORMONE–BASED TREATMENT

Progesterone

As noted previously, low progesterone levels or rapid withdrawal of progesterone may be a factor in the increased seizure frequency seen during the premenstrual and early follicular phase of women with catamenial epilepsy and normal ovulatory cycles, and during the entire luteal phase of women with anovulatory cycles.[1,16] Progesterone may be expected to be beneficial in these women.

Synthetic progestin therapy may be considered. Little or no benefits have been noted in a number of studies[87,88] with oral forms although occasional benefits have been described in single case reports. In one study of women with refractory partial seizures and normal ovulatory cycles, a medroxyprogesterone dose large enough to induce amenorrhea (i.e., 120–150 mg every 6–12 weeks intramuscularly or 20–40 mg orally daily) resulted in a 40% average seizure reduction.[87] We have found weekly doses of 400 mg of intramuscular depo medroxyprogesterone to be more effective. Potential side effects include depression, sedation, breakthrough vaginal bleeding, and delay in the return of regular menstrual cycles—the last side effect following only depo, not oral, medroxyprogesterone administration.

We have found natural progesterone to be a more effective treatment.[30] In a study of 25 women with catamenial exacerbation of complex partial seizures of temporal lobe origin, 14 with inadequate luteal phase or anovulatory cycles and 11 with normal cycles and perimenstrual seizure exacerbation, 72% of the women improved; there was a 55% decline in average seizure frequency.[30] Progesterone was administered as lozenges, 200 mg three times daily on days 23 through 25 of each menstrual cycle, for perimenstrual exacerbation; and on days 15 through 25 of each menstrual cycle, with taper over days 26 through 28, for exacerbations lasting throughout the entire luteal phase.[30]

Natural progesterone is available as soybean extract in lozenge, micronized capsule, cream, and suppository form. The usual daily regimen to achieve physiologic luteal-range serum levels is 100–200 mg three times daily.[30] The synthetic progestins are not equivalent because natural progesterone is metabolized to allopregnanolone, which has potent GABA-α mimetic and anticonvulsant action,[12,13] whereas synthetic progestins are not metabolized in this way. Potential side effects may include sedation, depression, weight gain, breast tenderness, and breakthrough vaginal bleeding—all readily reversible upon discontinuation of the hormone or lowering of the dose.

Clomiphene

Clomiphene citrate is an estrogen analog with both estrogenic and antiestrogenic effects that are dose-dependent. In its clinical use, it acts primarily as an antiestrogen at the hypothalamic and pituitary level to stimulate gonadotropin secretion, ovulation, and fertility. It exerts an anticonvulsant effect in rats in a dose-related fashion.[8] Remarkable reduction in seizure frequency has been reported in a number of isolated cases in both men and women.[78,79,89] In one series of 12 women who had complex partial seizures and menstrual disorders (polycystic ovarian syndrome or inadequate luteal phase cycles) and who were given clomiphene, 10 improved, often dramatically: They had an 87% average seizure frequency decline.[89] Improvement in seizure frequency was associated with normalization of the menstrual cycle and of luteal progesterone secretion. The only two women who did not improve continued to have menstrual abnormalities.[89] Side effects included one unwanted pregnancy, two cases of ovarian cysts, and three cases of transient breast tenderness and pelvic cramps.

Thus, clomiphene may be a useful adjunctive antiepileptic treatment in women with menstrual disorders. It is administered in doses of 25–100 mg daily on days 5–9 of each menstrual cycle in women and 25–50 mg daily in men. However, the possible endocrine reproductive side effects in women, particularly the potential for unwanted pregnancy and ovarian overstimulation syndrome, dictates caution in using clomiphene. It should not be administered in cases of suspected pregnancy or in the absence of adequate birth control measures unless it is used in conjunction with consultation with a gynecologist as part of a fertility program. Furthermore, seizure frequency may increase during the enhanced preovulatory rise in serum estradiol levels in some women. Additional studies are needed in establishing the role of clomiphene in the treatment of epilepsy.

Testolactone

We have reported notable improvement in seizures in a couple of patients whose AED-related hyposexuality was treated with testosterone and testolactone, an inhibitor of the enzyme aromatase that inhibits the conversion of estrogens and androgens.[77] Treatment with testosterone alone was ineffective. The successful treatment was associated with normalization of previously elevated estradiol levels, suggesting that the anticonvulsant effect of testolactone may be due to a reduction of the proconvulsant effects of estrogen.

LHRH Agonists

Lowering estrogen levels by inducing menopause could be expected to improve seizure control. Medical menopause can be achieved by chronic use of one of the long-acting LHRH analogs. Long-term suppression of gonadotropin and ovarian secretion develops after an initial 3- to 4-week-long phase of reproductive endocrine stimulation. One patient with severe refractory seizures that were exacerbated perimenstrually was reported to have improved markedly after treatment with the LHRH agonist goserelin.[90] Our observations in a few cases suggest that seizure control may improve but that seizure exacerbation during the first-month stimulation phase may preclude the use of LHRH analogs in some cases. Moreover, the immediate and long-term effects of hypoestrogenism need to be considered.

Adrenal Steroid-Based Treatments

Both corticotropin and prednisone have been used extensively in the treatment of refractory infantile spasms and other primarily generalized seizures of childhood (see Ref. 91 for review). They have been successfully used in another childhood epileptic syndrome, the Landau–Kleffner syndrome of acquired aphasia and seizures,[91] but not in other forms of partial epilepsy.

As mentioned previously, we have seen three patients with refractory seizures and hypercortisolemia whose seizures became controlled upon normalization of the patients' cortisol levels by ketoconazole.[65] Wider use of ketoconazole and other potential enzymatic inhibitors of cortisol synthesis has not been explored.

REFERENCES

1. Laidlaw J. Catamenial epilepsy. *Lancet.* 1956;271:1235–1237.
2. Herzog AG, Klein P. Three patterns of catamenial epilepsy. *Epilepsia* 1996;37:83.
3. Newark NE, Penry JK. Catamenial epilepsy: A review. *Epilepsia.* 1980;21:281–300.
4. Jones GS. The luteal phase defect. *Fertil Steril.* 1976;27:351–356.
5. Smith SS. Estrogen administration increases neuronal responses to excitatory amino acids as a long term effect. *Br Res.* 1989;503:354–357.
6. Hom AC, Buterbaugh GG. Estrogen alters the acquisition of seizures kindled by repeated amygdala stimulation or pentylenetetrazol administration in ovariectomized female rats. *Epilepsia.* 1986;27:103–108.

7. Logothetis J, Harner R. Electrocortical activation by estrogens. *Arch Neurol.* 1960;3:290–297.
8. Nicoletti F, Speciale C, Sortino MA, *et al.* Comparative effects of estradiol benzoate, the antiestrogen clomiphene citrate and the progestin medroxyprogesterone acetate on kainic acid-induced seizures in male and female rats. *Epilepsia.* 1985;26:252–257.
9. Woolley DE, Timiras PS. The gonad–brain relationship: Effects of female sex hormones on electroshock convulsions in the rat. *Endocrinology.* 1962;70:196–209.
10. Teresawa E, Timiras P. Electrical activity during the estrous cycle of the rat: Cyclic changes in limbic structures. *Endocrinology.* 1968;83:207.
11. Logothetis J, Harner R, Morrell F, *et al.* The role of estrogens in catamenial exacerbation of epilepsy. *Neurology.* 1959;9:35–360.
12. Majewska MD, Harrison NL, Schwartz RD, *et al.* Steroid hormone metabolites are barbiturate-like modulators of the GABA receptor. *Science.* 1986;232:1004–1007.
13. Paul SM, Purdy RH. Neuroactive steroids. *FASEB.* 1992;6:2311–2322.
14. Landgren S, Backstrom T, Kalistratov G. The effect of progesterone on the spontaneous interictal spike evoked by the application of penicillin to the cat's cerebral cortex. *J Neurol Sci.* 1978;36:119–133.
15. Backstrom T, Zetterlund B, Blom S, *et al.* Effects of intravenous progesterone infusions on the epileptic discharge frequency in women with partial epilepsy. *Acta Neurol Scand.* 1984;69:240–248.
16. Backstrom T. Epileptic seizures in women related to plasma estrogen and progesterone during the menstrual cycle. *Acta Neurol Scand.* 1976;54:321–347.
17. Shavit G, Lerman P, Korczyn AD, *et al.* Phenytoin pharmacokinetics in catamenial epilepsy. *Neurology.* 1984;34:959–961.
18. Rosciewska D, Buntner B, Guz I, *et al.* Ovarian hormones, anticonvulsant drugs and seizures during the menstrual cycle in women with epilepsy. *J Neurol Neurosurg Psychiatry.* 1986;49:47–51.
19. Lennox WG, Cobb S. Epilepsy. *Medicine.* 1928;27:105–290.
20. Knight AH, Rhind EG. Epilepsy and pregnancy: A study of 153 pregnancies in 59 patients. *Epilepsia.* 1975;16:99–110.
21. Schmidt D, Canger R, Avanzini G. Change in seizure frequency in pregnant epileptic women. *J Neurol Neurosurg Psychiatry.* 1985;46:751–755.
22. Sallusto L, Pozzi O. Relations between ovarian activity and the occurrence of epileptic seizures: Data on a clinical case. *Acta Neurol (Napoli).* 1964;19:673–681.
23. Beaussart M, Faou R. Evolution of epilepsy with rolandic (centrotemporal) paroxysmal foci. *Epilepsia.* 1978;19:337–342.
24. Panayiotopoulos CP. Benign childhood epilepsy with occipital paroxysms: A 15 year prospective study. *Ann Neurol.* 1989;26:51–56.
25. Longo LPS, Saldana LEG. Hormones and their influences in epilepsy. *Acta Neurol Latinoam.* 1966;12:29–47.
26. Rosciszewska D. The course of epilepsy at the age of puberty in girls. *Neurol Neurochir Pol.* 1975;9:597–602.
27. Diamontopoulos N, Crumrine PK. The effect of puberty on the course of epilepsy. *Arch Neurol.* 1986;43:873–876.
28. Lennox WG, Lennox MA. *Epilepsy and Related Disorders.* Boston: Little, Brown; 1960:645–650.
29. Carr BR. Disorders of the ovary and female reproductive tract. In: Wilson JD, Foster DW, eds. *Williams Textbook of Endocrinology.* Philadelphia: W.B. Saunders; 1992:733–799.
30. Herzog AG. Progesterone therapy in women with complex partial and secondary generalized seizures. *Neurology.* 1995;45:1660–1662.
31. Sharf M, Sharf B, Bental E, *et al.* The electroencephalogram in the investigation of anovulation and its treatment by clomiphene. *Lancet.* 1969;1:750–753.
32. Herzog AG, Seibel MM, Schomer DL, *et al.* Reproductive endocrine disorders in women with partial seizures of temporal lobe origin. *Arch Neurol.* 1986;43:341–346.

33. Dansky LV, Andermann E, Andermann F. Marriage and fertility in epileptic patients. *Epilepsia.* 1980;21:261–271.
34. Cummings LN, Giudice L, Morrell MJ. Ovulatory function in epilepsy. *Epilepsia.* 1995;36:353–357.
35. King JC, Anthony ELP, Fitzgerald DM, *et al.* Luteinizing hormone-releasing hormone neurons in human preoptic/hypothalamus: Differential intraneuronal localization of immunoreactive forms. *J Clin Endocrinol Lab.* 1985;60:88–97.
36. Drislane FW, Coleman AE, Schomer DL, *et al.* Altered pulsatile secretion of luteinizing hormone in women with epilepsy. *Neurology.* 1994;44:306–310.
37. Maeda K, Tsukamura H, Okhura S, *et al.* The LHRH pulse generator: A mediobasal hypothalamic location. *Neurosci Biobehav Rev.* 1995;19:427–437.
38. Canteras NS, Simerly RB, Swanson LW. Organization of projections from the medial nucleus of the amygdala: A PHAL study in the rat. *J Comp Neurol.* 1995;360:213–245.
39. Reynaud LP. Influence of amygdala on the activity of identified neurons in the rat hypothalamus. *J Physiol.* 1976;260:237–252.
40. Zolovnick AJ. Effects of lesions and electrical stimulation of the amygdala on hypothalamic–hypophyseal regulation. In: Eleftheriou BE, ed. *The Neurobiology of the Amygdala.* New York: Plenum Press; 1972:745–762.
41. Bilo L, Meo R, Valentino R, *et al.* Abnormal patterns of luteinizing hormone pulsatility in women with epilepsy. *Fertil Steril.* 1991;55:705–711.
42. Herzog AG. A relationship between particular reproductive endocrine disorders and the laterality of epileptiform discharges in women with epilepsy. *Neurology.* 1993;43:1907–1910.
43. Simerly RB, Chang C, Muramatsu M, *et al.* Distribution of androgen and estrogen receptor mRNA-containing cells in the rat brain: An in situ hybridization study. *J Comp Neurol.* 1990;294:76–95.
44. Morrell MJ, Guldner G. Self-reported sexual function in women with epilepsy. *Epilepsia.* 1994;35(S8):108.
45. Taylor DC. Sexual behavior and temporal lobe epilepsy. *Arch Neurol.* 1969;21:510–516.
46. Hierons R, Saunders M. Impotence in patients with temporal lobe lesions. *Lancet.* 1966;2:761–764.
47. Herzog AG, Seibel MM, Schomer DL, *et al.* Reproductive endocrine disorders in men with partial seizures of temporal lobe origin. *Arch Neurol.* 1986;43:347–350.
48. Blumer D. Changes of sexual behavior related to temporal lobe disorders in man. *J Sex Res.* 1970;6:173–180.
49. Bear DM, Fedio P. Quantitative analysis of interictal behavior in temporal lobe epilepsy. *Arch Neurol.* 1977;34:454–467.
50. Carter J, Tyson J, Tolis G. Prolactin-secreting tumors and hypogonadism in 22 men. *N Engl J Med.* 1978;299:847–852.
51. Molaie M, Culebras A, Miller M. Nocturnal plasma prolactin and cortisol levels in epileptics with complex partial seizures and primary generalized seizures. *Arch Neurol.* 1987;44:699–702.
52. Trimble MR. Serum prolactin in epilepsy and hysteria. *Br Med J.* 1978;2:1682.
53. Dana–Haeri J, Trimble MR, Oxley J. Prolactin and gonadotrophin changes following generalized and partial seizures. *J Neurol Neurosurg Psychiatry.* 1983;46:331–335.
54. Pritchard PB, Wannamaker BB, Sagel J, *et al.* Endocrine function following complex partial seizures. *Ann Neurol.* 1983;14:27–32.
55. Wyllie E, Luders H, Macmillan JP, *et al.* Serum prolactin levels after epileptic seizures. *Neurology.* 1984;34:1601–1604.
56. Sperling MR, Pritchard PB, Engel J, *et al.* Prolactin in partial epilepsy: An indicator of limbic seizures. *Ann Neurol.* 1986;20:716–722.
57. Reichlin S. In: Wilson JD, Foster DW, eds. *Williams Textbook of Endocrinology.* Philadelphia: W.B. Saunders; 1992:135–221.
58. Piva F, Marhini L, Motta M. A pharmacological analysis of the role of the amygdala in the control of gonadotropin and prolactin secretion. *Adv Biochem Psychopharmacol.* 1980;24:425–435.

59. Abbott RJ, Browning MCK, Davidson DLW. Serum prolactin and cortisol concentrations after grand mal seizures. *J Neurol Neurosurg Psychiatry.* 1980;43:163–167.

60. Aminoff MJ, Simon R, Wiedemann E. The hormonal responses to generalized tonic-clonic seizures. *Brain.* 1984;107:569–578.

61. Gallagher BB, Murvin A, Flanigin HF, et al. Pituitary and adrenal function in epileptic patients. *Epilepsia.* 1984;25:683–689.

62. Mandell AJ, Chapman LF, Rand RW, et al. Plasma corticosteroids: Changes in concentration after stimulation of hippocampus and amygdala. *Science.* 1963;139:1212.

63. Dunn JD, Whitener J. Plasma corticosterone responses to electrical stimulation of the amygdaloid complex: Cytoarchitectural specificity. *Neuroendocrinology.* 1986;42:211–217.

64. Gray TS, Carney ME, Magnusson DJ. Direct projections from the central amygdaloid nucleus to the hypothalamic paraventricular nucleus: Possible role in stress-induced adrenocorticotropin release. *Neuroendocrinology.* 1989;50:433–446.

65. Herzog AG, Sotrel A, Ronthal M. Reversible proximal myopathy in epilepsy-related Cushing's syndrome. *Ann Neurol.* 1995;38:306–307.

66. Woodbury DM. Effect of adrenocortical steroids and adrenocorticotropic hormone on electroshock seizure threshold. *J Pharmacol Exp Ther.* 1952;105:27–36.

67. Baram TZ, Hirsch E, Snead CO, et al. Corticotropin-releasing hormone-induced seizures in infant rats originate in the amygdala. *Ann Neurol.* 1992;31:488–494.

68. Woolley CS, Gould E, McEwen BS. Exposure to excess glucocorticoids alters dendritic morphology of adult hippocampal pyramidal neurons. *Brain Res.* 1990;531:225–231.

69. Toone BK, Wheeler M, Nanjee M, et al. Sex hormones, sexual activity and plasma anticonvulsant levels in male epileptics. *J Neurol Neurosurg Psychiatry.* 1983;46:824–826.

70. Isojarvi JIT, Pakarinen AJ, Ylipalosaari PJ, et al. Serum hormones in male epileptic patients receiving anticonvulsant medication. *Arch Neurol.* 1990;47:670–676.

71. Davidson JM, Camargo CA, Smith ER. Effects of androgens on sexual behavior in hypogonadal men. *J Clin Endocrinol Metab.* 1979;48:955–958.

72. Herzog AG. Hormonal changes in epilepsy. *Epilepsia.* 1995;36:323–326.

73. Kuhn–Velten WN, Herzog AG, Muller MR. Acute effects of anticonvulsant drugs on gonadotropin-stimulated and precursor-supported testicular androgen production. *Eur J Pharmacol.* 1990;181:151–155.

74. Isojarvi JIT, Repo M, Pakarinen AJ, et al. Carbamazepine, phenytoin, sex hormones and sexual dysfunction in men with epilepsy. *Epilepsia.* 1995;36:364–368.

75. Herzog AG, Levesque L, Drislane F, et al. Phenytoin-induced elevations of serum estradiol and reproductive dysfunction in men with epilepsy. *Epilepsia.* 1991;32:550–553.

76. Murialdo G, Galimberti CA, Fonzi S, et al. Sex hormones and pituitary function in male epileptic patients with altered or normal sexuality. *Epilepsia.* 1995;36:364–368.

77. Klein P, Jacobs AR, Herzog AG. A comparison of testosterone versus testosterone and testolactone in the treatment of reproductive/sexual dysfunction in men with epilepsy and hypogonadism. *Neurology.* 1996;46:177.

78. Herzog AG. Seizure control with clomiphene therapy: A case report. *Arch Neurol.* 1988;45:209–210.

79. Login IS, Dreifuss FE. Anticonvulsant activity of clomiphene. *Arch Neurol.* 1983;40:525.

80. Isojarvi JIT, Laatikainen TJ, Pakarinen AJ, et al. Polycystic ovaries and hyperandrogenism in women taking valproate for epilepsy. *N Engl J Med.* 1993;329:1383–1388.

81. Herzog AG. Polycystic ovarian syndrome in women with epilepsy: Epileptic or iatrogenic? *Ann Neurol.* 1996;39:559–561.

82. Isojarvi JIT, Laatikainen, Knip M, et al. Obesity and endocrine disorders in women taking valproate for epilepsy. *Ann Neurol.* 1996;39:579–585.

83. Margraf JW, Dreifuss FE. Amenorrhoea following initiation of therapy with valproic acid. *Neurology.* 1981;31:159.

84. Jones TH. Sodium valproate-induced menstrual disturbances in young women. *Hormone Res.* 1991;35:82–85.

85. Holmes GL. Carbamazepine: Toxicity. In: Levy RH, Mattson RH, Meldrum BS, eds. *Antiepileptic Drugs.* New York: Raven Press; 1996:567–579.

86. Isojarvi JIT, Pakarinen AJ, Ylipalosaari PJ, *et al.* Serum hormones in male epileptic patients receiving anticonvulsant medication. *Arch Neurol.* 1990;47:670–676.

87. Mattson RH, Cramer JA, Caldwell BV, *et al.* Treatment of seizures with medroxyprogesterone acetate: Preliminary report. *Neurology.* 1984;34:1255–1258.

88. Dana Haeri J, Richens A. Effect of norethisterone on seizures associated with menstruation. *Epilepsia.* 1983;24:377–381.

89. Herzog AG. Clomiphene therapy in epileptic women with menstrual disorders. *Neurology.* 1988;38:432–434.

90. Haider Y, Barnett D. Catamenial epilepsy and goserelin. *Lancet.* 1991;2:1530.

91. Snead OC. ACTH and prednisone: use in seizure disorders other than infantile spasms. In: Levy RH, Mattson RH, Meldrum BS, eds. *Antiepileptic Drugs.* New York: Raven Press; 1995:941–948.

CHAPTER 13

Epilepsy and the Elderly

Edward B. Bromfield, M.D.

It is a truism of modern American medicine that care of the elderly will demand an increasing share of resources as our population ages. Largely because of advances in the prevention and treatment of vascular disease, the longevity of both men and women continues to increase, putting them at risk for a variety of diseases and disorders, especially typically nonfatal ones, such as seizure disorders. The number of elderly persons continues to grow at a much faster rate than the general population; the number of people in the United States aged 75 and older, for example, comprised only 900,000 in 1900, reached 10 million by 1990, and is projected to exceed 13 million by 2000.[1] This demographic trend is magnified by the fact that the incidence of seizures and epilepsy increases above age 50. Furthermore, optimal care of older persons with epilepsy requires modifications in diagnostic, therapeutic, and psychosocial approaches.

HOW COMMON IS EPILEPSY IN THE ELDERLY POPULATION?

Epidemiologic studies of several populations[2-6] have shown that the incidence of seizures, epilepsy, or both is high within the first few years of life, stabilizes over the second through fifth decades, and then rises again, in some studies approaching or exceeding rates seen in infancy (Fig. 13.1). In the Rochester, Minnesota, population,[5] newly diagnosed epilepsy was seen in 139 of 100,000 persons aged 75 or older, versus 44 per 100,000 throughout the lifespan. Scheuer and Cohen[6] calculate, based on 1990 U.S. census data and incidence and prevalence data from the Mayo clinic, that in this country there are 331,000 persons aged 65 and older with epilepsy and that 41,700 of them have new-onset cases. These numbers are below those for stroke and dementia but comparable to those for such other age-related conditions as Parkinson's disease.[7]

WHAT ARE THE MOST COMMON CAUSES OF SEIZURES AND EPILEPSY IN OLDER AGE GROUPS?

Isolated seizures can be caused by nearly any condition that affects brain function, including such systemic insults as toxic-metabolic disturbances and acute

The Comprehensive Evaluation and Treatment of Epilepsy
Copyright © 1997 by Academic Press. All rights of reproduction in any form reserved.

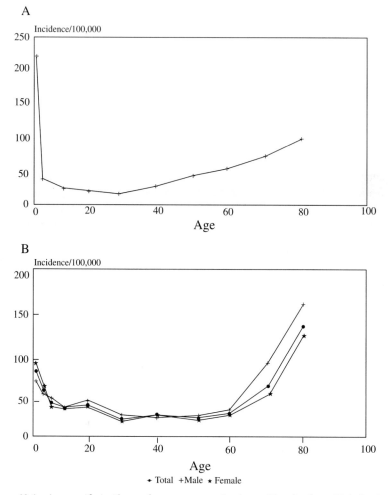

Figure 13.1   Age-specific incidence of acute symptomatic seizures (A) and epilepsy (B) in Rochester, Minnesota, 1935–1984. (Adapted from Hauser WA. Seizure disorders: The changes with age. *Epilepsia.* 1992;33:S6–S14.)[4]

neurologic conditions such as stroke or trauma. Among the former are disturbances in glucose or electrolytes, renal failure, and drug intoxication or withdrawal. Most metabolic conditions become more common with aging, as does the use of multiple prescription medications.[8] Offending drugs include theophylline and neuroleptics, as well as a variety of antidepressants[9] (Table 13.1). Sedative and alcohol withdrawal are also significant causes. Although these conditions may be recurrent, they are at least potentially preventable and, therefore, would not lead to a diagnosis of epilepsy.

Table 13.1

Commonly Used Drugs that May Lower Seizure Threshold

Category	Drug	Comment
Antiasthmatics	Aminophylline Theophylline	Especially but not exclusively above therapeutic levels
Antibiotics	Isoniazid Lindane Metronidazole Nalidixic acid Penicillins	Vitamin B$_6$ supplement may protect Especially with renal failure
Antidepressants	Tricyclics Serotonin-specific agents Bupropion	Rarely a practical problem; desipramine may be preferable
General anesthetics	Enflurane Ketamine	
Hormones	Insulin Prednisone Estrogen	By means of hypoglycemia By means of hypocalcemia Especially without progesterone
Immunosuppressants	Chlorambucil Cyclosporine A	
Local anesthetics	Lidocaine Bupivicaine Procaine	
Narcotics	Fentanyl Meperidine Pentazocine Propoxyphene	
Psychostimulants	Amphetamines Cocaine Methylphenidate Phenylpropanolamine	
Neuroleptics	Clozapine Phenothiazines Butyrophenones	1–4% of all patients, depending on dose Molindone, thioridazine, fluphenazine least likely
Other	Anticholinergics Anticholinesterases Antihistamines Baclofen Heavy metals Hyperbaric oxygen Lithium Mefenamic acid Oral hypoglycemics Oxytocin	 By means of water intoxication

Structural damage to the brain, on the other hand, even if functionally minor, can lead to permanent alterations in neuronal excitability and synchronization, resulting in a tendency toward recurrent unprovoked seizures—that is, epilepsy. Because recovery from central nervous system injury, at least on a cellular level, is usually incomplete, the accumulation of brain insults over time would lead to increased incidence and prevalence of epilepsy with aging.

Virtually every study of epilepsy in the elderly has found vascular disease, either acutely or remotely, to be responsible for the largest proportion of cases, in general the majority of those for which a cause is known (Table 13.2). Although the occurrence of seizures within a week or two after stroke does not necessarily indicate that epilepsy will develop, such early seizures increase the risk of later epilepsy.[8] The longer the interval between the insult and the first seizure, the more likely it is that the seizure represents a permanent change in neuronal connectivity predictive of further seizures if untreated.

After stroke, brain tumor (either metastatic or primary) is the next most common cause of epilepsy, reported in up to 28% of new-onset cases (Table 13.2). Structural causes of epilepsy other than vascular and neoplastic disease include trauma (which may not be recalled by the patient), degenerative disease, particularly senile dementia of the Alzheimer's type, and infectious causes such as meningitis or encephalitis. Alzheimer's disease, associated with seizures in perhaps 10% of cases,[22,23] will be an increasingly important cause in the future unless effective methods of prevention or treatment are found. It is important to recognize, however, that even in patients with structural lesions that could potentially cause

Table 13.2

Etiology of Seizures and Epilepsy in Selected Studies of Elderly Patients

Study	N	Vascular (%)	Tumor (%)	Other (%)	Unknown (%)
White et al., 1953[11]	107	41	9	28	22
Juul–Jensen, 1964[12]	78	69	15	7	9
Woodcock, 1964[13]	25	44	28	4	24
Carney et al., 1969[14]	92	18	22	28	32
Hildick–Smith, 1974[15]	48	44	10	24	22
Schold et al., 1977[16]	50	30	2	18	50
Gupta, 1983[17]	74	50	0	32	18
Luhdorf et al., 1986[18]	151	32	14	29	25
Sundaram, 1989[19]	67	22	24	20	34
Loiseau et al., 1990[20]	284	47	9	31	15
Hauser, 1992[4]	N/A	32	3	15	49
Ettinger, 1993[21]	80	54	8	31	8

N/A, Not applicable.

epilepsy, seizures can have a toxic-metabolic or other preventable cause, and these should be ruled out before assuming that epilepsy has developed.

WHAT TYPES OF STROKES ARE MOST LIKELY TO CAUSE SEIZURES?

Strokes are acute vascular insults; they may be divided into ischemic and hemorrhagic strokes. Ischemic strokes can be further subdivided into embolic, thrombotic, and small vessel ("lacunar"), and hemorrhagic strokes may be further subcategorized by location and etiology.[24] All the ischemic and most of the hemorrhagic causes show marked increases with aging. Some but not all studies have shown that embolic strokes have the greatest tendency to produce acute seizures as well as epilepsy,[25] perhaps because they are the most likely to involve the cortex directly and also often include at least a small hemorrhagic component; in experimental models, the direct application of iron increases cortical irritability. Overall, 4–14% of infarcts are associated with early seizures, usually defined as occurring within 1–2 weeks of the insult, whereas 3–10% are associated with later seizures.[25-30] As noted previously, Kilpatrick et al.[10] confirmed that early seizures were a risk factor for late seizures; late seizures developed in 10 of 31 patients with early seizures, in contrast to 3 of 31 matched stroke control patients without early seizures. Ng et al.[31] found an association between new-onset seizures and hypertension, presumably a marker for cerebrovascular disease, even in the absence of clinical or neuroimaging evidence of stroke. Transient ischemic attacks (TIAs) lasting less than 24 h have in some series been found to presage epilepsy, and Shinton et al.[32] found that elderly patients experiencing seizures had an increased incidence of vascular disease as compared with a control population. In addition, Annegers et al.[33] found a secular trend of declining incidence of idiopathic seizures in the elderly that paralleled the decline in cerebrovascular disease over the years 1935 to 1984. The preceding findings suggest that seizures may, in a sense, represent a marker for cerebrovascular disease in older patients.

The risk of seizures after hemorrhagic stroke is more strongly linked to mechanism and location than is ischemic stroke. Hypertensive hemorrhage is most often subcortical, decreasing the likelihood that seizures or epilepsy will result.[34] Faught et al.[35] found, however, that not just lobar hemorrhage but also basal ganglia hemorrhage involving the caudate was associated with a significant risk of acute seizures; Berger et al.[36] noted that 17% of hemorrhages, typically with cortical extension, were accompanied by seizures, all occurring at the onset of hemorrhage.

HOW DO SEIZURES PRESENT IN OLDER PEOPLE?

Information about specific seizures in the elderly varies among studies. Partial seizures, particularly if defined as in the International League against Epilepsy classification to include secondarily generalized seizures, are much more common than primarily generalized seizures, which usually have their onset in childhood or adolescence and often remit with maturity. However, retrospective studies have been inconsistent in their identification or classification of secondarily generalized seizures and have considered only one-third to two-thirds to be partial.[4–6,21] Electroencephalographic (EEG) data, when available, frequently shows focal abnormalities.[21,37] Anecdotally, manifestations of partial seizures in the elderly, reflecting the multiple areas of the brain vulnerable to largely vascular and neoplastic insults, are more varied than those in younger adults, the largest group of whom have partial seizures of mesial temporal origin. Although these limbic seizures can certainly begin late in life as a result of appropriately placed lesions, when present in the elderly they more commonly represent persistent cases dating back to childhood, adolescence, or early adulthood. Because mesial temporal lobe epilepsy (TLE) is often treatment resistant, the condition is likely to persist into old age. Although the prevalence of "typical" mesial TLE in the elderly is uncertain, complex partial seizures as a group have been found to be the most common seizure type in this population.[4]

Partial seizures with prominent motor manifestations, reflecting the low threshold of motor cortex to seizure generation,[38] are often seen after stroke, although it is not clear that these seizures are more common in older than in younger persons.[39] Reporting bias may affect these data, however, because motor seizures are more likely to be recognized and diagnosed in patients who may have diminished communicative skills than are seizures with only subjective manifestations. Visceral, visual, and somatosensory auras preceding complex partial or secondarily generalized seizures are probably not rare but must be carefully sought.[39,40] In the absence of a detailed history, seizures must be considered whenever there is a transient confusional state, unexplained loss of consciousness, or a fall without a clear environmental or medical explanation.[7,41]

As suggested earlier, classification of epilepsy syndromes in the elderly leans strongly toward the localization-related, symptomatic group; idiopathic syndromes would be represented by long-standing cases that have not remitted. Juvenile myoclonic epilepsy, for example, typically persists into adulthood and is often misdiagnosed, and may therefore on occasion present in old age. Hauser,[4] however, points out that most of these idiopathic syndromes are defined in part by age of onset, perhaps obscuring their identification in atypically older patients.

WHAT IS THE DIFFERENTIAL DIAGNOSIS OF TRANSIENT ALTERATIONS IN FUNCTION IN THIS POPULATION, AND WHAT TESTS BEST DISTINGUISH ONE DISORDER FROM ANOTHER?

Episodic neurologic dysfunction in the elderly has a wide differential diagnosis, certain conditions being much more strongly represented among older than younger patients. Disorders that can in some instances be difficult to distinguish from seizures include syncope, TIAs, migraine, sleep disorders, paroxysmal toxic-metabolic abnormalities, movement disorders, and psychiatric conditions.[42]

SYNCOPE

Syncope in the elderly is particularly important to recognize because it becomes both more common and potentially more ominous with aging. Mechanisms that can cause a sufficient decrease in cerebral perfusion to produce the loss of consciousness and postural tone that characterizes syncope include: (1) an inappropriate reflex-mediated decrease in heart rate, vascular tone, or both; (2) arrhythmias producing decreased cardiac output; (3) decreased cardiac output from other causes.[43] Typically, the mean blood pressure must drop suddenly and significantly, usually to less than 50 mm Hg.[44] Simple vasovagal fainting is the most common manifestation of reflex-mediated syncope. It usually follows a strong emotional stimulus and often but not always has a strong postural component. Although the most common cause of syncope in young people, it may account for only 1–5% of cases in the elderly.[44] Other reflex-mediated causes include carotid sinus syncope, micturition and defecation syncope, and syncope during and after eating.

Cardiac arrhythmias are essential to rule out, because they can lead to sudden death if untreated. Both bradycardias and tachycardias may result in syncope and frequently coexist in elderly patients.[43] The coexistence of an alteration in consciousness with a cardiac arrhythmia, however, can on occasion represent a seizure-induced arrhythmia.[45,46]

Additional potential causes of syncope include drugs that result in hypovolemia (e.g., diuretics), decreased venous tone (e.g., nitrates), or decreased systemic resistance (e.g., vasodilators and other antihypertensives). Nondrug causes of these phenomena, including fluid loss and autonomic neuropathy, are also common in the elderly. Syncope can also be caused by a sudden obstruction of blood flow from a pulmonary embolus, or more chronic obstruction from aortic stenosis in the setting of increased demand.

Historical elements that support the diagnosis of syncope include a postural component (although even vasovagal syncope can occur in the supine position with a sufficient emotional stimulus) and premonitory symptoms, such as palpitations, warmth, diaphoresis, fading vision and hearing, nausea, and diffuse weakness. Although all these symptoms may occur during partial seizure auras, in the case of syncope they are often of more gradual onset, and the nausea associated with syncope does not typically have the rising component that is so common in seizures of mesial temporal origin. Pallor is more often noted with syncope but may also occur during limbic seizures. Diffuse stiffening or frank clonic movements may occur with syncope, particularly if the person is maintained in the head-up position.[47] It is important to realize that in the vast majority of cases, convulsive syncope does not represent a cortical electrical seizure but occurs with cortical depression, usually manifested on the EEG by diffuse flattening.[48] The release of brainstem mechanisms from cortical inhibition is the hypothesized mechanism. Unlike a generalized tonic–clonic seizure, syncope, even if convulsive, is usually followed by little or no confusion or somnolence. Urinary incontinence and tongue biting are rare but may occur.

Physical examination should emphasize cardiovascular features, and orthostatic vital signs are sometimes revealing. Ancillary tests worthy of consideration include ECG (electrocardiogram), ambulatory ECG (Holter) monitoring, echocardiography, and in selected cases, tilt-table testing and cardiac electrophysiologic studies.[49]

TRANSIENT ISCHEMIC ATTACKS

Transient ischemic attacks (TIAs) are important to recognize because of the impact that treatment can have on the risk of future stroke as well as on myocardial infarction.[24,50] Although ischemia generally produces "negative symptoms" such as weakness or visual loss rather than "positive symptoms" such as stiffening, shaking, or visual hallucinations, there are many exceptions. Among the most dramatic, if not the most common, are the so-called limb-shaking TIAs associated with severe carotid disease contralateral to the involved limb.[50,51] These involve the leg, arm, or both, rarely bilaterally, and spare the face as well as spare cognition. Duration may be seconds to minutes, similar to that of seizures, but unlike motor seizures these TIAs are consistently postural and respond to endarterectomy rather than to antiepileptic drugs (AEDs). Conversely, seizures manifested by motor inhibition, amaurosis, and aphasia with preserved consciousness are rare but well documented, and can be difficult to distinguish from TIAs; EEG is invaluable in confirming the epileptic origin of these events.[52,53]

Historical features helping to diagnose TIAs include constellations of symptoms consistent with ischemia in either anterior or posterior circulations, or in a "lacunar" distribution, in the setting of prior vascular disease or known risk factors. Onset may be sudden or gradual, but resolution is usually much slower than for seizures, and duration is usually longer, up to several hours. Neurologic examination during symptoms usually confirms a vascular distribution. Bruits may be present. Neuroimaging studies can be extremely helpful in showing evidence of either prior vascular insults or an active lesion corresponding to the current symptoms. Vascular and cardiac studies may confirm a suspected location or mechanism. One must keep in mind, however, that an appropriately placed infarct could also provide the substrate for seizures; EEG may be helpful and, if recorded ictally, diagnostic.

MIGRAINE

Migraine can be difficult to distinguish from epilepsy, and the two processes can coexist. Although migraine is more common in younger than in older adults, the possibility that migraine may more often occur without headache in the elderly[54,55] complicates the picture. Migraine auras such as scintillating scotomata, hemianopia, or monocular blindness may be confused more readily with TIAs than with seizures. "Basilar migraine" symptoms, however, can include altered consciousness as well as vertigo, ataxia, and visual disturbances,[55] and can sometimes mimic a seizure or nonconvulsive status epilepticus.

SLEEP DISORDERS

Sleep disorders have been increasingly recognized in recent years. Obstructive sleep apnea is common in the elderly, affecting perhaps 5–10% or more of elderly persons, and may have significant consequences.[56] Excessive daytime somnolence is the most common consequence and may greatly affect functioning; in addition, nocturnal cardiac arrhythmias may increase the risk of cardiac or cerebral ischemia and of sudden death. Sleepiness can sometimes manifest itself as "microsleeps," which are brief periods of unresponsiveness because of sleep; these can be confused with partial seizures. Rarely, intermittent confusion or even apparent dementia can be a result of excessive sleepiness. Other causes of poor nocturnal sleep, such as periodic limb movement syndrome, can have similar daytime manifestations.[56] Occasionally, the limb movements themselves may be mistaken for seizure activity, although they are usually easy to distinguish, occurring as sustained 0.5–5-s movements at 20–60-s intervals rather than in a rapid rhythmic pattern.

The classic parasomnias of slow-wave sleep, somnambulism and night terrors, may be confused with seizures but are not found in and rarely persist to old age.[56,57] Nocturnal enuresis, raising the possibility of a nighttime convulsion, is also a condition of childhood, although the symptom may occur in the elderly as a consequence of a urinary tract infection or another urologic cause. Typically, however, daytime incontinence is also present. The narcolepsy–cataplexy syndrome generally appears in early adulthood, although it may not be diagnosed until later; obstructive sleep apnea is a more common cause of excessive daytime somnolence in the elderly, however, and may coexist with narcolepsy. Attacks of "paroxysmal nocturnal dystonia" are likely to represent frontal lobe seizures.[56]

Rapid eye movement (REM) sleep behavior disorder is a recognized parasomnia that occurs most commonly in elderly men. This disorder consists of sudden arousals from REM sleep that are immediately followed by complex and often violent behavior, at times appearing directed, although the patient is unresponsive and amnestic for these periods. There is a significant risk of injury to the patient or bed partner. These behaviors are often construed as defensive activity related to dreaming, with loss of the somatic atonia that is normally present during REM sleep and dreaming. There is great potential for misinterpreting these episodes as complex partial seizures or postictal agitation.[57]

Polysomnography is essential for the diagnosis of sleep apnea, periodic limb movements, and parasomnias. In most laboratories it is possible to perform a more complete EEG recording than the minimum needed for sleep staging, and this should be done when nocturnal seizures are under consideration. The multiple sleep latency test is a means of quantifying daytime sleepiness, which is essential in diagnosing narcolepsy, and which also can be helpful in assessing the effects of other sleep disorders on daytime alertness.

TOXIC-METABOLIC DISTURBANCES

Most toxic-metabolic disturbances produce a long-lasting confusional state that does not strongly suggest an isolated seizure, although nonconvulsive status epilepticus[58–60] or a prolonged postictal state should be considered. Myoclonus, which can occur in many electrolyte disturbances and intoxications as well as in uremia and sepsis, can further confuse the picture. The EEG may show sharp activity, although usually not frank spikes and not a dominant focus unless there is preexisting focal illness. The triphasic wave pattern, most strongly associated with hepatic encephalopathy, is also often seen in uremia and postanoxic coma as well as in other encephalopathies. At times, this pattern can be difficult to distinguish from the generalized sharp-slow or even frank spike-wave complexes of nonconvulsive generalized status epilepticus, which could clinically resemble a metabolic encephalopathy as well.[61] In doubtful cases, benzodiazepine infusion can be helpful if both the EEG and the patient improve, although this test is not always easy to interpret in practice.

Glucose abnormalities, particularly hypoglycemia in patients who are taking insulin or hypoglycemic agents, are notable in that the clinical manifestations may be brief. Typically, the patient exhibits anxiety, tremor, sweating, and tachycardia consistent with sympathetic nervous system activation, but at times loss of consciousness and even true convulsive seizures may occur. Nonketotic hyperglycemia can cause focal myoclonus and true focal or generalized seizures, as can uremia.

MOVEMENT DISORDERS

Movement disorders may be mistaken for motor seizures, but the former are associated with preserved consciousness, are usually bilateral, and are generally not episodic, although they may wax and wane. True paroxysmal kinesogenic choreoathetosis is primarily a condition of childhood and adolescence. It is notable that high doses of AEDs may actually produce movement disorders in some patients; valproate commonly causes a dose-related tremor, for example, and phenytoin rarely produces dystonia.

PSYCHIATRIC DISORDERS

Psychiatric disorders, particularly depression, are common in the elderly, but new-onset psychogenic nonepileptic seizures are probably rare, although this has not been carefully studied. Before making this diagnosis, it is essential that the physician rule out physiologic nonepileptic events such as those described earlier, as well as prove with video-EEG monitoring that there is no ictal or postictal EEG change.[62] Further, the physician must verify that the events do not resemble seizure types during which a negative surface EEG recording is common, such as simple partial or frontal lobe seizures. Placebo induction (see Chapter 9) may also have a place in diagnosis.

WHAT ARE THE MOST IMPORTANT ELEMENTS OF THE HISTORY AND PHYSICAL EXAMINATION, AND WHAT ANCILLARY DIAGNOSTIC TESTS SHOULD BE PERFORMED TO EVALUATE A FIRST SEIZURE?

As with younger patients, the most useful history is that provided by the patient, supplemented by a reliable observer for any period during which the patient was unconscious or confused. In the elderly, it is critical to inquire about any ongoing illnesses or medications, as well as position and activities at the time of the event, nature and rate of onset of symptoms, skin color changes, motor activity, and duration of ictal and postictal periods if identifiable. Any history of prenatal or perinatal difficulties; febrile seizures in childhood; staring spells or myoclonus in childhood or adolescence; inflammatory, vascular, or neoplastic disease; or head trauma should be elicited.

Physical and neurologic examinations should address mainly the issues of cardiovascular function, metabolic–endocrine status, and prior neurologic insults. In emergencies, metabolic studies (electrolytes, calcium, magnesium, glucose, and renal and liver function tests), a toxic screen, and a complete blood count should generally be performed. If symptoms or signs of infection are present, a lumbar puncture should be done, generally after a neuroimaging procedure. Noncontrast computed tomography is adequate to rule out hemorrhage or a large mass lesion, but magnetic resonance imaging is indicated in nonemergencies because of its high sensitivity to potentially treatable structural lesions, particularly small neoplasms.

Although the effects of electroencephalography on treatment may not always be obvious, it is a noninvasive, relatively inexpensive test that directly displays brain electrical activity and can provide additional data to support or refute the seizure diagnosis, help confirm the relevance of a minor structural lesion, demonstrate focality when no other localizing findings are seen on examination or neuroimaging, or, rarely, raise the possibility of late presentation of a primary generalized disorder. Although the EEG need not be obtained immediately, the yield of interictal epileptiform discharges and of diagnostic postictal slowing is maximal if the test is done sooner rather than later. In some situations, such as if encephalitis is suspected, the EEG can be crucial to early diagnosis.[61] Epileptiform findings on EEG, particularly periodic lateralized epileptiform discharges, are also predictive of the development of seizures after stroke even if no seizures have been observed before the study.[63] If diagnosis remains uncertain or frequent events are occurring despite treatment, long-term video-EEG monitoring, perhaps with additional ECG and sleep-related polygraphy, is indicated. In the acute setting, if full recovery does not follow promptly after the seizure apparently terminates, EEG is necessary to rule out ongoing nonconvulsive status epilepticus.[64] The electroencephalographer must be familiar with the effects of normal aging on the EEG, particularly regarding temporal slowing, which is often asymmetric (L>R), and with normal variants that could be mistaken for epileptiform abnormalities.[61,65]

WHEN SHOULD OLDER PATIENTS RECEIVE THERAPY AFTER A FIRST SEIZURE?

There is still controversy about the risks versus benefits of AED therapy after a first seizure at any age, and old age may sharpen the differences. First, a thorough evaluation should establish that the event was in fact a seizure, and should rule out a reversible or avoidable seizure precipitant. Alcohol withdrawal, for example, is not rare in older persons, and this history must be sought specifically. Acute treatment may be necessary to prevent status epilepticus in this situation, but in general AEDs are not used chronically except in those who have been shown to have seizures remote from heavy alcohol consumption.

Even if no precipitant is found, the seizure may not recur; the 2-year recurrence risk has been estimated at 23–71% in a meta-analysis of several studies.[66] Risk is highest in those with abnormal neurologic status and in those with a remote brain insult[66–68]; this would include the large proportion of elderly patients who experience a seizure after a stroke. Deciding whether or not to initiate treatment, however, depends on more than just recurrence risk. Patient activities, risk of injury with further seizures, coexisting illness, susceptibility to drug side effects, and attitudes toward taking medications must all be taken into account.[7,41,69] In addition, although a randomized study demonstrates that treatment decreases recurrence risk by approximately 50%,[70] it does not guarantee that no further seizures will not occur, and activities such as driving must be limited until it is clear that the risk of injury is sufficiently low. Furthermore, the elderly are more susceptible to adverse drug effects and to drug interactions (discussed later in this chapter). On the other hand, there have been rare reports of persistent worsening of stroke-related deficits after seizures, which would tend to favor treatment in this situation.[71]

It is not unusual for elderly persons to be taking more than three, and often ten or more, prescription medications.[8] In these cases, drug interactions are nearly inevitable, and the ability of many AEDs to induce or inhibit hepatic metabolizing enzymes makes pharmacokinetic interactions likely. Although the possibility of a seizure leading to a fall may drive the decision to treat, the physician must ensure that ataxia caused by excessive AED dosing or drug interactions does not in itself result in falling.

WHAT CONSIDERATIONS APPLY TO CHOICE OF AEDs IN THE ELDERLY? WHAT POTENTIAL ADVERSE EFFECTS AND DRUG INTERACTIONS ARE OF PARTICULAR CONCERN IN THE ELDERLY?

As discussed previously in this book, the drugs of first choice in the United States for the treatment of partial seizures remain phenytoin and carbamazepine. Some studies support the contention that valproate is equally effective and well tolerated,[72] especially for partial seizures that secondarily generalize, but other studies dispute this finding.[73] Valproate remains the preferred drug for primary generalized epilepsy, but as noted earlier, these syndromes are much less likely to appear in old age than partial epilepsies. Newer AEDs such as gabapentin and lamotrigine have advantages, but these agents have not yet been approved for monotherapy, which is still preferred to polytherapy, especially in the elderly. On the other hand, gabapentin in particular may be useful in this population because it appears to have minimal pharmacokinetic interactions with other drugs.

Several pharmacokinetic and pharmacodynamic aspects of widely used AEDs deserve special consideration in the elderly and may greatly influence drug choice. Table 13.3 lists some of the commonly used drugs that interact with AEDs. Enzyme induction raises the possibility of decreased concomitant drug effect when carbamazepine, phenytoin, or barbiturates are added; inducing properties of lamotrigine have not been fully worked out, although they seem to be less prominent than those of the other drugs listed. Warfarin is a particular problem if enzyme-inducing drugs are added, requiring more frequent checking of prothrombin time

Table 13.3

Common Drug Interactions with Antiepileptic Drugs

Drugs Whose Metabolism Is Induced by CBZ, PHB, PHT[a] (Decreased Drug Effect)	Drugs that Inhibit Metabolism of CBZ, PHB, LTG, and/or PHT[a] (Increased AED Effect)
Acetominophen	Amiodarone
Cyclosporine A	Chloramphenicol
Digoxin	Chlorpromazine
Disopyramide	Cimetidine
Furosemide	Ranitidine
Neuroleptics	Erythromycin
Propranolol	Imipramine
Quinidine	Ketoconazole
Steroids	Nifedipine
Theophylline	Trimethoprim
Tricyclics	Isoniazid
Warfarin	Phenylbutazone
	Verapamil

[a] CBZ, Carbamazepine; LTG, lamotrigine; PHB, phenobarbital; PHT, phenytoin.

to avoid loss of anticoagulant effect. Inducing drugs typically also lower folate and vitamin D levels, the latter being of particular importance in elderly women, who are already prone to osteopenia and associated fracture; vitamin D and calcium supplementation are generally indicated. Enzyme inhibition from other drugs, or withdrawal of an enzyme-inducing drug, presents the opposite risk. This is again a major issue particularly with warfarin, hemorrhage being a significant danger. Drugs with a high protein-binding fraction may displace and be displaced by other drugs that are highly bound, including such common medicines as aspirin. Typically, the displaced drug initially has a stronger effect as more free drug becomes available, and then an increased rate of metabolism tends to compensate. If aspirin is added to phenytoin, for example, transient toxicity may result until metabolism "catches up" to the higher free level. Because the free phenytoin fraction will be elevated as long as aspirin is taken, the patient's "therapeutic range" for total level falls. Direct measurement of free fraction may be helpful in this situation.

Several potential adverse effects of AEDs may be of particular concern in the elderly. Older patients are probably more sensitive than younger ones to sedation or paradoxical agitation from barbiturates and benzodiazepines.[7,69,74] Ataxia from several drugs may, as mentioned, result in falls and injury. Carbamazepine's ability to slow atrioventricular nodal conduction may pose a particular risk of bradyarrhythmias in elderly patients, especially those with cardiac conduction defects. The elderly may also be at increased risk for hyponatremia with carbamazepine, although the age relationship has not been confirmed. Valproate does not cause many of these adverse effects but may rarely induce thrombocytopenia or thrombocytopathy, of particular concern in patients who are taking antiplatelet agents or anticoagulants. Dose-related tremor may also be exacerbated in those with preexisting essential tremor or parkinsonism; parkinsonism itself, as well as dementia and hearing deficit, has also been reported with valproate.[75] Although gabapentin appears to be free from pharmacokinetic interactions, decreased renal function with aging may make elderly patients more sensitive to pharmacodynamic adverse effects and interactions, including sedation and ataxia. In general, AEDs should be started at lower doses in the elderly, titrated more slowly, and stabilized at lower doses and levels than in younger patients.

IN WHAT WAYS DO PHARMACOKINETIC FACTORS CHANGE WITH AGING? WHAT ARE THE IMPLICATIONS FOR THE WAY AEDs ARE USED IN OLDER PEOPLE?

Several aspects of drug pharmacokinetics change predictably with aging and are of variable clinical significance[74,76,77] (Table 13.4). Pharmacokinetics includes

Table 13.4

Pharmacokinetic Changes in Aging with Respect to Commonly Used Antiepileptic Drugs[77]

Phase	Function	Change (Up or Down)	Effect on Drug Action (Up, Down, Minimal)	Drugs Most Affected
Absorption	Gastric pH	Up	Minimal	
	Gastrointestinal motility	Down	Minimal	
	Splanchnic blood flow	Down	Minimal	
Distribution	Percentage of body fat	Up	Down	All
	Serum albumin	Down	Up (short term)	PHT, VPA, CBZ[a]
Metabolism	Hepatic mass	Down	Up	All except GP[a]
	Hepatic blood flow	Down	Up	All except GP[a]
Excretion	Renal blood flow	Down	Up	GP, PHB[a]
	Glomerular filtration	Down	Up	GP, PHB[a]

[a] CBZ, Carbamazepine; GP, gabapentin; LTG, lamotrigine; PHB, phenobarbital; PHT, phenytoin; VPA valproate.

the processes of drug absorption, distribution, and elimination via metabolism and excretion. Absorption of AEDs remains complete, unless calcium-containing antacids are taken. Gastric pH tends to increase, but this seems to have little effect. Drug distribution is affected by the decrease in lean body mass that occurs with aging, as well as by decreased albumin levels for drugs that are highly protein bound. These effects tend to oppose each other, since lipophilic AEDs would be distributed to tissues other than brain more than in younger people, but there is also more free drug to distribute. Drug elimination tends to be slower because of decreased hepatic enzyme activity and hepatic blood flow, as well as decreased renal clearance; the latter may affect excretion of barbiturates as well as gabapentin. The net result of these factors for most people and most drugs is to lower drug clearance,[8,74,77] which is another reason to start at lower doses and titrate more slowly than in younger patients.

WHAT IS THE PROGNOSIS OF EPILEPSY IN ELDERLY PATIENTS?

Although the response of seizures to treatment has not been studied systematically in the elderly, most retrospective series have reported that seizures are readily controlled in the majority of cases by a single AED.[6] However, compliance problems related to cognitive, sensory, and motor deficits and social isolation may interfere with successful treatment.[41,69]

Excess mortality over that expected for age appears to be related primarily to underlying illness such as cancer or vascular disease,[21] although there may also be an increased incidence of sudden death in epilepsy with aging.[78]

HOW SHOULD LONG-STANDING, APPARENTLY STABLE EPILEPSY IN THE ELDERLY BE TREATED? WHEN CAN AEDs BE WITHDRAWN IN THIS POPULATION?

As with any chronic condition, periodic reassessment is important, particularly when different caregivers are involved, either sequentially or simultaneously. Specific questioning about seizure frequency, including simple partial seizures, and potential adverse drug effects is essential.

Compliance should be verified, and obstacles such as those mentioned earlier should be addressed. Enlistment of family members or visiting nurses can be critical to ensuring compliance and adequate reporting of symptoms, because underreporting of symptoms has been well documented in the elderly.[1] It is important to inquire about any new drugs that can potentially interact with AEDs, as well as any other newly diagnosed conditions such as cardiac, renal, or hepatic disease. Periodic monitoring of blood chemistries and AED levels is probably of the most utility in this age group, in whom long-term changes in these parameters may be detected before they become symptomatic.

The possibility of adding or substituting one of the newer AEDs should be considered, although in general a change in therapy should be avoided if seizures are controlled without significant adverse drug effects. If it can be verified that the patient has been free from seizures for at least 2 years, the possibility of drug withdrawal can be raised; a prospective study[79] of the risk of seizure recurrence in this circumstance did not show advanced age to be a significant risk factor in a multivariate analysis. The use of electroencephalography has been of limited value in this setting. As at any age, an important issue is the risk of injury or social limitation (e.g., driving restriction) if a relapse occurs, as it does in one-third to one-half of cases under the best of circumstances.

IS SURGICAL TREATMENT FOR MEDICALLY INTRACTABLE EPILEPSY A POSSIBILITY IN ELDERLY PATIENTS?

Of several thousand patients nationwide who have received surgical treatment for intractable epilepsy, probably only a handful have been older than age 50. Cascino et al.[80] reported worthwhile outcomes in eight of eight patients, aged 50 to 60, after temporal lobectomy, with three becoming seizure free. Although the trend has been to operate earlier in childhood to minimize psychosocial limitations, many appropriate surgical candidates have never been referred for evaluation and may be first identified in old age. Increased risk of comorbidity and perioperative complications, as well as possibly decreased potential benefit from a successful outcome, should be considered. However, there are likely to be many patients who, despite these considerations, wish to pursue the possibility of living the rest of their lives with no or far fewer epileptic seizures. For patients with extratemporal lesional epilepsy, the same issues apply, although the likelihood of a progressive, histologically malignant lesion increases with age; in these cases the goal of resective surgery would be postponing disability and death rather than alleviating epilepsy. Arguments about increased risk and decreased benefit are more salient when applied to extratemporal, nonlesional epilepsy, which in most studies is associated with a lower success rate and a more demanding evaluation than for temporal lobe epilepsy, and usually requires invasive monitoring.

WHAT ARE THE CAUSES, MANIFESTATIONS, AND RISKS OF STATUS EPILEPTICUS IN THE ELDERLY, AND HOW SHOULD IT BE TREATED?

Both the incidence and complications of status epilepticus increase with aging. Morbidity and mortality increase steadily with age after age 20, mortality rates being in excess of 50% in patients over age 80[81,82] (see Fig. 13.2). To some extent this statistic both reflects and interacts with other mortality risk factors, including duration of status and, especially, etiology. The highest mortality rates are associated with anoxia, infection, metabolic dysfunction, trauma, tumor, and vascular disease, particularly hemorrhage.[82] Discontinuation of AED therapy, a major precipitant of status epilepticus among patients with known epilepsy, continues to have a relatively good prognosis, although prompt treatment is important to avoid systemic complications such as blood pressure lability, hypoxemia, acidosis, and rhabdomyolysis with renal failure.[83,84]

The classification and treatment of status epilepticus are discussed in detail in Chapter 8. Special considerations in the elderly include increased sensitivity to hypotensive and respiratory suppressant effects of intravenously administered AEDs, particularly phenytoin, barbiturates, and benzodiazepines. Careful monitoring of vital signs is mandatory, sometimes requiring slowing the rate of infusion despite

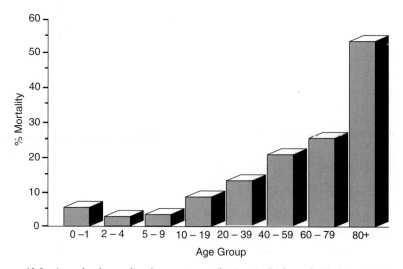

Figure 13.2 Age-related mortality due to status epilepticus in Richmond, Virginia, 1982–1989. (Adapted from DeLorenzo RJ, Towne AR, Pellock JM, *et al.* Status epilepticus in children, adults, and the elderly. *Epilepsia.* 1992;33:S15–S25.)[82]

the risk of prolonging status. Phenytoin, for example, should probably be infused at rates no greater than 25 mg/min. The decision to use pentobarbital coma in refractory status is particularly difficult; Yaffe and Lowenstein[85] documented increased complications related to both age beyond 40 and to the presence of multiple organ failure. There are insufficient data to determine whether the newer alternative of midazolam infusion will be safer, although anecdotally this may be true.[86] Finally, the possibility of nonconvulsive generalized[58,59] or partial[53,60] status epilepticus mimicking other neurologic or medical conditions was mentioned earlier.

WHAT ARE THE IMPLICATIONS OF EPILEPSY AND AED THERAPY FOR INDEPENDENT FUNCTION IN OLDER PERSONS?

Maximizing quality of life and, when possible, normalizing lifestyle in people with epilepsy have been made explicit goals of treatment. These goals remain paramount, if even more challenging, when the patient is facing the obstacles to full, independent function that aging may entail. Medical and psychosocial correlates of epilepsy in the elderly deserve careful attention, often through a multidisciplinary team including primary care providers, medical specialists, mental health professionals, social workers, and family members.[41,69] Increasing knowledge about aging, epilepsy, and their interaction will help to achieve these goals in the future.

REFERENCES

1. Katzman R, Rowe JW. *Principles of Geriatric Neurology*. Philadelphia: F.A. Davis; 1992:1–17.
2. Annegers JF. The epidemiology of epilepsy. In: Wyllie E, ed. *The Treatment of Epilepsy: Principles and Practice*. Philadelphia: Lea & Febiger; 1993:157–164.
3. Annegers JF, Hauser WA, Lee SR, *et al.* Incidence of acute symptomatic seizures in Rochester, Minnesota, 1935–1984. *Epilepsia*. 1995;36:327–333.
4. Hauser WA. Seizure disorders: The changes with age. *Epilepsia*. 1992;33:S6–S14.
5. Hauser WA, Annegers JF, Kurland LT. Incidence of epilepsy and unprovoked seizures in Rochester, Minnesota: 1935–1984. *Epilepsia*. 1993;34:453–468.
6. Scheuer ML, Cohen J. 1993. Seizures and epilepsy in the elderly. *Neurol Clinics*. 1993;11:787–804.
7. Tallis R. Epilepsy. In: Tallis R, ed. *The Clinical Neurology of Old Age*. New York: John Wiley & Sons; 1989:213–234.
8. Willmore LJ, Dulac O. Use of antiepileptic drugs in children and the elderly. In: Levy RH, Mattson RH, Meldrum BS, eds. *Antiepileptic Drugs, 4th Ed*. New York: Raven Press; 1995:231–242.
9. Gilmore R. Seizures associated with nonneurologic medical conditions. In: Wyllie E, ed. *The Treatment of Epilepsy: Principles and Practice*. Philadelphia: Lea & Febiger; 1993:667–677.
10. Kilpatrick CJ, Davis SM, Tress BM, *et al.* Epileptic seizures after acute stroke. *Arch Neurol*. 1990;47:157–160.
11. White PT, Bailey AA, Bickford RG. Epileptic disorders in the aged. *Neurology*. 1953;3:674–678.

12. Juul–Jensen P. A clinical and social analysis of 1020 adults with epileptic seizures. *Acta Neurol Scand.* 1964;40(suppl. 1):1–146.

13. Woodcock S, Cosgrove JBR. Epilepsy after age 40. *Neurology.* 1964;14:34–40.

14. Carney LR, Robert LH, Espinosa RE, *et al.* Seizures beginning after age 60. *Arch Intern Med.* 1969;124:707–709.

15. Hildick–Smith M. Epilepsy in the elderly. *Age Aging.* 1974;3:203–208.

16. Schold C, Yarnell P, Earnest MP. Origin of seizures in elderly patients. *JAMA.* 1977;238:1177–1178.

17. Gupta K. Epilepsy in the elderly: How far to investigate. *Br J Clin Pract.* 1983;37:259–262.

18. Luhdorf K, Jensen LK, Plesner AM. Etiology of seizures in the elderly. *Epilepsia.* 1986;27:458–463.

19. Sundaram MBM. Etiology and patterns of seizures in the elderly. *Neuroepidemiology.* 1989;8:234–238.

20. Loiseau J, Loiseau P, Duche B, *et al.* A survey of epileptic disorders in southwest France: Seizures in elderly patients. *Ann Neurol.* 1990;27:232–237.

21. Ettinger AB, Shinnar S. New onset seizures in an elderly hospitalized patient population. *Neurology.* 1993;43:489–492.

22. Hauser WA, Morris ML, Heston LL, *et al.* Seizures and myoclonus in patients with Alzheimer's disease. *Neurology.* 1986;36:1226–1230.

23. Romanelli MF, Morris JC, Ashkin K, *et al.* Advanced Alzheimer's disease as a risk factor for late-onset seizures. *Arch Neurol.* 1990;47:847–850.

24. Caplan LR. *Stroke: A Clinical Approach, 2nd Ed.* Boston: Butterworth–Heinemann; 1993:1–66.

25. Lesser RP, Luders H, Dinner DS, *et al.* Epileptic seizures due to thrombotic and embolic cerebrovascular disease in older patients. *Epilepsia.* 1985;26:622–630.

26. Louis S, McDowell F. Epileptic seizures in nonembolic cerebral infarction. *Arch Neurol.* 1967;17:414–418.

27. Olsen TS, Hogenhaven H, Thage O. Epilepsy after stroke. *Neurology.* 1987;37:1209–1211.

28. Kilpatrick CJ, Davis SM, Hopper JL, *et al.* Early seizures after acute stroke: Risk of later seizures. *Arch Neurol.* 1992;49;509–511.

29. Giroud M, Gras P, Fayolle H, *et al.* Seizures after acute stroke: A study of 1640 cases. *Epilepsia.* 1994;35:959–964.

30. Shinton RA, Gill JS, Melnick SC, *et al.* The frequency, characteristics, and prognosis of epileptic seizures at the onset of stroke. *J Neurol Neurosurg Psychiatry.* 1988;51:273–276.

31. Ng SKC, Hauser WA, Brust JCM, *et al.* Hypertension and the risk of new-onset unprovoked seizures. *Neurology.* 1993;43:425–428.

32. Shinton RA, Gill JS, Zezulka AV, *et al.* The frequency of epilepsy preceding stroke. *Lancet.* 1987;i:11–12.

33. Annegers JF, Hauser WA, Lee SR, *et al.* Secular trends and birth cohort effects in unprovoked seizures: Rochester, Minnesota, 1935–1984. *Epilepsia.* 1995;36:575–579.

34. Weisberg LA, Shansma MA, Elliot D. Seizures caused by nontraumatic parenchymal brain hemorrhage. *Neurology.* 1991;41:1197–1199.

35. Faught E, Peters D, Bartolucci A, *et al.* Seizures after primary intracerebral hemorrhage. *Neurology.* 1989;39:1089–1093.

36. Berger AR, Lipton RB, Lesser ML, *et al.* Early seizures following intracerebral hemorrhage: Implications for therapy. *Neurology.* 1988;38:1363–1365.

37. Daniele O, Mattaliano A, Tassinari CA, *et al.* Epileptic seizures and cerebrovascular disease. *Acta Neurol Scand.* 1989;80:17–22.

38. Van Ness P. Frontal and parietal lobe epilepsy. In: Wylie E, ed. *The Treatment of Epilepsy: Principles and Practice.* Philadelphia: Lea & Febiger; 1993:525–532.

39. Manford M, Hart YM, Sander JWAS, *et al.* National general practice study of epilepsy (NGPSE): Partial seizure patterns in a general population. *Neurology.* 1992;42:1911–1917.

40. Bromfield EB. Somatosensory, special sensory, and autonomic phenomena in seizures. *Semin Neurol.* 1991;11:91–99.
41. Lannon SL. Epilepsy in the elderly. *J Neurosci Nurs.* 1993;25:273–282.
42. Devinsky O. The differential diagnosis of epilepsy. *Semin Neurol.* 1990;10:321–327.
43. Dohrmann ML, Cheitlin MD. Cardiogenic syncope. *Neurol Clin.* 1986;4:549–562.
44. Maddens ME. Syncope. In: Barclay L, ed. *Clinical Geriatric Neurology.* Philadelphia: Lea & Febiger; 1993:121–133.
45. Epstein MA, Sperling MR, O'Connor MJ. Cardiac rhythm during temporal lobe seizures. *Neurology.* 1992;42:50–53.
46. Leidholm LJ, Gudjohsson O. Cardiac arrest due to partial epileptic seizures. *Neurology.* 1992; 42:824–829.
47. Lempert T, Bauer M, Schmidt D. Syncope: A videometric analysis of 56 episodes of transient cerebral hypoxia. *Ann Neurol.* 1994;36:233–237.
48. Stephenson JBP. *Fits and Faints.* Oxford, England: Blackwell; 1990:41–58.
49. Linzer M, Grubb B, Ho S, et al. Cardiovascular causes of loss of consciousness in patients with presumed epilepsy. *Am J Med.* 1994;96:146–154.
50. Feldmann E, Wilterdink J. The symptoms of transient ischemic attacks. *Semin Neurol.* 1991;11:135–145.
51. Baquis GD, Pessin MS, Scott M. Limb shaking—A carotid TIA. *Stroke.* 1985;16:444–448.
52. Engel J Jr. *Seizures and Epilepsy.* Philadelphia: F.A. Davis; 1989:312–321.
53. Wells CR, Labar DR, Solomon GE. Aphasia as the sole manifestation of simple partial status epilepticus. *Epilepsia.* 1992;33:84–87.
54. Fisher CM. Late-life migraine accompaniments as a cause of unexplained transient ischemic attacks. *Can J Neurol Sci.* 1980;7:9–17.
55. Ehrenberg BL. Unusual manifestations of migraine and "the borderland of epilepsy"—Re-explored. *Semin Neurol.* 1991;11:118–127.
56. Chokroverty S, ed. *Sleep Disorders Medicine.* Boston: Butterworth–Heinemann; 1994:401–416.
57. Labar DR. Sleep disorders and epilepsy: Differential diagnosis. *Semin Neurol.* 1991;11:128–134.
58. Thomas P, Beaumanoir A, Genton P, et al. "De novo" absence status of late onset. *Neurology.* 1992;42:104–110.
59. Guberman A, Cantu–Reyna G, Stuss D, et al. Nonconvulsive generalized status epilepticus. *Neurology.* 1986;36:1284–1291.
60. Tomson T, Svanborg E, Wedlund JE. Nonconvulsive status epilepticus: High incidence of complex partial status. *Epilepsia.* 1986;27:276–285.
61. Niedermeyer E, Lopes da Silva F. *Electroencephalography, 3rd ed.* Baltimore: Williams & Wilkins; 1993:405–418.
62. Rowan AJ, Gates JR. *Non-Epileptic Seizures.* Boston: Butterworth–Heinemann; 1993:1–7.
63. Holmes GL. The electroencephalogram as a predictor of seizures following cerebral infarction. *Clin Electroencephalogr.* 1980;11:83–86
64. Fagan KJ, Lee SI. Prolonged confusion following convulsions due to generalized nonconvulsive status epilepticus. *Neurology.* 1990;40:1689–1694.
65. Oken B, Kaye JA. Electrophysiologic function in the healthy, extremely old. *Neurology.* 1992;42:519–526.
66. Berg AT, Shinnar S. The risk of seizure recurrence following a first unprovoked seizure: A quantitative review. *Neurology.* 1991;41:965–972.
67. Hart YM, Sander JWAS, Johnson AL, et al. National general practice study of epilepsy: Recurrence after a first seizure. *Lancet.* 1990;336:1271–1274.
68. Hauser WA, Rich SS, Annegers JF, et al. Seizure recurrence after a first unprovoked seizure: An extended follow-up. *Neurology.* 1990;40:1163–1170.

69. Theodore WH. Epilepsy in the elderly. In: Barclay L, ed. *Clinical Geriatric Neurology*. Philadelphia: Lea & Febiger; 1993:134–142.

70. First Seizure Trial Group (FIR.S.T. GROUP principal investigators: Musicco M, Beghi E, Bordo B, Viani F). Randomized clinical trial on the efficacy of antiepileptic drugs in reducing the risk of relapse after a first unprovoked tonic-clonic seizure. *Neurology*. 1993;43:478–483.

71. Bogousslavsky J, Martin R, Regli F, *et al*. Persistent worsening of stroke sequelae after delayed seizures. *Arch Neurol*. 1992;49:385–388.

72. Callaghan N, Kenny RA, O'Neill B, *et al*. A prospective study between carbamazepine, phenytoin, and sodium valproate as monotherapy in previously untreated and recently diagnosed patients with epilepsy. *J Neurol Neurosurg Psychiatry*. 1985;48:639–644.

73. Mattson RH, Cramer JA, Collins JF, *et al*. A comparison of valproate with carbamazepine for the treatment of complex partial seizures and secondarily generalized tonic-clonic seizures in adults. *N Engl J Med*. 1992;327:765–771.

74. Troupin AS, Johannessen SI. Epilepsy in the elderly: A pharmacologic perspective. In: Smith DB, ed. *Epilepsy: Current Approaches to Diagnosis and Treatment*. New York: Raven Press; 1990:141–152.

75. Dreifuss FE. Valproic acid: Toxicity. In: Levy RH, Mattson RH, Meldrum BS. *Antiepileptic Drugs, 4th Ed*. New York: Raven Press; 1995:641–648.

76. Montamat SC, Cusack BJ, Vestal RE. Management of drug therapy in the elderly. *N Engl J Med*. 1989;321:303–309.

77. Parker BM, Vestal RE. Pharmacokinetics of anticonvulsant drugs in the elderly. In: Wyllie E, ed. *The Treatment of Epilepsy: Principles and Practice*. Philadelphia: Lea & Febiger; 1993:769–774.

78. Morrell MJ. Hormones and epilepsy through the lifetime. *Epilepsia*. 1992;33, S49–S61.

79. Medical Research Council Antiepileptic Drug Withdrawal Study Group. Randomized study of antiepileptic drug withdrawal in patients in remission. *Lancet*. 1991;337:1175–1180.

80. Cascino GD, Sharbrough FW, Hirschorn KA, *et al*. Surgery for focal epilepsy in the older patient. *Neurology*. 1991;41:1415–1417.

81. Hauser WA. Status epilepticus: Epidemiologic considerations. In: Leppik IE, ed. *Status Epilepticus in Perspective*. *Neurology*. 1990;40(suppl. 2):9–13.

82. DeLorenzo RJ, Towne AR, Pellock JM, *et al*. Status epilepticus in children, adults, and the elderly. *Epilepsia*. 1992;33:S15–S25.

83. Glaser GH. Medical complications of status epilepticus. In: *Status Epilepticus: Mechanisms of Brain Damage and Treatment*. In: Delgado–Escueta AV, Wasterlain C, Treiman DM, *et al.*, eds. *Advances in Neurology*. New York: Raven Press; 1983;(34):395–398.

84. Working Group on Status Epilepticus. Treatment of convulsive status epilepticus. *JAMA*. 1993;270:854–859.

85. Yaffe K, Lowenstein DH. Prognostic factors of pentobarbital therapy for refractory generalized status epilepticus. *Neurology*. 1993;43:895–900.

86. Kumar A, Bleck TP. Intravenous midazolam for the treatment of refractory status epilepticus. *Crit Care Med*. 1992;20:483–488.

CHAPTER 14

The Team Approach to the Treatment of Epilepsy

Donald L. Schomer, M.D.

WHAT IS THE TEAM APPROACH TO THE MANAGEMENT OF EPILEPSY?

Although epilepsy most often occurs in children and young adults, it can affect persons of any age, as well as of any psychosocial or educational background. Because epilepsy can prevent those who have the disorder from taking advantage of educational and vocational opportunities, it can adversely affect virtually every aspect of their sense of self. For these reasons, the successful management of epilepsy requires more than the services of a knowledgeable and compassionate physician. Patients whose seizures are somewhat or completely refractory to standard anticonvulsant therapy should be referred to centers that specialize in the management of this condition. Patients who have difficult behavioral, educational, or vocational problems as a result of their epilepsy should also be referred when these problems arise. Epilepsy centers should be able to address all these concerns as well as the medical and surgical aspects of treatment.

Three levels of epilepsy treatment programs exist. First-level programs are centered around a physician specialist in epilepsy (an epileptologist); these programs usually have a nursing staff with a similar degree of expertise. This first-level team is considered a good referral source for the epilepsy patient who has difficult medical or behavioral problems. The team can advise the referring physician on the use of additional antiseizure medications, combination therapy, or both. Team members are usually familiar with the newer anticonvulsants and their interactions and side effects. They also usually know about additional support services, such as psychiatry, social work, and educational or rehabilitative programs, although they do not work with specialists in these disciplines as a comprehensive team. In many cases, however, support services can be coordinated in a way that fully meets the needs and expectations of the patient and the patient's family.

Second-level programs are mostly found in major medical centers. These programs offer a more comprehensive and coordinated approach to patient care than first-level programs. Referral to these centers is usually made when the primary physician or epilepsy specialist in a first-level program thinks that the

The Comprehensive Evaluation and Treatment of Epilepsy
Copyright © 1997 by Academic Press. All rights of reproduction in any form reserved.

patient may be a good candidate for neurosurgery or may benefit from trials with experimental anticonvulsants. Also, patients may be referred to this type of program for behavioral problems. The patient's behaviors may be a part of the original disorder that led to the epileptic condition, such as birth-related injuries with retardation, progressive neurologic disorders, head injuries, or stroke. The referring physician may suspect that the patient's seizures are not epileptic in origin, in which case the patient is referred for further diagnostic studies. These second-level programs, in addition to having several physician and nurse specialists in epilepsy on staff, have psychiatrists, clinical psychologists or neuropsychologists, social workers, neurosurgeons, and radiologists on staff who are experienced in this field. This group of professionals works together as a team to provide a clinically coordinated approach to the management of epilepsy, which is often helpful in improving medical outcomes and is essential for patients who are considering surgery.

The highest-level team approach is found in third-level programs. These programs, which are few, are staffed with a concentrated group of specialists, as are second-level programs, but also offer comprehensive educational and rehabilitative services. Although many second-level centers have access to state or regionally funded rehabilitative services or units and state educational testing services, these resources are seldom an integral part of their epilepsy programs. In contrast, the staff in third-level programs includes rehabilitative and educational specialists with expertise in epilepsy-related concerns.

WHAT IS THE PHYSICIAN'S ROLE ON THE TEAM?

An epileptologist is the head of each patient's team. This person is a neurologist who has specialized experience and, often, specialized training in managing the myriad of problems that persons with epilepsy have. In most second- and third-level centers, this is a full-time position. The epileptologist needs to have extensive clinical experience with epilepsy, comprehensive knowledge about anticonvulsant medications and alternative therapies, and an understanding of the other team members' areas of expertise. Most important, however, the physician must be able to communicate his or her views and suggestions to patients and their families. Many of the patients who come to epilepsy centers are fearful about their disorder and its management or are misinformed about their condition. Others are unable fully to grasp information about their disorder because it was transmitted to them at times when their anxiety was heightened or their awareness was altered by seizures. A calm, direct, and patient-specific discussion with patients about their disorder and its treatment, presented at a level commensurate with their educational background and current clinical state, will often be effective in alleviating patients' anxieties. One especially important decision the epileptologist must make is when to stop advocating medications and to recommend a surgical evaluation. To make an informed judgment, the physician needs to be well versed in the electrophysiologic workup and clinical outcomes in order to guide patients through the various testing procedures that are required. These procedures include standard telemetry, with or without video and various minimally invasive electrodes, and more invasive techniques, which carry mortality and morbidity risks. The physician also needs to know which type of electrode array to use based on all the previously acquired data and how to advise patients so that they can direct their own care based on the information supplied by the physician. In determining whether surgery is likely to be successful in a given case, the physician reviews and interprets all electroencephalographic (EEG), radiologic, neuropsychologic, and psychiatric data pertaining to the patient. Such a decision must consider not only the outcome with respect to the patient's seizures but also the intellectual and psychologic impact that the surgery will have on the patient.

WHAT IS THE NURSE'S ROLE AS A MEMBER OF THE TEAM?

From a practical perspective, the clinical epilepsy nurse has the most demanding position of all the team members. The nurse is often the first person in the program to have contact with the prospective patient or referring physician. The nurse's attitude is often critical in the decision to go forward with appointments for the patient. Nursing consultations often emphasize the psychosocial impact the disorder has had on the patient and family. Patients are more likely to confide in nurses than in physicians concerning their true feelings about their disorder, and changes in their moods and behavior. Nurses who are aware of this phenomenon can often encourage patients to bring up topics that are of concern to them. Nursing staff members are also essential in the day-to-day management of patients with refractory epilepsy when they are followed regularly by a comprehensive team. Nurses in most programs review with patients the various procedures that they are going to undergo, thus providing an essential educational service. These procedures include not only routine EEG and neuropsychologic tests and radiologic studies but also invasive EEG tests, specialized radiologic tests such as the intracarotid sodium amytal test, and various types of surgical procedures. The nurse serves an important function by being aware of all aspects of management of the patient's epilepsy as well as by providing a consistent and informed source of educational materials and services.

WHAT ROLE DOES THE PSYCHIATRIST PLAY AS A MEMBER OF THE TEAM?

The psychiatrist on a dedicated epilepsy management team is well versed in the medical management of clinical epilepsy and is aware of the cognitive and psychiatric impact of the various medications used to treat it. This role requires a strong primary psychiatry background that enables the psychiatrist to understand the psychosocial impact that epilepsy, as a chronic illness, can have, and how epilepsy-related cognitive deficits may affect patients' educational and employment opportunities and hence their sense of control and independence. The psychiatrist may need to consult with the patient about disturbed relationships that may develop within the family or between spouses as a result of the dependent positions in which many patients find themselves. Another responsibility of the psychiatrist is to identify any primary or secondary psychiatric disorders that patients may have, such as personality disorders or disorders of affect or mood. Some of these disturbances may require additional medical treatment, and the psychiatrist needs to know how various psychotropic medications may interact with antiepilepsy medications. In the evaluation of patients who will undergo a surgical workup, the psychiatrist plays a key role in assessing not only the patients' competence but their ability to manage themselves postoperatively.

WHAT IS THE PSYCHOLOGIST'S OR NEUROPSYCHOLOGIST'S ROLE AS A MEMBER OF THE TEAM?

The psychologist or neuropsychologist has several roles on a comprehensive team. He or she provides both diagnostic and therapeutic services. The first aspect of diagnosis is to determine what parts of the brain are not working properly and why, through the use of various standardized tests of cognition, memory, and function that are described earlier in this book. The second aspect of diagnosis, which is based in part on the person's clinical experience, may include identifying the structural component of the disorder, if one exists; the presence of subclinical seizure equivalents; medication effects; and unrelated and independent learning disabilities. The psychologist is also called upon to assist with or organize the intracarotid amytal procedure, also referred to as the Wada test. In most comprehensive centers, the psychologist also provides consultative support for patients who need it. These services include individual standard short- or long-term counseling and specialized counseling related to more unusual presurgical tests or longer-term cognitive rehabilitation. The psychologist may conduct group sessions to help with family relationships, education-related problems, or work-related opportunities.

Whether or not the psychologist performs these functions depends on his or her professional training, time availability, and interest in supporting such services within the program.

WHAT IS THE SOCIAL WORKER'S ROLE ON THE TEAM?

The social worker provides a unique service because of his or her knowledge of the availability of support services and ability to direct the patient or family to these services. Often local or regional services are available through state, federal, or local agencies. The social worker has the training and experience to minimize the paperwork involved in applying for some of these services. This person sometimes also participates in the counseling process with the psychiatrist or neuropsychologist, depending on his or her clinical training and available time.

WHAT ROLE DOES THE NEUROSURGEON PLAY ON THE TEAM?

In many programs, the epileptologist is also the neurosurgeon on the team. In the past, several centers developed around the surgical approach to medically intractable epilepsy and, therefore, the leaders of these programs were (and still are) neurosurgeons. Most programs now recognize that there is a pressing need for both medical and surgical physician specialists on the team. The advent of many new anticonvulsants and the expectation of still more has resulted in most programs having a medically oriented physician as the head of the team but with neurosurgical expertise readily available. In either case, the neurosurgeon in a comprehensive epilepsy program must be fully versed in the medical aspects of the disorder as well as a recognized expert in the surgical management of epilepsy. The neurosurgeon on the team will have acquired his expertise in a specialized training program in which various types of epilepsy surgery are routinely performed.

WHAT PRACTICAL AND ECONOMIC ADVANTAGES DO COMPREHENSIVE EPILEPSY MANAGEMENT TEAMS OFFER?

Although it may appear to referring physicians that most patients in comprehensive epilepsy treatment centers receive attention from representatives of all the disciplines on the team, not every patient who is referred to a comprehensive team needs to interact with all the participating specialists. The epileptologist will determine the patient's needs, willingness, and readiness to be a part of a multidisciplinary team approach.

Evidence is mounting that most patients who participate in a multidisciplinary clinical program function at higher and more independent levels than patients who do not. As an example, one of the major complaints voiced by patients with medically intractable epilepsy is a loss of control because of the seizures themselves and the dependency fostered by standard medical practices. Patients who are frequently seen by physicians in their offices or in emergency rooms may begin to regard themselves as chronically ill. This attitude tends to lead to excessive use of medical facilities, a practice that can often be reversed by returning to patients control over their own care. Through the educational process, patients become more adept at deciding how and when to engage the medical team.

Comprehensive programs are most successful with three particular groups of patients. The first group consists of patients who are undergoing presurgical evaluation. Patients who are good surgical candidates and do in fact have surgery stand an excellent chance of being cured or gaining control over their epilepsy. When that happens, many of these patients return to normal, productive lives. The second group of patients is composed of those who have had significant improvement in their seizure control because of improved diagnostic and therapeutic techniques. Often, reducing the number of medications that a patient takes or switching to medications that are more appropriate for the patient's type of epilepsy will lead to better seizure management and to improved memory and greater independence on the patient's part. Neuroendocrinologic approaches may occasionally help the patient with medically refractory epilepsy to lead a more independent and productive life. The third group of patients often helped by referral to comprehensive centers constitutes those whose events are not epileptic in origin. The differential diagnosis of "epileptic-like events" is discussed in Chapter 9. By identifying those patients whose signs and symptoms have been misdiagnosed as epilepsy and who have been treated with anticonvulsants, physicians on the team can offer appropriate treatments that may produce startlingly good results. Among the disorders that may masquerade as epilepsy are cardiac rhythm disturbances, complicated migraine, hypotension, and certain psychiatric disorders. However, it remains an unproven supposition that this type of comprehensive team approach is cost effective for those patients that do not segregate into one of the previously mentioned groupings. For these cases, epilepsy centers still need to do well-designed prospective comparative studies to prove their cost effectiveness.

INDEX